PHYSICS FOR THE ANAESTHETIST

PHYSICS

FOR THE

ANAESTHETIST

INCLUDING A SECTION ON

EXPLOSIONS

SIR ROBERT MACINTOSH

D.M., F.R.C.S.E., F.F.A.R.C.S., Hon. F.F.A.R.A.C.S., M.D.(h.c.), Buenos Aires and
Aix-Marseilles, D.Sc.(h.c.) Wales

Nuffield Professor of Anaesthetics, University of Oxford

WILLIAM W. MUSHIN

M.A., M.B., B.S., F.F.A.R.C.S.
Hon. F.F.A.R.A.C.S., F.F.A.R.C.S.I., F.F.A.(S.A.)

*Professor of Anaesthetics, Welsh National School of Medicine,
University of Wales
Formerly First Assistant, Nuffield Department of Anaesthetics,
University of Oxford*

H. G. EPSTEIN

M.A., Ph.D., F.F.A.R.C.S.

*First Assistant, Nuffield Department of Anaesthetics,
University of Oxford*

Illustrated by Miss M. McLarty and Miss M. Beck.

*THIRD EDITION
FOURTH PRINTING*

BLACKWELL SCIENTIFIC PUBLICATIONS

OXFORD   LONDON   EDINBURGH   MELBOURNE

ISBN 0 632 02690 1

First Edition 1946
Reprinted 1947
Second Edition 1958
Third Edition 1963
Reprinted 1968, 1970, 1972
First German Edition 1961
First Russian Edition 1962
First French Edition 1968

Printed in Great Britain by
WILLIAM CLOWES AND SONS, LIMITED, London, Beccles and Colchester
and bound at KEMP HALL BINDERY, Oxford

To

THE RIGHT HONOURABLE

THE VISCOUNT NUFFIELD

G.B.E., F.R.S., M.A., F.R.C.S., D.C.L., LL.D., D.L.

Honorary Fellow of the Faculty of Anaesthetists of the Royal College of Surgeons of England

Honorary Fellow of the Association of Anaesthetists of Great Britain and Ireland

whose generous concern for the advancement of medical science in general has included a particular interest in anaesthetics which has made possible the establishment, in the University of Oxford, of the first Chair and Department of Anaesthetics to be set up in Europe

PREFACE

In recent years there has been a tendency for the anaesthetist to concentrate on technique and to overlook the value of the basic sciences on which our speciality is founded. During the war anaesthetists had to be turned out in short time to meet the demand for numbers. It was inevitable that stress should be laid on a few tricks of the trade, such as how to put needle into vein or theca, or tube into trachea. The importance of technique in what, after all, is predominantly an art, cannot be over-stressed; nevertheless a little book knowledge should not come amiss, and should, in fact, make progress in our speciality less a matter of trial and error—always an expensive method of advance.

We disclaim any pretence at being physicists. We are practising anaesthetists who have had our fair share of teaching. We are not unaware of the limitations in our knowledge of physics, but these are not more marked than those of post-graduate anaesthetists who have attended here on courses. We sympathize with their observations that a book is not available from which they can readily brush up their knowledge or obtain the information they want. It is true that there are books on medical physics, but these do not make light reading for the anaesthetist weary after a hard day in the operating-theatre, nor is it always easy for someone, not himself a physicist, to extract from these text-books answers to straightforward questions.

Our task has been to gather such applications of physics to anaesthetics as we meet with and discuss during our routine work. Many of these are elementary for we are not unmindful of the practitioner who turns to anaesthetics comparatively late in life, when physics is remembered only as a hurdle in the pre-medical curriculum. For the same reason we have striven after simplicity rather than precision. Precise definitions of fundamental terms and processes are notoriously difficult. The ones we give are accurate enough for the purpose for which they are intended—the teaching of physics to practising anaesthetists and to other doctors and dentists interested in the relation of elementary physics to their particular job.

It has been our great good fortune to enlist the interest and guidance of our colleague, Dr. H. G. Epstein. His wide knowledge of physics has allowed us almost to dispense with reference books. He has pointed out the errors which attend attempts at over-simplification, and he has revealed other pitfalls into which those who trespass outside their own speciality can so easily tread. We are grateful to him for revising our manuscript, for supervising our diagrams and for carrying out a host of experiments in the laboratory which give the answers to questions long discussed amongst anaesthetists.

We are fortunate again in having the services of Miss McLarty. She holds that in an illustration art lies in bringing out clearly the point the authors wish to make. Like a previous effort of ours this book largely tells its story in pictures. Any economy in time or effort on the part of the reader in acquiring the ideas is not reflected in the time taken to present them. Just as a paragraph may have to be re-written several times before it brings out an idea concisely, so too we have found that even an apparently simple drawing may have to be altered several times before all that is inaccurate or irrelevant is eliminated.

It is a pleasure to acknowledge the very able secretarial help so willingly extended by Miss Marjorie R. Gibson.

R. R. M.

W. W. M.

PREFACE TO SECOND EDITION

It has often been said that teaching is the best way of learning. Twelve years ago anaesthetists visiting this Department often propounded questions involving the application of physics to our Specialty. When we didn't know the answers we found it a helpful discipline to clarify our minds by referring to the proper sources. Our difficulty often turned out to be reconciling scientific accuracy with simplicity and brevity. A statement accurate enough to satisfy the scientist might be too ponderous for the clinician whose previous training had not prepared him to digest such unpalatable fare. Eventually we felt pen should be put to paper, and in this book we set out to increase the anaesthetist's appetite for knowledge by making the diet more attractive.

Despite a reprint the book has been out of print for nearly five years. We realized it needed revision and enlarging, but the promotion of my co-author to the Chair of Anaesthetics in the University of Wales, and the post-war demands on the free time of both of us, made it impossible to spend the necessary tranquil evenings together on the project. Dr. H. G. Epstein, with his expert knowledge, has come to our help again, this time by joining us as a third author, in the preparation of this new edition.

The bulk of the book has been kept at an elementary standard, but we might have been kinder to the occasional reader if some of the new material had been added in the small print traditionally used to suggest that its message is not so urgent, nor so easily assimilated. It was difficult, however, to decide what parts, if any, could be relegated with advantage to smaller type. Credit (or responsibility!) for the alterations and additions, including new chapters on reducing valves and explosions, belongs almost entirely to Dr. Epstein and Professor Mushin.

Although throughout this book the intermediate steps of calculation have been carried out accurately, we have thought it adequate to round off the results to either two or three significant figures. By the same token, we have not thought it necessary in the interest of accuracy to differentiate between cm^3 and ml.

ROBERT MACINTOSH

NUFFIELD DEPARTMENT OF ANAESTHETICS,
OXFORD
January, 1958

CONTENTS

CHAPTER I

DENSITY OF GASES

The Structure of Matter

AN element, however much it is subdivided by chemical or mechanical means, remains the same substance; its properties remain unaltered. Examples—hydrogen, helium, carbon, nitrogen, oxygen, chlorine.

A *compound* is composed of two or more elements, chemically united to form a substance differing in properties from those of the individual elements composing it. At a certain stage of subdivision a compound loses its identity and is resolved into its constituent elements. This is seen, for example, in the case of ether which is compounded of carbon, hydrogen and oxygen; or in the case of nitrous oxide, a compound of nitrogen and oxygen.

A *molecule* is the smallest particle of a substance which still possesses the distinctive properties of that substance. Thus a compound can be divided into molecules without losing its identity; but if division proceeds beyond this, each molecule is found to consist of 'atoms' of elements. That the atom can be split is common knowledge, but for our purposes it suffices to define the *atom* as the smallest part into which an element can be subdivided. The atoms of certain elements, for example, helium, exist in the free state as separate entities. There is no difference between the atom and the molecule of helium. Atoms of many other elements, for example, oxygen, hydrogen, nitrogen, do not exist in the free state, but are found united with other atoms to form molecules. Thus an oxygen atom when joined to its fellow forms a molecule of oxygen, as is indicated by the formula O_2. The gaseous oxygen with which we are all familiar consists of a multitude of oxygen molecules. If the oxygen atom is joined to atoms of other elements a molecule of a new substance is formed. For example, the molecule of ether is a compound of 1 atom of oxygen with 4 atoms of carbon and 10 atoms of hydrogen. This is shown by its formula $(C_2H_5)_2O$.

Molecular Movement

The fact that the densities of solids and liquids considerably exceed those ·of gases at atmospheric pressure is accounted for by the small intermolecular distances in solids and liquids compared to gases.

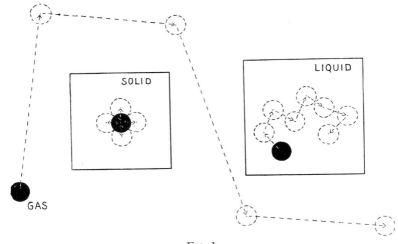

FIG. 1

The molecules of which matter is composed are in a state of incessant motion, and the magnitude of the movement and the ability of the molecules to alter their position vary according to whether the substance is in the solid, liquid or gaseous state. In the following example we consider the same substance in the three states of aggregation at the same temperature (fig. 1). In the solid state the molecules cannot alter their relative positions and merely oscillate about a fixed point. The molecules in the liquid state are mobile and gradually shift their position throughout the whole liquid. The free path of a molecule in the liquid, however, is very short before it collides with its neighbours. In the gas state* the molecules have a much greater degree of mobility, and travel longer distances before colliding with others.

The speed at which the molecules move at any given temperature is approximately the same whether the substance is in the solid, liquid or

---

* Fig. 1 gives only a rough picture of the actual situation. A nitrogen molecule, for instance, has a diameter of about 3 Å (Å = Ångstrom unit, see Ch. XXIV). If the gas is under a pressure of 1 atmosphere, the 'mean free path' between collisions would be a bout 1000 Å. In this case the length of the path between two collisions would have to be drawn 300 times the diameter of the small discs representing the molecules.

gaseous state. However, by reason of the fewer collisions in a given time, the molecules in a gas travel a greater distance in any given direction than they do in a liquid. Owing to the mobility of its molecules, a fluid, liquid or gas, has no fixed shape. All gases, and many liquids, mix readily with their fellows.

Atomic Weight

The atomic weight of oxygen is used as the basis from which the atomic weights of the other elements are determined. The atomic weight of oxygen is given the value of 16, and since hydrogen, the lightest of all elements, is 16 times lighter than oxygen, its atomic weight is 1.

The carbon atom is $\frac{3}{4}$ the weight of the oxygen atom and 12 times as heavy as the hydrogen atom. The atomic weight of carbon is therefore said to be 12. Examples of atomic weights:

Hydrogen	1·0	Sulphur	32·1
Helium	4·0	Chlorine	35·5
Carbon	12·0	Potassium	39·1
Nitrogen	14·0	Argon	39·9
Oxygen	16·0	Calcium	40·1
Fluorine	19·0	Iron	55·8
Sodium	23·0	Bromine	79·9
Phosphorus	31·0	Xenon	131·3

Molecular Weight

The 'molecular weight' of a substance, solid or fluid, is the sum of the atomic weights of the element or elements of which it is composed. Thus oxygen with a formula of O_2 has a molecular weight of 32, and ether with a formula of $(C_2H_5)_2O$, or $C_4H_{10}O$, has a molecular weight of

$$(4 \times 12) + (10 \times 1) + 16 = 74$$

Nitrous oxide (N_2O) is readily found to have a molecular weight of 44.

From the above it is seen that the weight of one molecule of ether is to the weight of one molecule of nitrous oxide as 74 is to 44; equally that 74 grams of ether contain the same number of molecules as 44 grams of nitrous oxide.

The term 'mole' is an abbreviation for 'gram molecular weight'. The gram molecular weight of a substance is its molecular weight expressed in grams. Thus one mole of ether is 74 grams. The gram molecular weights of all substances contain the same number of molecules.

Avogadro's Hypothesis states that equal volumes of gases at the same temperature and pressure contain equal numbers of molecules. It is known by experiment and inference that a mole of any gas at the same temperature and pressure occupies the same volume. At 0 °C and 760 mmHg pressure (referred to as normal temperature and pressure, or **N.T.P.**) this volume is 22·4 litres. The weight of 22·4 litres of any gas at N.T.P. is therefore that of a gram molecule of that gas.

Fig. 2—illustrates the above statement in the case of 3 substances in the gaseous state. The weight of the containers is disregarded. In each case the weight of 22·4 litres of the substance gives its molecular weight in grams.* At room temperature and on the assumption that the gas behaves like an 'ideal' gas (p. 114), this volume is increased to approximately 24 litres.

Throughout this book whenever the conditions of temperature and pressure are those in an average room (20 °C and 760 mmHg) we have referred to them as 'room' conditions; unless otherwise stated N.T.P. is implied.

An estimate of the number of molecules in 1 cm³ of an ideal gas at N.T.P. was first made by **Loschmidt**[1] in 1865. Recent estimates give a value of $2 \cdot 68 \times 10^{19}$ molecules/cm³.

The number of molecules contained in 1 gram molecular weight of any element or compound is known as Avogadro's number; its value is $N = 6 \cdot 02 \times 10^{23}$.

Density

The 'density' of a gas is usually expressed as the weight in grams of one litre of that gas.

Since the weight of 22·4 litres of a gas is that of a gram molecule of that gas

1 litre of a gas weighs: $\dfrac{\text{molecular weight}}{22 \cdot 4}$ g

The molecular weight of ether is 74

∴ the weight of 1 litre of ether vapour** $= \dfrac{74}{22 \cdot 4}$ g $= 3 \cdot 31$ g

---

* The lowermost figure illustrates a hypothetical state of affairs, since pure ether vapour does not exist under conditions of N.T.P. (See p. 10.)
** See previous footnote.

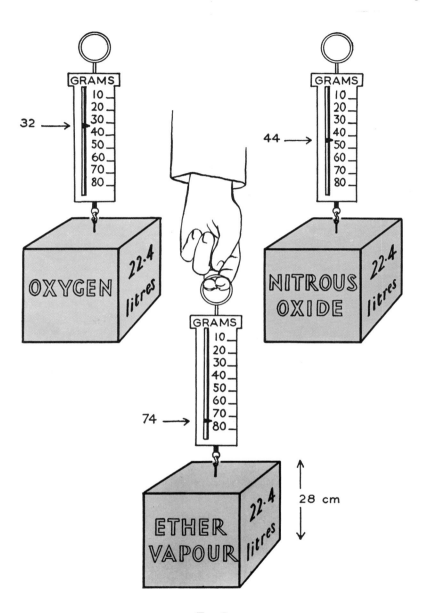

FIG. 2

It is customary to express this by stating that the density of ether vapour is 3·3 grams per litre.

The density of nitrous oxide (mol. wt. 44) is $\frac{44}{22·4} = 1·96$ g/l

The density of chloroform vapour (mol. wt. 119) is $\frac{119}{22·4} = 5·31$ g/l

For practical purposes air* consists of a mixture of 1 volume of oxygen and 4 volumes of nitrogen.

At N.T.P. the weight

of $\frac{1}{5}$ litre of oxygen   is $\frac{32}{22·4} \times \frac{1}{5}$ g $= 0·29$ g

of $\frac{4}{5}$ litre of nitrogen   is $\frac{28}{22·4} \times \frac{4}{5}$ g $= 1·0$ g

∴ the weight of 1 litre of air

is 0·29 g $+$ 1·0 g $= 1·3$ g

The density of air is 1·3 g/l

It is seen that—

nitrous oxide   is 1½ times as heavy as air
ether vapour   is 2½   „   „
chloroform vapour is 4   „   „

The density of a gas is often expressed relatively to the density of air which is given the value of 1. Thus the relative density—or *specific gravity*—of nitrous oxide is 1½, of ether vapour 2½ and of chloroform vapour 4.

Although the word *density* has been used in the popular sense to denote the weight of a given volume of gas, the proper scientific term is '*specific weight*'.

The following nomenclature may be of use:

Specific weight: weight per unit volume†

Specific gravity: (a) LIQUIDS: ratio of specific weight of the liquid at any given temperature to that of water at 4 °C.

(b) GASES: ratio of specific weight of the gas to that of air; both are usually given at N.T.P.

---

* The correct values for dry air are: $N_2 = 78·1\%$; $O_2 = 20·9\%$; Argon $= 0·9\%$; $CO_2 = 0·03\%$.

† For example: g/l or lb/gal.

The Waller Chloroform Balance*

Waller[2] made use of the principle of Archimedes in utilizing the different densities of air and chloroform vapour as a means of estimating and regulating the concentration of chloroform vapour in the chloroform/air mixture being delivered to a patient.

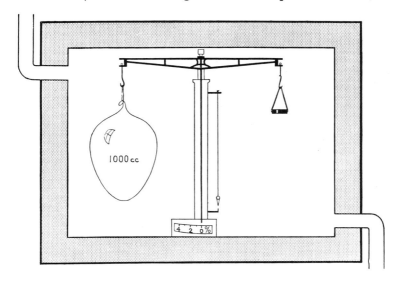

FIG. 3

Fig. 3—The essential part of the apparatus consists of an accurate balance enclosed in a gas-tight case. A sealed glass bulb of 1000 cm^3 capacity is suspended from one arm of the balance and is exactly counterbalanced by a *small* weight suspended from the other. When the balance case is full of air the indicator points to zero. Two ports are provided, one opening into and the other leading from the case. The chloroform/air mixture enters through the top one and passes out through the other to the patient.

The concentration of chloroform vapour can be varied by the control tap on the bottle seen on the left of the balance on fig. 5.

* See also footnote, p. 280.

Fig. 4—The chloroform/air mixture on its way to the patient passes through the balance case. The air is displaced and the bulb is now further buoyed up by the heavier chloroform/air mixture. The small balance weight is also buoyed up, but this effect is so small that it can

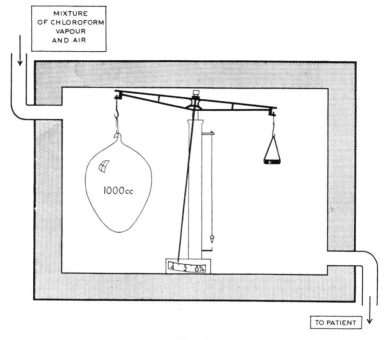

MIXTURE OF CHLOROFORM VAPOUR AND AIR

1000cc

4   2   0%

TO PATIENT

Fig. 4

be ignored, since the volume of the weight compared to that of the glass bulb is negligible. The net result is that the balance indicator swings to the left.

The scale is easily calibrated to show the percentage of chloroform in the mixture passing through the case.

The apparent difference in weight of the glass bulb when it is weighed first in air and then in a chloroform/air mixture is equal to the difference in weight between the 1000 cm³ of the chloroform vapour mixture and the 1000 cm³ of air it displaces. The principle of Archimedes is recognized.

$$
\begin{aligned}
&1000 \ cm^3 \ air && \text{weigh } 1 \cdot 3 \ g \\
&1000 \ cm^3 \ CHCl_3 \ vapour && ,, \quad \underline{5 \cdot 3 \ g} \\
&&& \text{difference } \overline{4 \cdot 0 \ g}
\end{aligned}
$$

The apparent reduction in weight of the glass bulb
when weighed in 100% $CHCl_3$ vapour is therefore   4 g†

  „ „ 10% „ „ „ 400 mg†

  „ „ 2% „ „ „ 80 mg

  „ „ 1% „ „ „ 40 mg

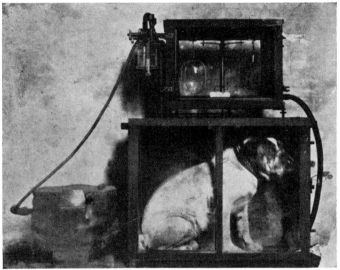

FIG. 5

With the case full of air and the weight of the sealed glass bulb just
balanced by the small weight, the indicator points to 0. A 40 mg weight
is now added to the original weight. The point on the scale where the
indicator comes to rest is marked 1. An 80 mg weight gives the mark
for 2, and a 160 mg weight the mark for 4. The scale is now calibrated
to indicate the percentages of chloroform vapour in air, commonly used
in clinical practice.

Fig. 5—Waller's original balance. Air is pumped by the foot bellows
through a chloroform bottle into the balance case, whence the anaesthetic mixture is led into the chamber below. Inside the latter is
'Jimmie', Waller's friend and subject of many an experiment.[3]

Density of a Vapour

At atmospheric pressure the volume of a given weight of a substance
is many hundred times greater when the substance is in the gaseous

† These concentrations at room conditions (or N.T.P.) represent a hypothetical
state of affairs.

state than when it is liquid. From this it follows that the density of a vapour at 1 atm is very much less than that of its corresponding liquid.

The density of liquid ETHER is 0·72, that is, 0·72 g is the weight of 1 cm³ of liquid ether.

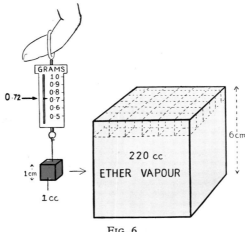

FIG. 6

We have seen that 3·3 g is the weight of 1000 cm³ of ether vapour

∴ 0·72 g is the weight of $\frac{1000}{3\cdot3}$ × 0·72 cm³ ether vapour = 220 cm³

From this it will be seen that 1 cm³ of liquid ether volatilizes into 220 cm³ of ether vapour at N.T.P. (fig. 6). Under room conditions this figure is increased to 230.

Since the boiling-point of ether is 34·6 °C, undiluted ether vapour cannot exist under room conditions. For purposes of calculation, however, ether vapour is treated as though it could exist as an undiluted gas under these conditions. That this is justifiable is shown by the fact that if 1 cm³ of ether is volatilized in sufficient air at room temperature to make a 50% mixture of ether vapour in air, the volume occupied by the mixture is 460 cm³, twice the hypothetical volume it would occupy as an undiluted vapour.

Density of liquid CHLOROFORM is 1·5.

We have seen that 5·3 g is the weight of 1000 cm³ chloroform vapour

∴ 1·5 g is the weight of $\frac{1000}{5\cdot3}$ × 1·5 cm³ = 280 cm³ chloroform vapour

1 cm³ of liquid chloroform volatilizes into 280 cm³ of chloroform vapour at N.T.P.

Density* of liquid NITROUS OXIDE at 20 °C and 51 atmospheres $= 0.80$
44 g is the weight of 24 litres of N_2O gas at room conditions

$\therefore 0.80$ g is the weight of $\dfrac{24}{44} \times 0.80$ l.

$= 440 \text{ cm}^3$

1 cm³ of liquid N_2O at 20 °C and 51 atmospheres volatilizes into 440 cm³ of N_2O gas at room conditions.

Practical application

Probably the most accurate method of administering the vapour of a liquid anaesthetic in any desired concentration is to volatilize a calculated volume of the liquid in a known volume of air, and to deliver the resultant mixture to the patient. This method was used in animal experiments a hundred years ago by Snow[4] and later was employed clinically by Clover.[5]

Clover's Chloroform Apparatus

The molecular weight of chloroform ($CHCl_3$) is 119.

119 g of chloroform when in the gaseous state occupy 22.4 l at N.T.P. The weight of 1 cm³ of liquid chloroform is 1.5 g, from which it is easily calculated that 1 cm³ of the liquid volatilizes to 280 cm³ of chloroform vapour. At room temperature this volume is increased to approximately 300 cm³.

In order to produce a 4% mixture of chloroform vapour in air, pure chloroform vapour must be diluted with 24 times its own volume of air. Thus 1 cm³ of liquid chloroform, which volatilizes into 300 cm³ of vapour, mixed with (300 × 24) cm³ of air, gives 7500 cm³ of 4% chloroform vapour in air.

Fig. 7—A concertina bag with a capacity of 7200 cm³ is shown being filled with air. The syringe holds 1 cm³ of liquid chloroform. The centre of the vaporizing chamber is occupied by a hot water container, covered on its outside by blotting-paper. The vaporizing chamber is connected to the very large reservoir bag by wide-bore rubber tubing.

* See tables, p. 421, column 10, row a′.

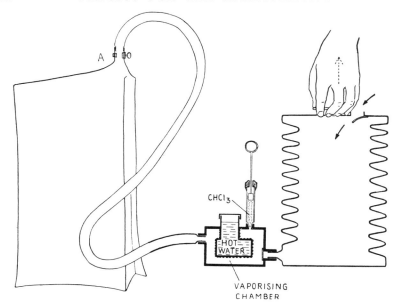

FIG. 7

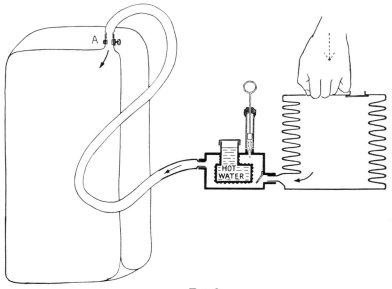

FIG. 8

Fig. 8. (See also fig. 9)—The concertina bag is now slowly compressed. Unidirectional valves ensure that the 7200 cm³ of air pass through the vaporizing chamber, into which 1 cm³ of chloroform is slowly dropped. A 4% chloroform vapour accumulates in the reservoir

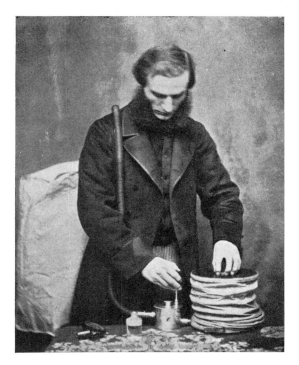

FIG. 9

bag. The process is repeated until the reservoir bag is fully charged. The tap (A) is closed and the wide-bore rubber tubing is disconnected from the vaporizing chamber and connected to the facemask, shown in fig. 10.

The size of the concertina bag actually used by Clover (fig. 9) was 1000 cubic inches; the contents of the syringe, 40 minims of liquid chloroform.

Fig. 9—Compare with fig. 8.

Fig. 10—The facemask has two short tubes; one of these connects to the flexible tubing from the reservoir bag, the other contains Clover's spring-loaded expiratory valve.

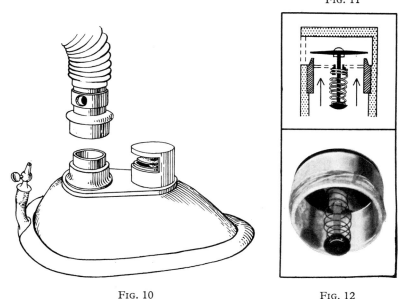

FIG. 11

FIG. 10   FIG. 12

At the end of the flexible tube near the facemask is a side aperture for the admission of diluting air; it can be varied in size by rotating a ferrule. When the aperture is completely closed, the chloroform mixture inhaled by the patient is that contained in the bag, that is, 4%. This device for diluting the potent mixture in the bag served both to render induction less unpleasant, and later to regulate the maintenance dose.

By 1862 the facemask was already equipped with an inflatable rim!

Fig. 11—illustrates the construction of the valve.

The valve disc was made from an ebonite-like substance. A pin attached to the centre of the disc passes through a bearing which is fixed on a crossbar inside the tube. The lower end of the pin carries a small knob which forms a rest for a light compression spring. The other end of the spring rests against the crossbar.

The complete valve assembly was pushed into the short tube on the facemask.

Fig. 12—is a photo of one of Clover's original valves.

Fig.13—Clover himself is administering chloroform—hand on pulse! The tap (A, fig. 8) is of course open. Inspiratory and expiratory valves on the facemask prevent rebreathing.

Fig. 14—Clover's chloroform apparatus packed into a small box and was readily transportable.

Here the empty black reservoir bag is seen folded in the background.

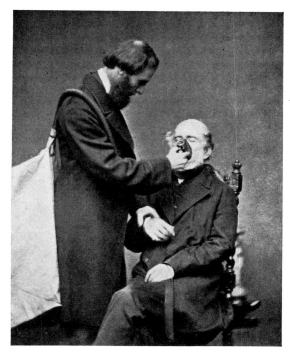

FIG. 13

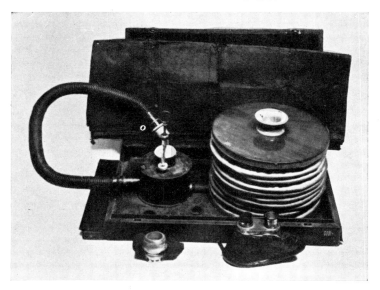

FIG. 14

Further examples

(1) 2 cm³ of liquid ether are added to 10 l of air and completely vaporized. What percentage of ether vapour will there be in the resultant mixture?

At room conditions 2 cm³ liquid ether vaporize into 460 cm³ ether vapour

$$\text{Air added} \qquad . \qquad . \qquad . \qquad \underline{10000} \text{ cm}^3$$

$$\text{Total volume} \qquad . \qquad . = 10460 \text{ cm}^3$$

$$\text{Percentage of ether vapour is } \frac{460}{10460} \times 100 = 4{\cdot}4$$

(2) 1 cm³ liquid divinyl ether is vaporized in 10 l of air. What percentage of divinyl ether vapour will there be in the resultant mixture?

$$\text{Divinyl ether—formula} \qquad . \qquad (CH_2CH)_2O$$
$$\text{molecular weight} . \qquad . \qquad 70$$
$$\text{density} \qquad . \qquad . \qquad . \qquad 0{\cdot}77 \text{ g/cm}^3$$

At room temperature

70 g is the weight of 24 l   of divinyl ether vapour

$$1 \text{ g} \quad \text{,,} \qquad \text{,,} \quad \frac{24}{70} \text{ l} \qquad \qquad \text{,,} \qquad \text{,,} \qquad \text{,,}$$

$$0{\cdot}77 \text{ g} \quad \text{,,} \qquad \text{,,} \quad 0{\cdot}77 \times \frac{24}{70} \times 1000 \text{ cm}^3 \text{ ,,} \qquad \text{,,} \qquad \text{,,}$$

$$= 260 \text{ cm}^3$$

1 cm³ liquid divinyl ether vaporizes into   260 cm³ vapour

Air added   .   .   .   .   .   10000 cm³

$$\therefore \text{ percentage of divinyl ether vapour} = \frac{260}{10260} \times 100 = 2{\cdot}5$$

(3) A mixture of 5 litres of nitrous oxide and 2 litres of oxygen per minute, on their way to the patient, pass through an ether bottle. In the course of one hour 3 oz. liquid ether are used. What is the average concentration of ether vapour in the mixture?

$$3 \text{ oz} = 3 \times 28 \text{ cm}^3$$
$$3 \times 28 \text{ cm}^3 \text{ liquid ether} = 3 \times 28 \times 230 \text{ cm}^3 \text{ vapour}$$
$$7 \text{ l/min} = 7 \times 1000 \times 60 \text{ cm}^3/\text{h}$$

∴ average concentration of ether vapour

$$\text{in mixture is (approx.)} \qquad \frac{3 \times 28 \times 230}{7 \times 1000 \times 60} \times 100 = 4{\cdot}6\%$$

REFERENCES

[1] Loschmidt, J. (1865). *S. B. Akad. Wiss. Wien*, **52**, 395–407.
[2] Waller, A. D., and Geets, V. (1903). *Brit. med. J.* i, 1421.
[3] Waller, Miss Mary, B.Sc., Ph.D. Personal communication.
[4] Snow, J. (1858). *On chloroform and other anaesthetics*, p. 80. Lond.
[5] Traer, J. R. (1862). *Med. Times Gaz.* ii, 148–9; cf. p. 149.

Chapter II

SPECIFIC HEAT

It is necessary to draw a clear distinction between heat and temperature. Heat can be given to a substance or abstracted from it. Temperature is the thermal state of a substance which determines whether it will give heat to or receive heat from another substance when brought in contact with it.

Calorie. The unit of heat is the calorie (cal), and this is defined as the quantity of heat required to raise the temperature of 1 g of water by 1 °C.

Example

How much heat is required to raise the temperature of 1 litre (approx. 1000 g) of water from 18 °C to 37 °C?

The temperature of   1 g of water is raised   1 °C by   1 cal

,,   1000 ,,   ,,   ,,   1 °C by   1000 cal

,,   1000 ,,   ,,   ,,   19 °C by 19000 cal

                                        = 19 kcal

The larger heat unit, the kilocalorie (Cal or kcal) is used to express the caloric value of foodstuffs.

Specific Heat

To raise the same weight of different substances through any given range of temperature requires different quantities of heat. The specific heat of a substance is the number of calories required to raise the temperature of 1 g of that substance by 1 °C. Since the temperature of 1 g of water is raised 1 °C by 1 calorie, it follows that the specific heat of water is 1. It is interesting to note that no other substance in common use has a specific heat higher than 1.

The specific heat of ether* is 0·5 cal/g. This means that 0·5 cal are required to raise the temperature of 1 g of ether by 1 °C.

It is often useful to use a slightly different definition of specific heat and refer it to 1 cm³ of a substance, instead of to 1 g.

---

* The specific heat of a substance depends on whether it is in the gaseous or the liquid state. In the case of ether the difference is small and we have disregarded it. The correct values are 0·54 cal/g for liquid and 0·44 cal/g for gaseous ether at room conditions; see tables on p. 419, column 3, rows h & h'.

Since the specific weight of ether is 0.72 g/cm^3, the specific heat related to the unit *volume* of the liquid is given by:

$$0.5 \times 0.72 = 0.36 \text{ cal/cm}^3$$

1 cm^3 of liquid ether volatilizes to 230 cm^3 of vapour

$\therefore$ the specific heat of ether vapour is $\dfrac{0.36}{230}$

$$= 0.0016 \text{ cal/cm}^3$$

1 gm of ether may exist in the

form of either (1) $\dfrac{1}{0.72}$ cm^3 liquid ether

$$= 1.4 \text{ cm}^3 \text{ liquid ether}$$

or (2) $\dfrac{1}{0.72} \times 230$ cm^3 ether vapour

$$= 320 \text{ cm}^3 \text{ ether vapour}$$

Thus we may say that

(i) The specific heat of liquid ether is 0.5 cal *per g*

or (ii)   „   „   „   „ $\dfrac{0.5}{1.4}$ cal *per cm^3*

$$= 0.36 \text{ cal } per \ cm^3$$

and (iii)   „   „   of ether vapour is $\dfrac{0.5}{1.4} \times \dfrac{1}{230}$

$$= 0.0016 \text{ cal } per \ cm^3$$

We have seen that under room conditions the volume of a given weight of a substance is many hundred times greater in the gaseous state than in the liquid. From this and from the definition of specific heat given above, it follows that the specific heat per cm^3 of a gas is many hundred times less than that of a cm^3 of the corresponding liquid.

Specific heat is generally expressed in calories *per g* weight of a substance, but as anaesthetists invariably talk about volumes of liquids or gases we think it more profitable to consider the problem in terms of specific heat *per cm^3* of a substance, liquid or gas.

Since 1 cm^3 of water weighs very nearly 1 g, the number of calories required to raise the temperature of 1 g or 1 cm^3 of water by any number of degrees is the same.

The difference in the amount of heat required to raise the temperature by 1 °C of 1 g and of 1 cm^3 of a substance is very great in the case of gases under room conditions. Thus with ether vapour the figures expressed in calories are 0.5 and 0.0016.

In the case of air the difference is more marked still. The specific heat of air is 0·24 cal *per g*.

1 gm of air at N.T.P. occupies $\dfrac{1}{1\cdot3}$ litres = 770 cm³

∴ the specific heat* of air may be expressed as $\dfrac{0\cdot24}{770}$ cal *per cm³*

$$= 0\cdot0003 \text{ cal } per\ cm^3$$

Thus 0·0003 cal are required to raise the temperature of 1 cm³ of air by 1 °C.

but 0·24 cal are required to raise the temperature of 1 g of air by 1 °C.

Example

What is the specific heat of a 10% mixture of ether vapour in air?

Specific heat of ether vapour = 0·0016 cal/cm³

„ „ air = 0·0003 „

∴ specific heat of

10% ether vapour in air = $(\dfrac{1}{10} \times 0\cdot0016) + (\dfrac{9}{10} \times 0\cdot0003)$

$$= 0\cdot00016 + 0\cdot00027$$

$$= 0\cdot0004 \text{ cal/cm}^3$$

This is only $\dfrac{1}{1000}$ of the specific heat per cm³ of liquid ether.

TABLE 1

Substance	Specific heat cal/cm³
Water	1
Liquid ether . .	0·36
Ether vapour . .	0·0016
10% ether vapour in air	0·0004
Oxygen . . .	0·0003
Air	0·0003

* From the definition of specific heat it is apparent that its unit should be: cal/(g × degC). For convenience of printing the unit of temperature interval (degree Celsius) has been omitted and the unit written as: cal/g.

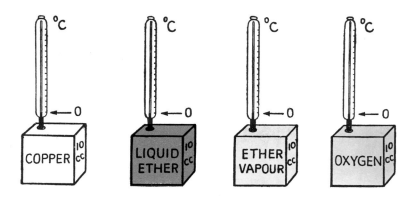

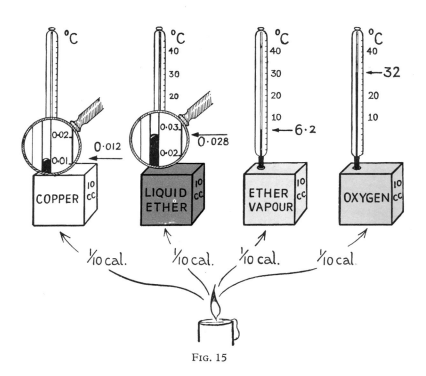

FIG. 15

Fig. 15—Here the same volumes (10 cm³) of copper, liquid ether, ether vapour and oxygen are used to compare the specific heat *per cm³* of a solid, liquid, vapour and gas.

Owing to the wide variation in these, only a minute amount of heat ($\frac{1}{10}$ cal) is used so that the rise in temperature can be recorded on similar thermometers.

It will be seen that although this minute amount of heat raises the temperature of the oxygen by 32 °C, the temperature of the copper rises only 0·012 °C. The temperature rise of the liquid ether is 0·028 °C and that of the same volume of ether vapour is 6·2 °C.

The temperature rises of the copper and of the liquid ether are so small that a magnifying glass is used to read the thermometer.

From these experiments the following specific heats can be calculated:

copper	.	.	. 0·80	cal/cm³
liquid ether		.	. 0·36	,,
ether vapour		.	. 0·0016	,,
oxygen	.	.	. 0·0003	,,

The experiments of fig. 15 show the great divergence in temperature rise when equal volumes of various substances are heated by the same amount of heat. The following experiments illustrate the great divergence in volumes of various substances which are raised to the same temperature by a given amount of heat.

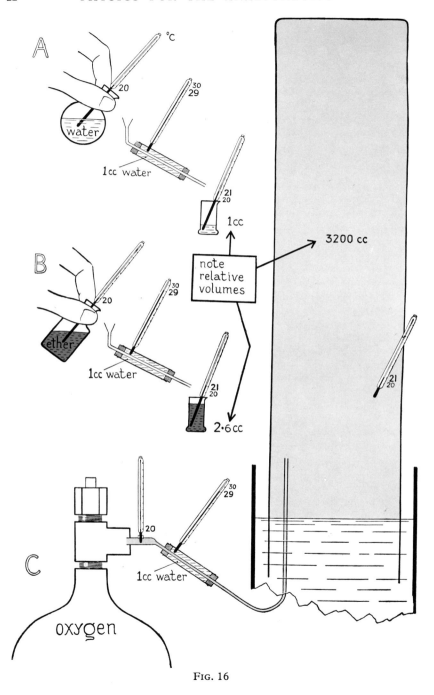

FIG. 16

Fig. 16—Here three substances, water, liquid ether and oxygen, all at 20 °C are passed through a tube surrounded by 1 cm³ of warm water until 1 calorie has been extracted from the surrounding water as is shown by the fall in the temperature of the water from 30 °C to 29 °C. It is found that 1 calorie is sufficient to raise the temperature of 3200 cm³ of oxygen from its initial temperature by 1 °C. In the case of liquid ether, the volume is only 2·6 cm³, whilst with water (specific heat = 1) the volume, of course, is 1 cm³.

An everyday example of the low specific heat of a gas is seen in the lighted cigarette. The glowing tip is at a temperature of several hundred degrees centigrade. Yet after travelling less than three inches, the inhaled hot gases have already cooled sufficiently not to burn the lips or tongue of the smoker.[1]

It will be appreciated from these experiments that the temperature of a gas can be raised with the expenditure of a comparatively minute amount of heat. Conversely, the heat content of a gas under normal pressure is small and is quickly depleted if the gas is brought in contact with a colder environment.

An appreciation of this fact will remove a common misconception in anaesthetic practice. It is still generally believed that warming the anaesthetic gases as they enter the standard breathing tubes results in the mixture arriving at the mask 'warm', that is, above room temperature. It is a fact, however, that in the case of the semi-open circuit (e.g. Boyle's Apparatus) whatever the temperature of the gases when they enter the familiar corrugated breathing tube they arrive at the facemask substantially at room temperature (p. 43).

The total quantity of heat required to raise the temperature of a given volume of a substance by a certain number of degrees is given by the formula:

volume (cm³) × specific heat (cal/cm³ × degC) × temperature rise (degC)

Examples

(1) What quantity of heat is required to raise the temperature of 1 fluid ounce (28 cm³) of liquid ether by 10 °C ?

volume (28 cm³) × specific heat (0·36 cal/cm³) × temp. rise (10 degC)
$$= 28 \times 0·36 \times 10$$
$$= 100 \text{ cal}$$

The contrast between the number of calories required to heat the same volume of (*a*) a liquid and (*b*) a gas through the same range of temperature is appreciated from the following two examples:

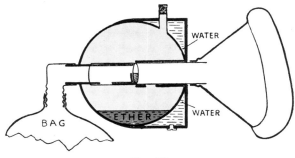

FIG. 17

(2) How much heat is required to raise the temperature of 1 litre of water from 18 °C to 37 °C?

$$a = 1000 \times 1 \times 19 = 19000 \text{ cal}$$

(3) How much heat is required to raise the temperature of 1 litre of a 10% mixture of ether vapour in air from 18 °C to 37 °C?

$$b = 1000 \times 0.0004 \times 19 = 7.6 \text{ cal}$$

Practical applications

In anaesthetic apparatus the high specific heat of water is sometimes used to prevent a rapid fall in temperature of liquid ether. One example of the way in which this is done is described on p. 32. Another way is exemplified by Clover's inhaler.

Fig. 17—One half of the ether chamber in Clover's original ether inhaler[2] is surrounded by a sealed water compartment. The water serves as a source of heat supply to vaporize the ether. The way in which this is effected may involve two separate physical processes. The heat capacity of the water in cooling from room temperature to freezing-point is an obvious source of heat supply. When the temperature falls to zero this source of heat (the heat capacity of the water) is exhausted. If the water now begins to freeze, the latent heat of crystallization (p. 56) of water becomes available without further drop in temperature. The inhaler then behaves in a way similar to the Oxford Vaporiser, with crystalline water (ice) serving the function of the crystalline calcium chloride in the Oxford Vaporiser as a reservoir of heat.

The water container holds 80 cm³
Specific heat of water is 1.
Amount of heat given off when the temperature of the water falls from 20 °C to 0 °C is

$$80 \times 1 \times 20 = 1600 \text{ cal}$$

Latent heat of crystallization of water is 80 cal/g
Amount of heat given off if 80 c.c. of water at 0 °C is transformed into ice at 0 °C is

$$80 \times 80 = 6400 \text{ cal}$$

Total heat available without temperature falling below 0 °C

$$= 8000 \text{ cal}$$

Since the latent heat of evaporation of ether is 65 cal/cm³, 8000 calories are sufficient to vaporize 120 cm³ of ether. It must be remembered, moreover, that there are other sources of heat supply to the ether in the inhaler. Clover's apparatus is made of metal and there is a rapid transfer of heat from the anaesthetist's hand; and since the system is a closed one, a further considerable supply of heat comes from the condensation of the water vapour of the patient's expirations.

The steadying effect of a water jacket on temperature fluctuations has been utilized both in the 'Emotril' apparatus[3] for trichloroethylene analgesia and in the 'E.M.O.' inhaler[4] for ether anaesthesia.

REFERENCES

[1] HARLOW, E. S. (1956). *Science*, 123, 226.
[2] CLOVER, J. T. (1877). *Brit. med. J.* i, 69–70.
[3] EPSTEIN, H. G., and MACINTOSH, R. R. (1949). *Brit. med. J.* ii, 1092–4.
[4] EPSTEIN, H. G., and MACINTOSH, SIR ROBERT (1956). *Anaesthesia*, 11, 83–8.

CHAPTER III

VAPORIZATION

THE molecules in a liquid are in a constant state of movement, but the liquid does not disintegrate because of the strong mutual attraction of the closely-packed molecules. Some, in the surface layer, move vertically with sufficient speed to overcome the force with which their neighbours tend to pull them back into the liquid. They escape into the surrounding atmosphere, where they form what is termed the vapour of the liquid. The more the liquid is heated the more violently do the molecules move and the greater the number which escape into the atmosphere above the liquid.

In a closed container evaporation ceases when the concentration of vapour above the liquid reaches a certain value for any given temperature. After equilibrium is established as many molecules enter the liquid from the vapour as leave the liquid in order to become vapour. The higher the temperature the greater the final concentration of the vapour above the liquid. Conversely as the temperature of the liquid falls there is a corresponding diminution in the concentration of vapour in the atmosphere above it (p. 69).

The process of evaporation entails an expenditure of energy, since the natural tendency of the molecules of a liquid towards cohesion must be overcome. This loss of energy, the latent heat of vaporization, is taken either from (a) an outside source, or (b) from the liquid itself.*

(a) This can be appreciated by evaporating a few drops of water or ether on the hand, or more readily by spraying ethyl chloride on to the skin (fig. 18). The heat necessary to vaporize the liquid is taken from the tissues and cooling is soon apparent. In the case of ethyl chloride, a liquid which because of its low boiling-point evaporates readily, the

---

* The cooling of a liquid during evaporation can be explained in terms of molecular theory. Since only the fastest moving molecules in the surface layer of the liquid escape, the average speed of the remaining molecules is reduced. The average molecular speed of the liquid is a measure of its temperature; as the speed diminishes the temperature falls.

latent heat of vaporization extracted from the tissues is sufficient to cause refrigeration.

(*b*) This is shown in the experiment on p. 35.

The phenomena of latent heat of vaporization are seen also when a

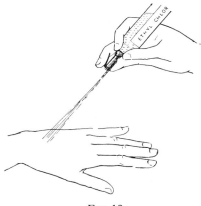

FIG. 18

cylinder of liquid nitrous oxide is turned on and the gas allowed to escape freely. The rapid transformation of liquid nitrous oxide into the gaseous nitrous oxide results in a sharp fall in temperature of the liquid.

Fig. 19—the cylinder was opened and the nitrous oxide allowed to escape freely as an experiment. The marked cooling of the liquid nitrous oxide and of the cylinder has resulted in condensation and freezing of the water vapour in the air immediately surrounding the cylinder.

The formation of snow occurs initially round the bottom of the cylinder, particularly if this was partly emptied before the start of the experiment. The localization of the snow is partly due to the tilting of the cylinder bringing the cold liquid to the lower end, and also to the good heat transfer at the top where it is screwed to the yoke.

The latent heat of vaporization of a liquid is defined as the number of calories required to change 1 *g* of the liquid into vapour *without change of temperature*. Since anaesthetists refer to volumes rather than weights of liquids, we think it more helpful to use the term *latent heat* *of vaporization per cm³* of a liquid. This denotes the number of calories required to convert 1 *cm³* of a liquid into vapour without change of temperature.

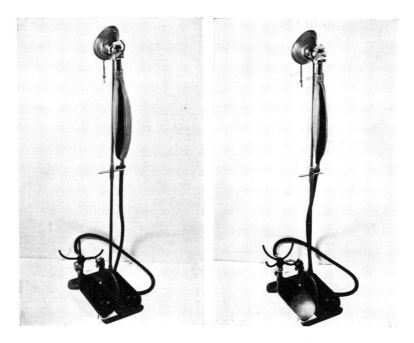

FIG. 19   FIG. 20

Examples

(*a*) Approximately 580 calories are required to convert 1 cm³ of water into water vapour without change of temperature. Conversely when water vapour condenses to liquid water, 580 calories are liberated for each cm³ of water condensed, and the surroundings correspondingly warmed. It is of interest to note that water has a much higher latent heat of vaporization than any other liquid.

(*b*) The latent heat of vaporization per cm³ of liquid ether is 63, that is, 63 calories are required to convert 1 cm³ of liquid ether into ether vapour at the same temperature (fig. 21).

Thus to evaporate 1 oz. (28 cm³) of liquid ether, without change of temperature, $28 \times 63 = 1800$ calories are required.

Fig. 21—A test tube containing 2 cm³ of liquid ether is placed in a bowl holding 63 cm³ of water. The cork is removed, and when 1 cm³ of ether has evaporated, it is found that the temperature of the water has fallen by 1 °C.

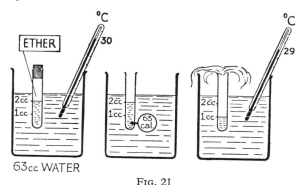

FIG. 21

Perhaps the magnitude of the latent heat of evaporation of ether can be appreciated by realizing that the amount of heat necessary to vaporize any given volume of liquid ether, without change of temperature, is of the same order as the amount of heat required to raise the temperature of the same volume of lukewarm water (say at body temperature) to boiling-point.

Heat of vaporization as function of temperature

The latent heat of vaporization of a given liquid varies with the temperature of the liquid. The colder the liquid the greater is the amount of heat necessary to convert a given quantity into vapour without change of temperature. The latent heat of evaporation becomes smaller with increase in temperature of the liquid until at the critical temperature (p. 93) of the substance the latent heat of vaporization is nil. At its critical temperature a liquid changes spontaneously into vapour without heat being required for the change. Above this temperature the substance cannot exist in the liquid state.

Fig. 22—Shows that the latent heat of evaporation of liquid N_2O is 59 cal/g at 0 °C and 41 cal/g at 20 °C. From this latter point the curve continues to descend sharply until at 36·5 °C, the critical temperature, the latent heat of evaporation is nil.

It will be noticed that when a cylinder of nitrous oxide is used in clinical practice at a constant rate of, say, 8 litres per minute, it frequently takes a long time before it becomes cold enough to condense and freeze the water vapour in the contiguous air. It is noticed, too, that when condensation and freezing do commence, they progress rapidly. If the temperature of the cylinder when it is first used is 20 °C,

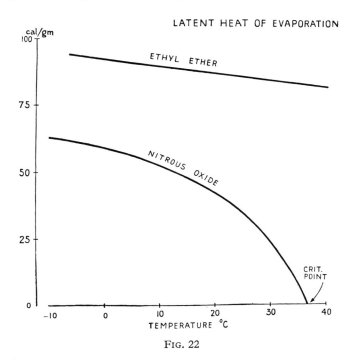

LATENT HEAT OF EVAPORATION

FIG. 22

he latent heat of evaporation of the liquid nitrous oxide is only 41 calories per gram. As the cylinder gradually cools, the latent heat of evaporation of the liquid gradually increases until at 0 °C it is 59 calories per gm. Evaporation now is accompanied by a heat loss 50% greater than when the cylinder was at room temperature. In very warm climates condensation of water vapour and freezing on a cylinder of nitrous oxide do not occur*. Above room temperature the latent heat of evaporation is small; above 36 °C it is nil.

The latent heat of evaporation of ether is also plotted on fig. 22. It is seen that within the range of temperatures at which ether is used in clinical practice, there is no significant variation in the latent heat of

* Cooling effects due to expansion of the compressed gas escaping through the cylinder valve are neglected in this discussion.

evaporation. Thus at 0 °C and 20 °C the figures are 92 and 87 calories per gram respectively.

Fig. 23—of academic interest only, shows the curves for these two agents plotted for a range of temperatures which includes the critical

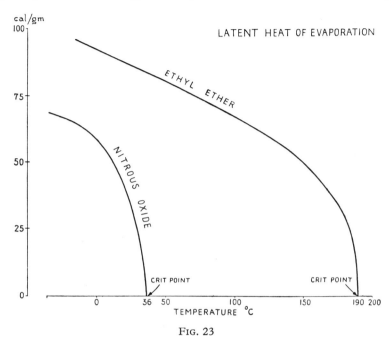

FIG. 23

temperature of ether, 190 °C, at which the latent heat of evaporation of ether is, of course, 0.

Temperature decrease of evaporating liquid

If air or other gas flows over the surface of a liquid, the vapour of the liquid is carried away, and is replaced by fresh vapour. This continuous process of vaporization is accompanied by a corresponding loss of heat (fig. 26). This is seen, also, in a Boyle's apparatus in which nitrous oxide and oxygen are diverted through the liquid ether. As ether evaporates heat is consumed. In fig. 28 (p. 37) where the outside source of heat is very small heat is taken from the liquid ether itself as the fall in temperature testifies. With the fall in temperature of the liquid ether there is a corresponding decrease in the speed of evaporation. If, as in fig. 32, the ether bottle is surrounded by a container of

warm water, there will not be such a rapid fall in temperature of the
liquid ether. Here the water acts as an outside supply of heat. The
same amount of heat is still required to vaporize the same amount of
ether, but in this case there is not a rapid and marked fall in temperature

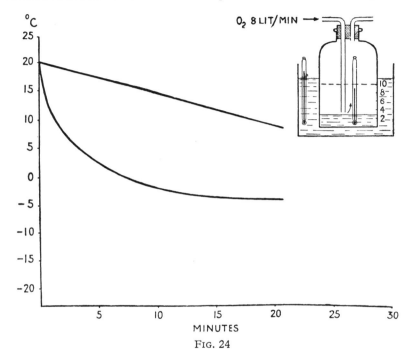

FIG. 24

of the liquid ether. The heat in this instance is supplied largely by the
surrounding water and is transferred through the glass bottle to the
ether. Water has a high specific heat and is therefore a good reservoir
of heat. The rapidity of transfer of heat here from water to the ether is
not striking since glass is a bad conductor.

Fig. 24—Lag in heat transfer through glass can be shown by surrounding the bottle of liquid ether with water at the same temperature,
in this case 20 °C. As in fig. 32 oxygen is bubbled through the ether
at a rate of 8 litres per minute. If the transfer of heat through the glass
were rapid the temperature of the ether (lower line) and the water
(upper line) would fall at substantially the same rate. In the experiment
it was found that after twenty minutes 7 oz (200 cm³) of ether had been
evaporated. The temperature of the ether had fallen to — 4 °C, that of

the water at its periphery to 9 °C, a difference of 13 °C occasioned by the lag in heat transfer not only through the glass, but also through the water from the periphery inwards.

That water is a poor conductor of heat is a daily observation. If hot water is added to a lukewarm bath, transfer of heat is not effective unless the water is mixed by stirring.

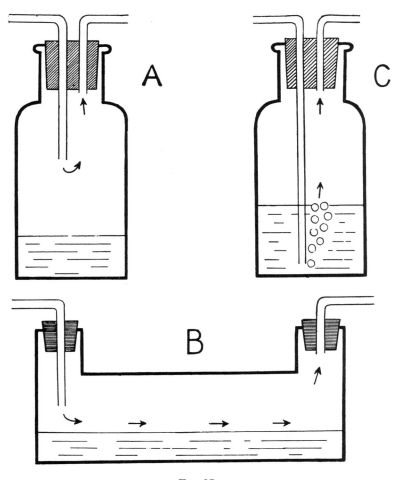

FIG. 25

Bubbling gases through a liquid

When oxygen is blown over the surface of the ether, the percentage of vapour delivered from the bottle depends not only on the temperature of the liquid but on the time during which each unit volume of oxygen is in contact with the liquid ether. If the time is prolonged indefinitely the maximum percentage of ether vapour for that particular temperature is delivered. In actual practice no vaporizer delivers anything near this theoretical maximum.

The only device in production which yields practically saturated vapour is the 'copper kettle' by L. E. Morris.[1] This is a plenum-vaporizer in which a slow flow of oxygen (usually less than 1 l/min) is passed through a porous, sintered metal plate at the bottom of the compartment containing the liquid anaesthetic. The gas rises in numerous, fine bubbles through the liquid and becomes fully saturated with its vapour. The highly concentrated mixture is diluted with oxygen or other anaesthetic gases supplied through accurate flowmeters. The use of a heavy copper container reduces temperature changes due to evaporation and assists in transfer of heat from the anaesthetic trolley to which it is attached. A smaller compartment for liquid can be inserted if the copper vaporizer is to be used with halothane.[2]

In A (fig. 25) the surface area of the ether exposed to the oxygen is small, so that the time of contact with the flowing oxygen is small.

In B the surface area of the ether is increased and the time of contact with the gas passing over it prolonged. The increased time of contact allows a concentration of ether vapour nearer the maximum possible to be picked up. In order to be efficient such a vaporizer would have to be of large dimensions.

C shows a more practical way of increasing the area of contact between the ether and the oxygen by bubbling the oxygen through the liquid. The sum of the surface areas of the individual bubbles is of considerable magnitude, and the contact between the ether and the oxygen may exceed that of B.

REFERENCES

[1] MORRIS, L. E. (1952). *Anesthesiol.*, **13**, 587-93.
[2] FELDMAN, S. A. & MORRIS, L. E. (1958). *Anesthesiol.*, **19**, 650-55.

CHAPTER IV

EXPERIMENTS ON ETHER VAPORIZATION

ON each occasion an ether bottle from a standard Boyle's gas/oxygen machine was filled with 10 fl. oz (285 cm³) of liquid ether at room temperature. 8 litres per minute of oxygen were blown through the bottle. The standard glass bottle has a threaded neck which screws into the cap containing the control lever which was always left in the 'ON' position. The bottle is 12 cm high with an internal diameter of 8 cm; the 10 fl. oz mark is approximately halfway up. In the illustrations a simple glass bottle is depicted.

Figs. 26 and 27—The oxygen passes over the surface of the ether.

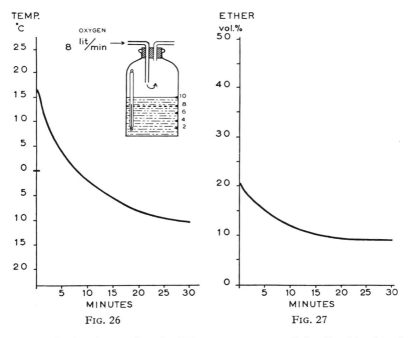

FIG. 26

FIG. 27

No water jacket is employed. The temperature of the liquid ether is taken at frequent intervals, and the ether concentration in the mixture

35

leaving the bottle is measured every five minutes. At first the ether concentration is high, in fact half the saturation concentration at that temperature (fig. 66). Since there is no efficient outside source of heat supply, most of the heat required for the vaporization of the liquid ether is taken from the liquid itself, which cools rapidly. Thus we see that by the end of ten minutes its temperature has fallen below 0 °C and by the end of thirty minutes to — 10 °C. There is a corresponding fall in the concentration of ether vapour leaving the bottle. At the end of thirty minutes 2 oz of liquid ether have been vaporized (note broken line, inset bottle).

Only a very small amount of heat is transmitted from the surrounding atmosphere to the ether through the glass bottle. The effect of this is negligible at the beginning of the experiment when the temperature gradient from the adjacent atmosphere to the liquid ether is small, that is, when the temperature of the liquid ether and the surrounding atmosphere is practically the same. Later in the experiment when there is a pronounced fall in the temperature of the liquid ether, say to — 10 °C, the temperature difference may be as much as 30 °C. The temperature gradient is now considerable, and sufficient heat is transferred to vaporize the small amount of ether now leaving the bottle. The heat supply from the atmospheric air in the room is small, but uniform and inexhaustible. In addition, the heat capacity of the stream of oxygen, radiation from warm objects in the room and condensation of water vapour on the outside of the bottle, all supply additional small amounts of heat. These account for the flattening of the curves after the experiment has been carried on for some time. Towards the end of the experiment the temperature of the liquid ether and the percentage of ether vapour given off remain practically constant.

Figs. 28 and 29—Here the oxygen bubbles through the ether; there is a greatly increased surface contact with the liquid (p. 34). Early in the experiment a high concentration of vapour is obtained. The cooling effect is correspondingly more pronounced. Thus at the end of five minutes the temperature falls to — 5 °C and at the end of thirty minutes to below — 20 °C. The marked fall in temperature is reflected in the fall in the concentration of ether vapour leaving the bottle. At the start of the experiment a high concentration of vapour is delivered. Owing to the fall in temperature the curve falls steeply, but soon flattens out as in the previous experiment, and for the same reasons. At the end of thirty minutes 5 oz of ether have been vaporized.

Clinical Notes

The low temperatures which were recorded in the above experiments actually occur in clinical practice. Condensation of water vapour from the warm humid operating theatre air is commonly seen, and this

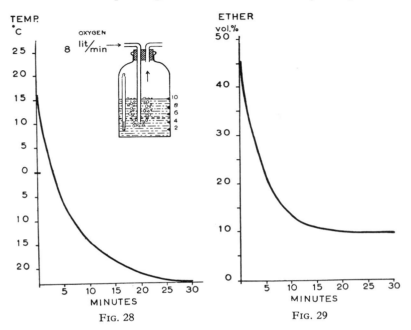

FIG. 28   FIG. 29

condensed water may even freeze into a firm coating of ice on the ether bottle.

These experiments demonstrate that the increased vapour strength produced by bubbling the gases through the liquid ether is maintained for only a short time. The concentration then falls rapidly to the level which it would have reached, had the gases been merely passed over the surface. The inexperienced anaesthetist is sometimes surprised that his patient does not get more deeply anaesthetized when the gases bubble through the ether. Warming the ether by putting some luke-warm water in the outer jacket, or better still, adding some fresh ether at room temperature, would have produced a much more marked effect.

In the experiments shown in figs. 30–33 the ether bottle is surrounded by a water jacket, containing water initially at 27 °C. The temperature of the ether at the start of these two experiments also is 27 °C.

Figs. 30 and 31—Oxygen is blown over the surface of the ether. Since the temperature of the ether is higher than in experiments 26 and 27, the rate of vaporization is higher, and the concentration of ether vapour in the mixture leaving the bottle is higher.

The water surrounding the bottle is a source of supply of heat, and is placed there so that it shall supply some of the latent heat of vaporization of the ether. Glass, however, is a poor conductor of heat (p. 32), and at the beginning the liquid ether loses heat faster than it can be replaced by the surrounding water. At the end of ten minutes the temperature of the ether is 7 °C. The difference between the temperatures of the water and the ether is now great enough to effect the transfer of heat across the glass almost quickly enough to compensate for the heat loss from evaporation. From now onwards the temperature of the liquid ether and the concentration of the vapour delivered falls only very slightly. This tendency is due to the gradual exhaustion of the heat capacity of the water jacket. At the end of thirty minutes 4 oz of ether have been used.

We must emphasize that *water put into the jacket* surrounding the ether bottle *should never* in clinical practice *be more than lukewarm*, say 28 °C (82 °F).

If the ether bottle is surrounded with too hot water and the control tap is turned off, a high vapour pressure will develop inside the ether bottle. A leak of vapour easily occurs past the tap which is not constructed to hold back vapours under pressure greater than atmospheric, and ether in considerable quantity may mix with the gases going to the patient unknown to the anaesthetist. This may be a cause of explosion.

In any case, hot water in the jacket may cause excessively high concentrations of ether vapour to be delivered to the patient causing powerful reflex reactions when they may be least expected, or even lead to gross overdose.

Figs. 32 and 33—The previous experiment is repeated except that here the oxygen is bubbled through the ether. In the early stages high concentrations of ether vapour are delivered. There is a corresponding rapid fall in temperature of the liquid, since there is a lag in the transfer of heat through the glass bottle from the surrounding water. After some fifteen to twenty minutes the percentage of ether vapour delivered has fallen to a level where the heat loss from evaporation is replaced from the surrounding water. At the end of the experiment the temperature

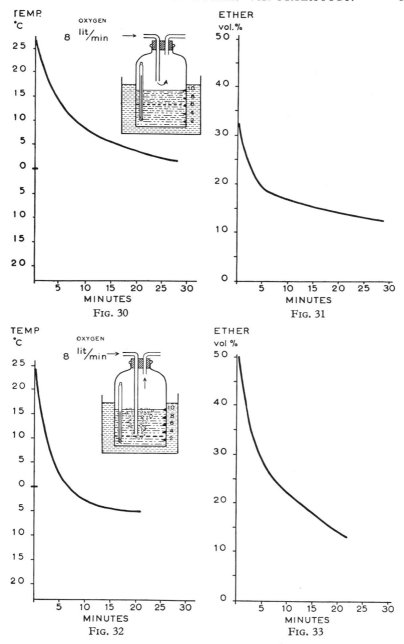

FIG. 30

FIG. 31

FIG. 32

FIG. 33

curve flattens out at a time when the curve showing the percentage of ether delivered is still falling, although gradually. The discrepancy in this experiment is due partly to the rapid drop in the level of the liquid ether, and hence to the shorter distance travelled by the bubbles of O_2 through the liquid. The experiment was abandoned at the end of twenty minutes since the ether level had fallen below that of the oxygen inlet tube. At the end of twenty minutes 7 oz of ether have been evaporated.

The preceding four laboratory experiments bring out physical facts connected with the vaporization of ether. Such striking variations in the range of temperatures and concentrations over such short periods are, of course, not seen in the operating-room, where patients are never exposed to such high initial concentrations of ether vapour.

Temperature of gases passing through ether bottle and breathing tube

The next experiments were carried out during an investigation to see whether warming a liquid anaesthetic has any effect on the temperature of the vapour after it passes through a standard breathing tube.

Experiments 26–33 are repeated in a standard Boyle's bottle with metal cap. In addition to observing the temperature of the ether in the bottle (t_1), the temperature of the gas mixture is taken immediately after it leaves the bottle (t_2), and near the mask (t_3) after it has traversed a standard corrugated rubber breathing tube of one yard (90 cm) length, such as is used in clinical anaesthesia. Throughout the following experiments the room temperature is 18 °C.

The various temperatures were recorded with fine thermocouples, although mercury thermometers are shown on the drawings.

Fig. 34—At the beginning of the experiment the temperatures of the liquid ether, the gas mixture immediately after leaving the bottle and the gas mixture after passing through the corrugated breathing tube, are all practically at room temperature (18 °C). As the experiment proceeds there is a rapid fall in the temperature of the liquid ether (t_1), and by the end of half an hour it has fallen to $-$ 10 °C. The temperature of the gas mixture leaving the bottle (t_2) falls too, but gradually. The straight line (t_3) brings out the striking fact that whatever the temperature of the gas mixture may be on leaving the bottle, the mixture has warmed up to room temperature by the time it reaches the mask end of the breathing tube. This is easily accounted for. The specific heat

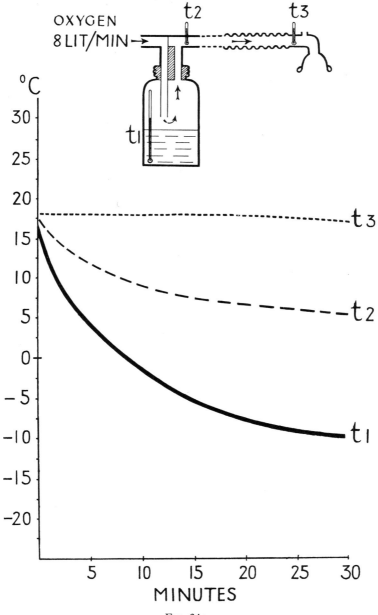

Fig. 34

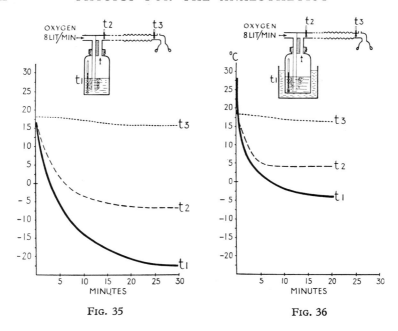

FIG. 35   FIG. 36

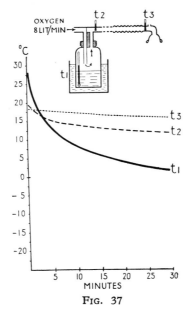

FIG. 37

per cm³ of the gas mixture is so small (approximately 0·0004 cal/cm³ or 0·4 cal/l) that the temperature of quite a large volume is raised by only a small supply of outside heat. The small amount of heat used in warming up the gas mixture flowing through this tube is

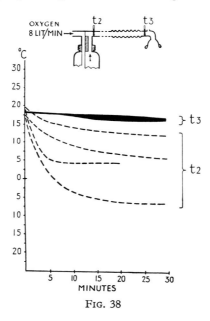

FIG. 38

readily available from the tube itself and the surrounding air. It may be justifiable here to emphasize the difference in the specific heat per cm³ of gases and liquids by pointing out that cold water (specific heat = 1) passing through a similar rubber tube in similar circumstances would emerge with its temperature unchanged. The specific heat per cm³ of water is approximately 2500 times greater than that of the gas mixture used in this experiment.

The experiments illustrated in figs. 35, 36, and 37, show that although the gas mixture may leave the bottle with a temperature as low as — 7 °C, it arrives at the mask substantially at room temperature.

Fig. 38 is a composite of the four previous ones. The four dotted lines record the wide variation in the temperatures of the gas mixtures leaving the bottles. The range is from 20 °C to — 7 °C. The thick line (t₃) covers the temperatures at which these mixtures reached the mask; the range is only between 18 °C and 16 °C.

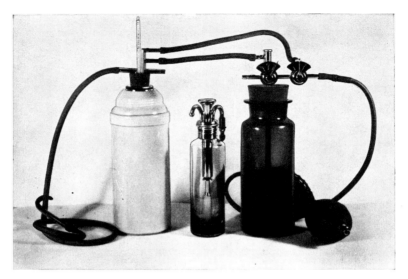

FIG. 39

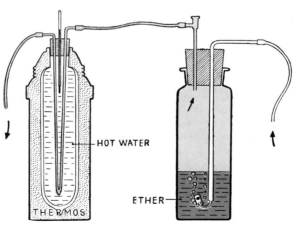

HOT WATER

THERMOS

ETHER

FIG. 40

Experiment with Shipway's Apparatus

By means of a hand bellows air is blown at varying rates through the ether bottle of a Shipway's apparatus, figs. 39, 40. The chloroform bottle has been omitted in the drawing for the sake of clarity. The ether/air mixture passes through the metal U-tube immersed in hot water in a thermos flask. The temperature of the hot water and of the mixture leaving the thermos flask was 80 °C (175 °F).

After passing through the thirty inches (75 cm) of rubber tubing supplied with the apparatus, the temperature of the mixture had fallen to room temperature, as was only to be expected from the experiments just cited.

We were, in fact, unable to reproduce with this model of Shipway's apparatus the results published by the inventor.[1]

This experiment shows that whatever the merits of this apparatus may be, they are not attributable to the ether vapour reaching the patient above room temperature. It has been alleged that the 'warm' ether vapour delivered by Shipway's apparatus accounts for a smoothness of anaesthesia not found when ether is administered by other methods.[2] It is well to bear in mind that this apparatus incorporates a chloroform bottle, the judicious or surreptitious use of which can be of great value in ironing out some of the difficulties which may be encountered with ether, 'warm' or otherwise!

'Warm' anaesthetic vapours

It is worth recording that the claims made for the Oxford Vaporiser did not include delivery of warm ether vapour to the patient. Until recent years the virtues and drawbacks of warm ether vapour were freely discussed. Those who favoured it claimed that it facilitated smooth anaesthesia and that post-operative complications were diminished, whilst the opposition held that warming the ether was responsible for post-operative 'chests', particularly bronchitis.

Although in apparatus like Boyle's and Shipway's warm ether vapour is a myth in the sense that ether vapour does not reach the patient above room temperature, cool ether vapour (as from an open mask) is a fact, although the effect of this on the patient is a subject for discussion. The condensation and freezing of water vapour, so commonly seen on an open mask when ether is administered by this method, shows that the temperature of the gauze has fallen to 0 °C or lower. Since the ether/air mixture travels such a short distance from the gauze to the face it reaches the patient at a temperature well below that of the room.

This chapter demonstrates that little advantage is to be gained by warming the vapours going to the patient if they have to pass through a length of uninsulated tubing after having been warmed. Many attempts have been made in the past to warm vapours of which Shipway's apparatus is but one example.

REFERENCES

[1] SHIPWAY, F. E. (1916). *Lancet*, i, 70–4.
[2] WILSON, S. R., and PINSON, K. B. (1921). *Ibid.* i, 336.

CHAPTER V

HEAT LOSS DURING ANAESTHESIA

THERE are two causes of heat loss through the respiratory tract:

(1) Inhaling gases at a temperature below that of the body. Expired gases are, of course, practically at body temperature, and the difference in heat content between the inspired and the expired gases must be supplied by, and is lost to, the patient.

(2) Inhaling gases with a water vapour content below that of the expired gases. The amount of water vapour in the inspirations varies, but is always below that in the expirations which are saturated with water vapour at body temperature. The difference is made good by water from the body, and for every cm^3 of water vaporized into water vapour for this purpose 580 cal must be supplied by the patient (p. 28).

Heat Loss During the Inhalation of Ether by Various Methods

There are five common methods by which ether is administered by inhalation: (a) open mask, (b) 'semi-open', for example, from Boyle's apparatus, (c) Oxford Vaporiser and 'E.M.O.' Inhaler, (d) carbon dioxide absorption—circle or 'round the houses' and (e) carbon dioxide absorption—Waters' or 'to-and-fro'. Each of these methods will be considered in so far as they influence loss of heat from respiration.

For purposes of uniformity the patient in each case will be assumed to have a respiratory minute volume of 8 litres per minute, and to be breathing a mixture containing 10% ether vapour.

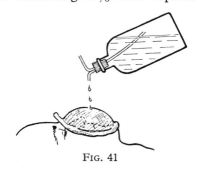

FIG. 41

Open Ether

Frequently as much as 8 fluid oz of ether are poured on the mask within the hour. The amount of heat necessary to volatilize 8 oz.

47

(1 oz $= 28$ cm^3) of ether is $8 \times 28 \times 63 = 14000$ cal approximately. Since the sources of supply of heat are so limited it is little wonder that the temperature of the outside of the mask quickly falls to zero. Assuming that the temperature of the inspired ether/air mixture passing through the mask falls to 0 °C, any water vapour in the mixture condenses on the mask. The inspired mixture, therefore, is practically dry.

The patient draws through the gauze the cold dry mixture, and inspires this, mixed with the gases already under the mask. His expirations, however, continue warm and moist. What effect have these two factors on heat loss?

Respiratory minute volume $= 8000$ cm^3
Temperature of inspired gases $=$ say 0 °C
       ,,   expired   ,, $=$,, 37 °C
Specific heat of 10% ether/air mixture $= 0.0004$ cal/cm^3
(p. 19, Table 1)
Heat loss per minute from this cause
$$8000 \times 37 \times 0.0004 = 120 \text{ cal}$$

Water vapour content of inspired gases at 0 °C, say 0·5% (fig. 70)
      ,,   ,,   expired   ,,   37 °C, say 6%
Loss of water vapour per minute $= 5\frac{1}{2}\%$ of 8000 cm^3 $= 440$ cm^3
At body temperature 1 cm^3 of liquid water is transformed to 1400 cm^3 of water vapour*, and the heat needed for the transformation is 580 cal.
∴ the heat required to furnish 440 cm^3 of water vapour

$$= \frac{440}{1400} \times 580$$

$$= 180 \text{ cal.}$$

With a respiratory minute volume of 8 litres, the heat loss by the patient when ether is administered by the open drop method is of the order of 300 cal/min.

---

* For the sake of uniformity in this, as in many other calculations, we have made use of a fictitious vapour (p. 10) with a pressure of 1 atmosphere at temperatures *below* the boiling-point of the liquid.
If the actual vapour is considered the calculation is carried out as follows:
Specific vol. (p. 97) of saturated water vapour at   0 °C $= 210$ l/g
at 37 °C $= 23$ l/g
Assuming the respired gases are saturated with water vapour:
Water content of 8 litres of inspired air at 0°C $= \dfrac{8}{210} = 0.04$ g
of expired air at 37 °C $= \dfrac{8}{23} = 0.35$ g
∴ loss of water each minute $= (0.35 - 0.04) = 0.31$ g
The latent heat of evaporation of water is 580 cal/g
∴ 0·31 g of water represent a heat loss of $580 \times 0.31 = 180$ cal/min.

Semi-Open Administration

In the Boyle's apparatus, so popular among British anaesthetists, the gases reach the patient at room temperature (p. 43). The amount of heat which has to be supplied by the patient to heat

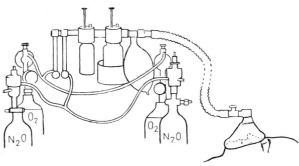

FIG. 42

these gases up to body temperature is therefore smaller than when ether is given by the open method. The nitrous oxide and oxygen which are used as the vehicle to convey ether vapour to the patient are entirely deficient in water vapour, since the gases are dried perfectly before they are compressed into cylinders. The heat lost in saturating the dry gases with water vapour at body temperature is therefore of the same order as when ether is given by the open method.

Respiratory minute volume	$= 8000$ cm³
Temperature of inspired gases	$=$ say 20 °C
„ expired „	$=$ „ 37 °C
Specific heat of inspired mixture	$= 0 \cdot 0004$ cal/cm³
∴ heat loss per minute from this source	$= 8000 \times 17 \times 0 \cdot 0004$
	$= 54$ cal
Water vapour content of inspired gases	$=$ nil
„ „ expired gases at 37 °C	$=$ say 6%
∴ loss of water vapour per minute	$= 6\%$ of 8000 cm³
	$= 480$ cm³

To transform 1 cm³ of liquid water to 1400 cm³ of water vapour requires 580 cal

∴ the heat required to furnish 480 cm³ of water vapour

$$= \frac{480}{1400} \times 580 = 200 \text{ cal}$$

Assuming a respiratory minute volume of 8 litres per minute, the heat lost by the patient when a mixture of gas, oxygen, ether is given from a Boyle's machine is of the order of 250 calories per minute.

The Oxford Vaporiser and the E.M.O. Inhaler

The temperature of the air/ether mixture leaving the Oxford Vaporiser is about 30 °C, but the temperature of the mixture by the time it reaches the mask is practically that of the room, say 20 °C.

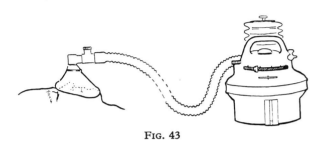

FIG. 43

Since air in the theatre is the vehicle which conveys the ether vapour, the water vapour content of the inspired ether/air mixture is practically the same as that of the air in the operating-theatre, say 1%.

Respiratory minute volume $= 8000$ cm³
Temperature of inspired gases $=$ say 20 °C
    „ expired „ $= $ „ 37 °C
Specific heat of inspired mixture $= 0·0004$ cal/cm³
∴ heat loss per minute from this
  source

$= 8000 \times 17 \times 0·0004$
$= 54$ cal

Water vapour of inspired gases $=$ say 1%
  „   „ expired „ $= $ „ 6%
∴ loss of water vapour per minute $= 5\% \times 8000$ cm³
$= 400$ cm³
The heat required to furnish this $= \dfrac{400}{140} \times 580$ cal
$= 165$ cal

Assuming a minute volume respiration of 8 litres per minute, the heat lost by the patient when ether is given by the Oxford Vaporizer is approximately 220 calories per minute.

In the latest type of draw-over inhaler* ('E.M.O.'), the temperature in the vaporizing compartment may fall below that of the room. However, the temperature of the air/ether mixture leaving this inhaler and passing into the breathing tube to the patient is again at room temperature. The account of the heat lost by the patient which was set out above for the Oxford Vaporiser, applies also to this new inhaler.

Carbon Dioxide Absorption

(a) Circle method

When the ether vapour is confined to a closed circuit as little as 2 oz

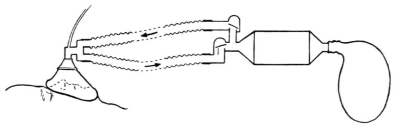

FIG. 44

may suffice for prolonged deep anaesthesia. There is quite a large heat supply from the soda lime, yet some heat is still lost by the patient. Although the soda lime canister may be warm, or even hot, it is remote from the patient (fig. 44). The gases cool down as they pass through the rubber tubing, and by the time they reach the patient are at room temperature. Condensation of water is a feature of closed circuit anaesthesia. The water vapour comes from the patient's expirations and from the soda lime.

The temperature of the inspired gases will rise very gradually with passage of time above that of the surroundings. This is due to condensation of water in the breathing tubes and to the heat produced by the reaction of carbon dioxide with soda lime. However, with fresh soda lime and during the length of an average operation this rise in temperature is unlikely to be great unless the theatre temperature is high.

For the following calculation the inspired gases are considered to be saturated with water vapour at room temperature.

* See p. 25

Minute volume respiration $= 8000 \text{ cm}^3$

Temperature of inspired gases $= \text{say } 20 \text{ °C}$

„   expired   „ $= \text{„} \quad 37 \text{ °C}$

Specific heat of inspired mixture $= 0\cdot0004 \text{ cal/cm}^3$

∴ heat loss from this source $= 8000 \times 17 \times 0\cdot0004$

$= 54 \text{ cal}$

Water vapour of inspired gases at 20 °C $= 2\%$

„   „   expired   „   37 °C $= 6\%$

Loss of water vapour per minute $= 4\% \times 8000 \text{ cm}^3$

$= 320 \text{ cm}^3$

The heat required to furnish this $= \dfrac{320}{1400} \times 580 \text{ cal}$

$= 130 \text{ cal}$

Assuming a respiratory minute volume of 8 litres per minute (in fact, the minute volume seldom attains this magnitude in closed circuit anaesthesia), the heat lost by the patient when ether is given by the circle method is of the order of 180 calories per minute.

(b) To-and-fro method

In this method suggested by Waters[1] the patient breathes through a soda lime canister situated close to the face. Absorption of carbon dioxide by the soda lime soon results in the temperature of the canister rising well above body temperature. After this no heat loss is entailed in warming up the gases. An abundance of water vapour is available from the soda lime and from the expirations; the inspired gases are saturated with water vapour at a temperature well above that of the body. The heat loss by the patient during anaesthesia by this method is negligible, if any.

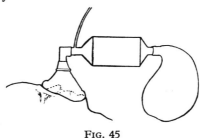

FIG. 45

There is a general feeling that patients anaesthetized with Waters' canister fare better than when the same anaesthetic is given by other means. The improvement, if any, can be accounted for by conservation of body heat.

Humidification of inspired gases

It is worth remarking that heat loss occurs as a result of respiration at all times. It occurs during normal life, and, of course, during an intravenous or a local anaesthetic. The patient breathes the ordinary air in the operating-theatre, say with 1% water vapour, at 20 °C. The factors influencing heat loss and the magnitude of this loss are almost identical with those discussed in connection with the Oxford Vaporiser.

During unconsciousness and anaesthesia, muscular activity, the main source of body heat, is in abeyance. The tendency is for the body temperature to fall.

Any differences in heat loss due to the various methods of giving anaesthetics are probably of little importance if the patient is reasonably fit. In theory, and we think too in practice, the difference is enough to matter when the shocked patient is being anaesthetized. Here heat production has been depressed for some time and every effort must be made to conserve heat.

In order to eliminate heat loss due to respiration we carried out a series of experiments in which the anaesthetic vapours were delivered to the patient at body temperature, and saturated with water vapour at this temperature.

Two different types of humidifiers were made, either of which can be used in conjunction with a Boyle's machine or a draw-over inhaler. Both types of humidifier are equally effective in supplying to the patient gases at body temperature and saturated with water vapour.

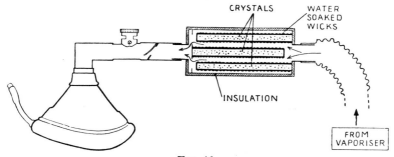

FIG. 46

In both humidifiers, wicks soaked in warm water serve to heat and moisten the gases passing to the patient. The one illustrated in fig. 46

is small because it is attached to the facemask. The heat required to keep the wicks warm and to humidify the inspired gases is supplied by the latent heat of crystallization of an appropriate substance incorporated in the humidifier. Prior to use the crystals are melted by immersing the apparatus in hot water.

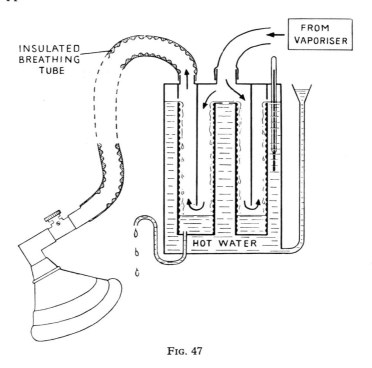

FIG. 47

The second humidifier (fig. 47) is situated remote from the facemask. On this account size is not a consideration. The heat required is supplied from a large volume of hot water which surrounds the wick chamber through which the gases pass on their way to the patient. Overflow from the hot water jacket keeps the wicks moist. In this apparatus there is a certain heat loss through the breathing tube even though it is insulated. To ensure that the gas mixture reaches the patient saturated with water vapour at body temperature, the humidifier is kept at a higher temperature than the previous one.

To assess the effect of abolishing heat loss by the respiratory route various tests were made, but no convincing data were obtained. For example, rectal temperatures showed similar variations to those observed in anaesthesia where humidifiers were not used.

Most anaesthetists have a clinical impression that the results of ether given in a CO_2 absorption apparatus are better than when given by the 'open' method. If this is so it can be accounted for only by conservation of heat.

However, in attempting to minimize heat and water loss, there is evidence of danger in overdoing it. The patient may then suffer from hyperthermia[2] and water intoxication. Such a state of affairs has been blamed as the cause of convulsions during anaesthesia.

REFERENCES

[1] WATERS, R. M. (1924). *Curr. Res. Anesth.* 3, 20–2.
[2] CLARK, R. E., ORKIN, L. R., and ROVENSTINE, E. A. (1954). *J. Amer. med. Ass.* 154, 311–9.

CHAPTER VI

LATENT HEAT OF CRYSTALLIZATION

IT is well known that if heat is given to, or abstracted from, a vessel containing both ice and water, the temperature remains constant until either all the ice has been converted into water, or all the water con-

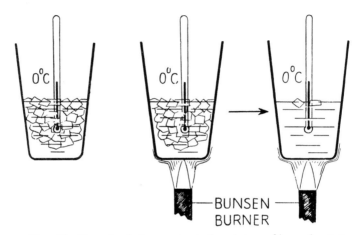

FIG. 48. Alteration in heat content of a mixture of ice and water does not result in temperature changes as long as both ice and water are present.

verted into ice. When heat is added some of the ice melts, and when heat is abstracted some of the water freezes.

The latent heat of crystallization of a substance is the amount of heat given out when 1 gm of the substance is changed from the liquid to the solid state, without alteration of temperature.

In the reverse process—**melting**—the same amount of heat must be supplied to 1 gm of the solid substance to change it into liquid without alteration of temperature. This heat is referred to as the *latent heat of melting*.

If a container of calcium chloride hexahydrate is heated, the temperature of the calcium chloride rises until it begins to melt. Just as in the case of any other crystalline substance (for example, ice) the temperature then remains constant in spite of the addition of more heat, until all the crystals have melted.

In fig. 49 the process of melting is indicated by the horizontal part of the heavy line.

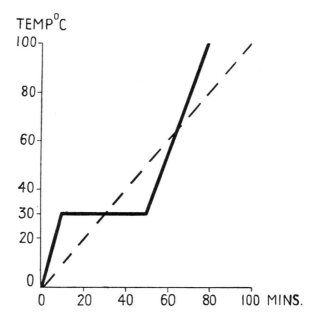

FIG. 49. The effect on the temperature of 1 gram of calcium chloride (continuous line) compared with the effect on the temperature of 1 gram of water (dotted line) when heat is supplied at the rate of 1 calorie per minute.

The melting point of the substance is 30 °C, the latent heat of crystallization is 40 cal/g. The addition of further heat after all crystals have melted results in the temperature rising again steadily.

The steepness of the first and third segment of the heavy line gives an indication of the specific heats of solid and of molten calcium chloride hexahydrate. These can be compared to the specific heat of water indicated by the steepness of the broken line.

The utilization of the latent heat of crystallization of water to replace the heat loss when ether is evaporated has been mentioned in the case of Clover's inhaler (p. 24). On the following pages the use of the calcium chloride in the Oxford Vaporiser is discussed.

Fig. 50—A. Container with calcium chloride at 18 °C (room temperature).

B. The container is heated. Five minutes later the temperature has risen to 30 °C and melting begins.

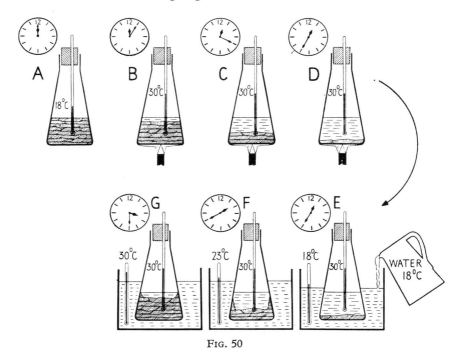

FIG. 50

C. Despite continued heating the temperature remains constant.

D. At the end of thirty-five minutes the bulk of the crystals has melted. Throughout this period heat has been absorbed but the temperature remains unaltered.

E. The container of molten calcium chloride is placed in cool water at 18 °C, and the heat recently given to the calcium chloride is now abstracted from it, and the water round it is warmed. The calcium chloride begins to recrystallize but its temperature remains constant (F) until it has all crystallized. During this time it gives out the heat which it had, so to speak, in storage.

G. This transfer of heat continues for three hours, by which time crystallization is almost complete, and the heat store almost exhausted.

The temperature of a container of partially molten calcium chloride must be 30 °C. If the container is brought into contact with another substance it will tend to make the temperature of the second substance 30 °C. If the temperature of the second substance is higher than 30 °C heat will be abstracted from it and more crystals of calcium chloride

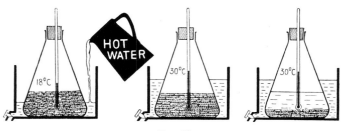

FIG. 51

will melt. If the temperature of the second substance is below 30 °C it will absorb heat from the calcium chloride, some of the liquid of which crystallizes.

In the previous experiment heat is supplied to the crystalline calcium chloride by a Bunsen burner. Another way is to immerse the container with calcium chloride in hot water (fig. 51). Again, once it begins to melt the temperature of the calcium chloride remains constant, until it is all molten.

In the Oxford Vaporiser[1] use was made of the latent heat of crystallization of calcium chloride in order to keep uniform the temperature of ether in an adjoining container, despite heat loss by evaporation. This ensures a fixed concentration of ether vapour being available to the patient for any one setting of the control tap. Calcium chloride hexahydrate proves suitable since amongst other things its melting-point is sufficiently high to ensure a strong concentration of ether vapour within the apparatus.

REFERENCE

[1] MACINTOSH, R. R., and BANNISTER, F. B. (1952). *Essentials of general anaesthesia*, 5th ed., chap. 32. Oxford.

Chapter VII

PARTIAL PRESSURE

THE pressure of a gas is a measure of the molecular bombardment on each unit area of the wall of its container in unit time. The closer the molecules the greater the number which strike each unit area, and therefore the greater the pressure exerted.

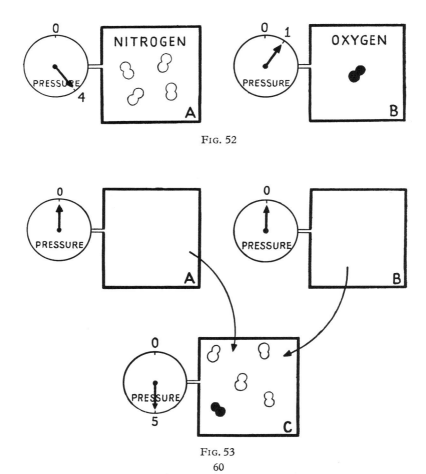

FIG. 52

FIG. 53

Fig. 52—A closed jar (A), the walls of which have unit area, contains 4 molecules of nitrogen. The effect of the bombardment on the walls of the jar by these molecules is called the pressure of the nitrogen. If each molecule striking the wall produces 1 unit of pressure, the pressure in A is 4 units. An identical jar (B) contains 1 molecule of oxygen. The pressure in B is 1 unit.

Fig. 53—If the nitrogen and oxygen molecules are now transferred into a third container of similar dimensions (C), the molecules still continue to bombard the walls in the same way as they did before. There are now 5 molecules in the jar and the total pressure is 5 units.

We have seen on page 3 that at the same temperature and pressure the same number of molecules of any gas occupies the same volume. Since 5 molecules occupy the volume of the jar, the molecule of oxygen occupies the equivalent* of $\frac{1}{5}$ of the volume, and exerts $\frac{1}{5}$ of the total pressure. The pressure of the oxygen is referred to as its partial pressure, and is the same proportion of the total pressure as its volume is of the total volume.

In describing a mixture of gases one can refer to its percentage composition by volume, or, when the total pressure exerted by the mixture is known, to the partial pressure exerted by its component gases. Thus in the above example the mixture can be said to contain 80% nitrogen, or nitrogen exerting a partial pressure of 4 units out of a total of 5.†

From this example it can be seen that

(*a*) In a mixture of gases each gas exerts the same pressure which it would if it alone occupied the container (**Dalton's** Law).

(*b*) In a mixture of gases the pressure each gas exerts is called its partial pressure, and the total pressure of the mixture is the sum of the partial pressures of the constituent gases.

(*c*) In a mixture of gases each constituent gas exerts the same proportion of the total pressure as its volume is of the total volume.

---

* By this is meant that if the oxygen were isolated and compressed until it exerted the same pressure as the original mixture, its volume would be only $\frac{1}{5}$ of the original mixture.

† For simplicity small numbers are used. For the laws relating to partial pressure to be true these would have to represent many billions of molecules

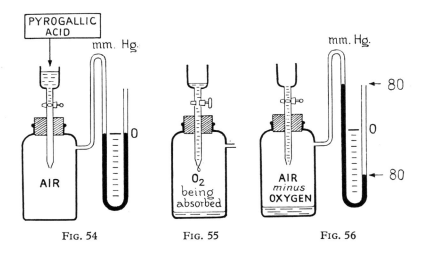

FIG. 54   FIG. 55   FIG. 56

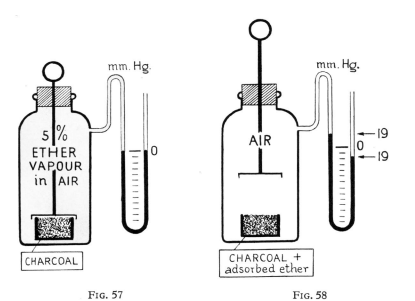

FIG. 57   FIG. 58

Experiments.

(i) To determine (*a*) the partial pressure, (*b*) the percentage by volume of oxygen in the atmosphere.

Figs. 54 and 55—Pyrogallic acid is run into a jar containing air at atmospheric pressure.

Fig. 56—The tap is now closed. When the oxygen has been absorbed the difference in the levels of the mercury in the manometer U-tube is 160 mm. The partial pressure of oxygen in the atmosphere is therefore 160 mmHg .

Total atmospheric pressure $= 760$ mmHg
Partial pressure of oxygen $= 160$ mmHg
Percentage of oxygen in atmosphere $= \dfrac{160}{760} \times 100 = 21$

(ii) To determine the partial pressure exerted by ether vapour in a mixture of 5% ether vapour in air at sea level.

Figs. 57 and 58—The lid of the charcoal container is raised, and the ether vapour is adsorbed by charcoal. It is found that the pressure in the jar falls by 38 mmHg . This is therefore the partial pressure of the ether vapour. *N.B.* 38 is 5% of 760.

These experiments illustrate a principle widely used in the analysis of gases. From a mixture in a closed container one component is absorbed and the resultant fall in pressure in the container gives the volume per cent of this component in the original mixture. A well-known example of an apparatus utilizing this principle is the Van Slyke method for the analysis of blood gases.

Significance of partial pressure for the diffusion of gases

If a gas exists on either side of a membrane,* the direction of its diffusion is determined not by any difference in its amount but by any

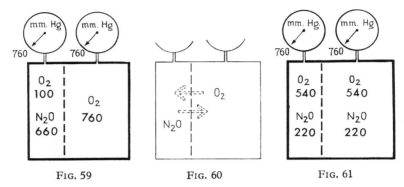

| FIG. 59 | FIG. 60 | FIG. 61 |

difference in the partial pressures which it exerts on either side of the membrane. A gas diffuses from a place where it is at high partial pressure to a place where it is at a lower partial pressure, even though the latter may contain a larger volume of the gas (see also Chap. xviii).

Fig. 59—Two containers are separated by a permeable membrane. The total pressures within the containers are identical. One is filled with oxygen only, the other with a mixture of nitrous oxide and oxygen. The partial pressure of the gases are indicated.

Fig. 60—Oxygen diffuses from the right container where it is at a higher partial pressure, and similarly nitrous oxide diffuses into the right container where initially it was absent.

Fig. 61—The total pressure in each container remains unchanged. The individual gases are in equilibrium. The partial pressure of oxygen (and that of nitrous oxide) on either side of the membrane is identical. If the container volumes are in the ratio of 1 : 2, the final oxygen pressure is given by:

$$\frac{1}{3} \times 100 + \frac{2}{3} \times 760 = 540; \text{ that of nitrous oxide becomes } 220.$$

* In this and the following examples a permeable membrane is postulated, which, although preventing the transfer of gases in bulk, allows them to diffuse through it. This process is a molecular one and takes place through the microscopic pores of the membrane.

In the alveoli the percentage of oxygen is 14; the partial pressure this gas exerts, therefore, is 14% of 760 mmHg $= 100$ mm Hg . The tension of oxygen (p. 241) in the venous blood in the capillaries of the lungs is known to be approximately 40 mmHg . The thin alveolar

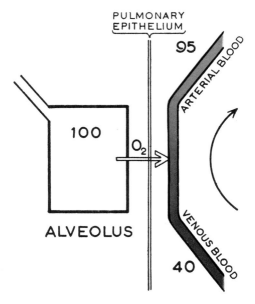

FIG. 62. The slight discrepancy between the values of the partial pressure of oxygen in the alveoli and the tension of oxygen in the arterial blood is discussed on p. 67 and in a footnote on p. 241.

membrane is readily permeable to oxygen, and allows oxygen to diffuse from the place of high partial pressure, the alveoli, to the place where it is at lower tension, venous blood. This process of diffusion raises the tension of oxygen in the arterial blood leaving the alveoli to 95 mmHg .

The composition and therefore the partial pressures of the component gases in the alveoli are maintained practically constant by respiration. At least 15-20 times a minute about 400 cm^3 (approximately one-twelfth of the total lung content) of fresh air is distributed throughout the lungs, and an equal volume of gases, high in CO_2 content, is carried away. Although breathing is an intermittent act, the composition of alveolar air can be regarded as constant.

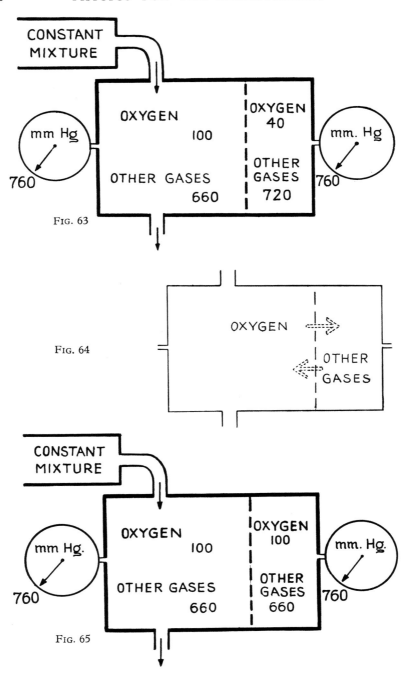

Fig. 63

Fig. 64

Fig. 65

These three figures illustrate the change from venous to arterial blood by the diffusion of gases across the alveolar membrane.

Fig. 63—The left hand chamber represents the alveoli, the right the venous blood. The total pressures in both are the same, but the partial pressure of oxygen is much higher in the alveoli than in the venous blood.

In life complete equilibrium is not attained, since a part of the lungs may be quiescent during respiration, as a result of which blood flowing through remains unoxygenated.

Transfer of oxygen across a membrane is in no way comparable to the flow of a gas through a tube from a region of high pressure to one of lower. The total tension of the gases in the blood is virtually the same as the total pressure of gases in the alveoli (760 mmHg). During respiration oxygen can pass across the alveolar membrane only by diffusion and not 'in bulk' as in the 'flow' of gas.

Fig. 64—Oxygen diffuses into the venous blood. Carbon dioxide diffuses into the alveoli.

While respiration is intermittent, diffusion proceeds continuously.

Fig. 65—Equilibrium has been reached. The partial pressure of oxygen is the same on both sides of the membrane. The right hand chamber represents arterial blood. The composition of the gases in the chamber representing the alveoli remains unaltered.

CHAPTER VIII

VAPOUR PRESSURE

JUST as in any other gas the molecules of a vapour (p. 95) are continually in violent movement. The bombarding force which they exert on each unit area of the walls of their containing vessel, or on a measuring instrument, is called the pressure of that vapour. When the space above a liquid is in communication with the outer air, the total pressure of the mixture of vapour and air equals the atmospheric pressure.

The molecules of, say, ether vapour occupy space and have weight just as have molecules of, say, oxygen or nitrogen. The expression '5% mixture of ether vapour in air' is meaningless unless it is known whether the percentage refers to weight or to volume of the components. It can be calculated that a 5% mixture of ether vapour in air by volume (v/v) differs considerably from the same percentage by weight (w/w). A 5% ether vapour (v/v) is, in fact, equivalent to 12% (w/w).

When present-day anaesthetists speak of 5% ether vapour in air they mean by volume, that is, 5% of the volume of the mixture is ether vapour, the remaining 95%, air. We follow this practice, and when we refer to the percentage composition of gas mixtures we mean percentage by volume (v/v).*

A mixture of gases exerts a pressure on the walls of its container. That part of this total pressure which is exerted by any one of the vapours—the partial pressure of that vapour—bears the same proportion to the total pressure as the volume of the vapour bears to the volume of the mixture. 5% ether vapour in air at sea level exerts a pressure of 5% of 760 mmHg = 38 mmHg .

When a liquid at a given temperature is in a closed container, the number of vapour molecules ultimately re-entering the liquid becomes

---

* The same considerations apply to liquids. It was common practice to mix liquid chloroform and ether in the same drop bottle. A favourite mixture, the so-called 'C$_2$E$_3$' mixture consists of 2 volumes of chloroform mixed with 3 volumes of ether. There is a marked difference in the specific gravities of chloroform (1·5) and of ether (0·72). In fact, a 'C$_2$E$_3$' mixture (v/v) has the same composition as a 'C$_3$E$_2$' mixture (w/w); the chloroform content are 40% (v/v) or 60% (w/w).

A mixture of 25% Vinesthene and 75% ether (w/w) is on sale under the name of Vinesthene/Ether mixture. Since the specific gravities of these two liquids are very similar, a practically identical mixture can be made by mixing 25 volumes of Vinesthene and 75 volumes of ether.

exactly equal to the number leaving it. A state of equilibrium is reached; no increase in the vapour occurs. The 'saturated vapour' now above the liquid is the strongest vapour it is possible to have at that particular temperature. Any stronger concentration at that temperature would

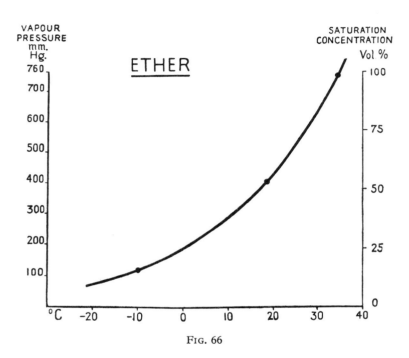

FIG. 66

result in condensation of surplus vapour to liquid. With any increase in temperature more molecules leave the liquid and a higher concentration of vapour results. Conversely, when the temperature falls some of the vapour molecules return to the liquid state with a corresponding fall in the concentration of the vapour.

Fig. 66—shows how the concentration of ether vapour over liquid ether varies with the temperature. Such a graph, the 'vapour pressure curve' of a liquid, shows the relationship between temperature and the pressure of a saturated vapour, that is, a vapour in equilibrium with its own liquid.

Fig. 67—The vapour pressure curves of liquids commonly used by the anaesthetist.

When the pressure of the vapour of a liquid which is in communication with the outer air becomes equal to the atmospheric

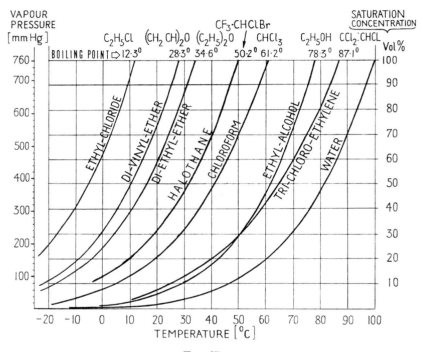

FIG. 67

pressure, the vapour occupies 100% of the space immediately above the liquid, that is, the vapour is undiluted with air. At this pressure, that is, atmospheric pressure, or very slightly above, bubbles of vapour form in the interior of the liquid and the liquid is said to 'boil'. There is rapid transformation of the liquid into vapour. The *boiling-point* of any given liquid is the temperature at which its vapour pressure equals the pressure of the atmosphere.

The above figure shows that at 20 °C the percentage of saturated **water** vapour in the atmosphere is very small. It shows, too, that the *maximum* volume percentage of **trichloroethylene** vapour available at this temperature from a saturated Schimmelbusch mask is of the order of 6. This theoretical maximum percentage is, of course, never realized in clinical practice. Not only is the vapour constantly being removed by respiration through the mask, but the concentration of vapour available is soon reduced still further by cooling. This explains why the open mask method of administration is unsuitable for this drug.

Air saturated with **chloroform** at room temperature contains 20% chloroform vapour by volume, a percentage very much greater than the 4·5% which is commonly accepted as the maximum ever justifiable in clinical practice.

At room temperature the maximum percentage of **di–ethyl ether** vapour is very high. Under experimental conditions such high concentrations when inhaled have proved to be alarmingly potent. In fact, breathing even a 40% mixture of ether vapour in air rapidly results in respiratory arrest. In clinical practice, however, as for example on an open mask or in a Boyle's bottle (p. 35), evaporation leads to a rapid fall in temperature with a corresponding fall in the volume percentage of vapour. Unless the liquid ether is warmed by external means, concentrations above 15% are rarely obtainable.

Halothane ('Fluothane', or trifluoro-chloro-bromo ethane) has a boiling point of 51 °C. At room temperature its vapour pressure lies between that of chloroform and ether. Care in its administration and the use of quantitative vaporizing devices are therefore indicated in order that the patient does not inhale concentrations in excess of the clinical range of, say, 4%.

The vapour pressure curve of **di–vinyl ether** is not far removed from that of di-ethyl ether. Its high vapour pressure at room temperature makes the open mask an easy means of administering this agent. Its low boiling point (28·3 °C) accounts for the fact that from time to time unopened bottles are found empty, if they have not been perfectly stoppered.

Ethyl chloride is supplied in sealed bottles. Its boiling-point is 12·5 °C, therefore at room temperature the pressure of the vapour over the liquid exceeds 760 mmHg . If the bottle is inverted and the tap opened, a stream of liquid ethyl chloride is forced out.

We have attempted unsuccessfully to use the vapour of ethyl alcohol as a general anaesthetic. At room temperature it will be seen that the vapour pressure of this agent is even less than that of trichloroethylene. Its use on an open mask is quite ineffective and its administration through an Oxford Vaporiser does not take the patient beyond a state of mild drunkenness.

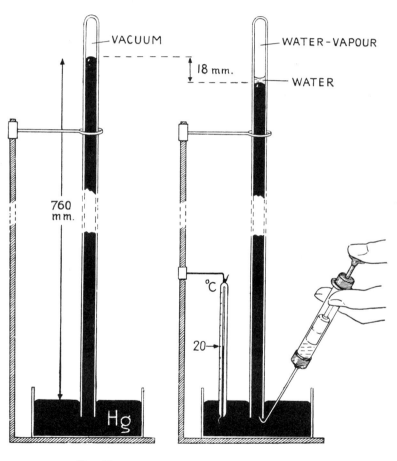

FIG. 68   FIG. 69

Water Vapour Pressure

To determine the pressure of water vapour at room temperature.

Fig. 68—The atmospheric pressure at sea level supports a column of mercury 760 mm high.

Fig. 69—A little water is introduced into the mercury tube. The level of the mercury is depressed to 742 mm by the pressure of the water vapour above it. The pressure of saturated water vapour at 20 °C is therefore 18 mmHg . For water vapour to exert this pressure when mixed with air, its concentration must be $\frac{18}{760} \times 100 = 2\cdot4\%$.

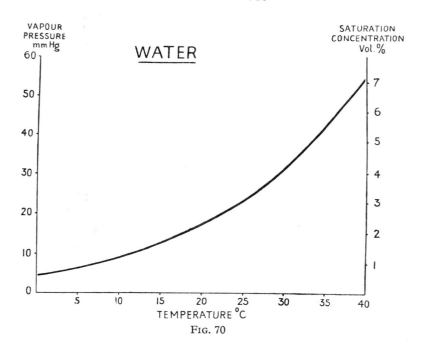

FIG. 70

Fig. 70—Vapour pressure curve for water from 0 °C to 40 °C. This curve shows the partial pressure of saturated water vapour over a range of temperatures from 0 °C to 40 °C, and also the volume percentage of water vapour to which these pressures correspond.

If air is saturated with water vapour at a given temperature, it is said to have a relative humidity of 100%. Thus a relative humidity of 50% means that the partial pressure of water vapour is half the saturation pressure at that temperature.

In the open air the relative humidity varies with the temperature and other weather conditions, and ranges between the extremes of 0% and 100%; the air may be quiet dry or it may be saturated with water vapour.

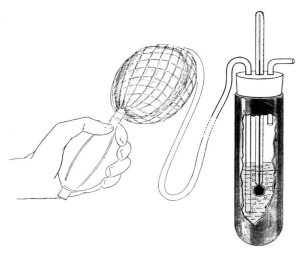

Fig. 71. Regnault's hygrometer

The humidity in the operating-theatre is increased by proximity to sterilizers, especially if the ventilation is poor. In these circumstances it may exceed 60%, but it may be reduced to any desired figure by air conditioning. Although reduction of the humidity of the air in the operating-theatre increases the comfort of the operating team,[1] it is not without its hazards in certain circumstances. The drier the atmosphere the more conducive it is to static electricity, one of the causes of anaesthetic explosions.

Methods of Measuring the Humidity of the Air

Fig. 71—The apparatus consists of a thin silver tube containing ether and a thermometer to show the temperature of the ether. As air is pumped through the ether evaporation takes place. The temperature of the ether falls and that of the silver tube (an excellent conductor of heat) falls with it. The air in contact with the tube chills. Cooling continues until the water vapour in the contiguous outside air is saturated, and condenses as a mist on the bright silver. The temperature at which this takes place is known as the 'dew point', and represents the saturation temperature of the water·vapour in the room.

Example. To determine the humidity of a room.

Using Regnault's hygrometer the silver tube became misty when the temperature fell to 5 °C.

Fig. 70 shows that the saturation pressure of

water vapour at 5 °C = 6·5 mmHg

This, therefore, is the partial pressure of the water vapour in the room.

Temperature of room = 20 °C

Saturation pressure of water at

20 °C = 18 mmHg

∴ relative humidity $= \dfrac{6·5}{18} \times 100$

$= 36\%$

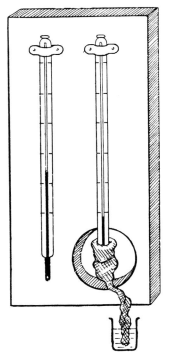

Fig. 72—The apparatus consists of two similar thermometers mounted side by side. The bulb of one is covered by a muslin bag kept constantly wet by dipping into a small container of water. If the atmosphere is not already saturated with water vapour, some of the water on the muslin evaporates, with resulting cooling of the thermometer bulb enclosed by the muslin. There is now a lower reading on the 'wet' thermometer than on the dry one. This difference depends on the rate of evaporation, and this in turn on the amount of water vapour in the atmosphere. On a humid day there will be little difference between the two readings, while the converse holds on a dry day. With each instrument a table of figures is supplied which gives at once the relative humidity of the atmosphere for any pair of wet and dry thermometer readings.

FIG. 72.

Wet and dry bulb thermometer

A short abstract of such a table is given below. The 'wet bulb depression' is the difference between the wet and the dry bulb readings.

TABLE 2

Wet Bulb Depression (t_d-t_w) °C	RELATIVE HUMIDITY (%) When the Dry Bulb Temperature (t_d) is			
	10 °C	20 °C	30 °C	40 °C
1	88	91	93	94
2	77	83	86	88
3	66	74	79	82
4	55	66	73	77
6	34	51	61	67
8	15	37	50	57
10	—	24	39	48

The meaning of *absolute humidity* and its importance for problems of humidification will be discussed on pages 397–402.

REFERENCE

[1] WYNNE, R. L. (1947). *Brit. med. J.*, i, 528–9.

CHAPTER IX

ATMOSPHERIC PRESSURE

THE air is compressed by the weight of air above it. At ground level this compression results in the molecules of the component gases being packed together so that they exert a pressure of 760 mmHg (or 760 Torr; see p. 422). Some idea of the magnitude of this pressure will be grasped

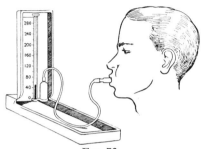

FIG. 73

when it is realized that the fit adult blowing hard can force mercury up a tube only about 50 mm,—approximately 1/15 atmospheric pressure (fig. 73).

At heights above sea level the weight of overlying air is less. The molecules are less closely packed so that they now exert less pressure. At 10000 feet, for example, the pressure is sufficient to support a column of mercury only 520 mm high (p. 86). The pressure of the atmosphere is a molecular effect and is exerted in all directions.

Examples

1. What is the partial pressure at sea level of
    (*a*) oxygen in air?
    (*b*) ether vapour in a mixture of 5% ether vapour in air?

(*a*)   Percentage of oxygen in air is   21
    ∴ at sea level partial pressure

of oxygen is $\dfrac{21}{100} \times 760 = 160$ mmHg

(*b*)   Percentage of ether is   5
    ∴ at sea level partial pressure

of ether vapour is $\dfrac{5}{100} \times 760 = 38$ mmHg

2. What is the partial pressure (*a*) of oxygen in air, and (*b*) of ether vapour in a mixture of 5% ether vapour in air, when the atmospheric pressure is 600 mmHg corresponding to an altitude of about 6000 feet?

(*a*) The percentage composition of the atmosphere remains unchanged irrespective of the height above sea level.

Percentage of oxygen   = 21

∴ the partial pressure of

$$\text{oxygen} = \frac{21}{100} \times 600$$

$$= 126 \text{ mmHg}$$

(*b*)   Percentage of ether vapour = 5

∴ partial pressure of

$$\text{ether vapour} = \frac{5}{100} \times 600$$

$$= 30 \text{ mmHg}$$

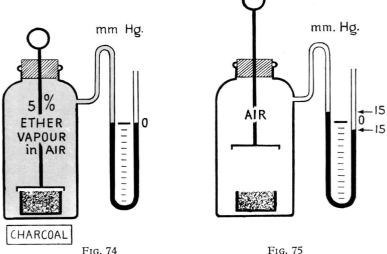

FIG. 74   FIG. 75

Figs. 74 and 75. Experiment at 6000 feet.

Compare with figs. 57 and 58 (p. 62).

The transfer of ether vapour between the lungs and the blood depends on the difference in the partial pressures of ether vapour in the alveoli and in the blood.

5% ether vapour at ground level exerts a pressure of 38 mmHg, and at a height of 6000 feet, 30 mmHg . It is obvious that a patient at sea level breathing 5% ether vapour is exposed to a slightly more potent anaesthetic mixture than the same percentage breathed at 6000 feet.

As long as a flask remains open to the atmosphere the total pressure

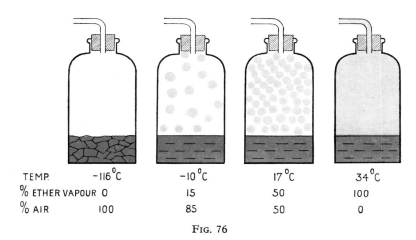

TEMP	−116 °C	−10 °C	17 °C	34 °C
% ETHER VAPOUR	0	15	50	100
% AIR	100	85	50	0

FIG. 76

within it remains equal to atmospheric. At sea level the pressure exerted by the atmosphere is 760 mmHg . At this level air can be described either as '100% air' or as 'air exerting a pressure of 760 mmHg'. If liquid ether is now poured into the flask ether vapour will displace some of the air, but the combined pressures exerted by the ether vapour and the air remain 760 mmHg .

Fig. 76—The partial pressure exerted by the ether vapour within the bottle depends on the temperature of the liquid ether. Thus in the extreme case of the ether being frozen (a condition never met with clinically, since ether freezes at − 116 °C) the pressure exerted by the minute amount of ether vapour above it is negligible, and we can describe the state of affairs by saying that the pressure of the ether vapour is 0, or that the percentage of ether vapour in the bottle is 0.

When the temperature of the ether is − 10 °C , a situation common in practice, the pressure exerted by the ether vapour in the flask is 110 mmHg, the remaining 650 mmHg being exerted by the air. The composition of the gas in the flask would be equally well described by the anaesthetist as a 15% mixture of ether vapour in air; this follows from: $\frac{110}{760} \times 100 = 15$.

If the liquid ether is warmed evaporation takes place into the space above the liquid. There is a rise in vapour pressure at the expense of the partial pressure exerted by the air. The vapour pressure curve of ether (fig. 77) shows at a glance the pressure exerted by saturated ether

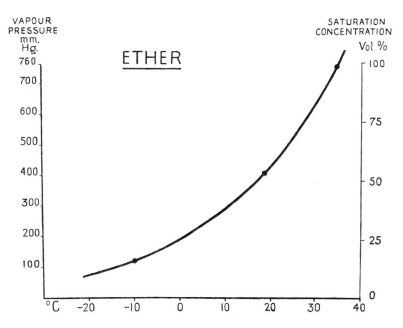

Fig. 77—The dots on the vapour pressure curve represent the conditions in three of the bottles of fig. 76.

vapour at any given temperature, and the scale on the right shows the corresponding percentage composition. When liquid ether is heated to 35 °C the pressure exerted by its vapour exceeds 760 mmHg . At this temperature air is entirely displaced and the atmosphere above the liquid ether consists of 100% ether vapour (fig. 76). At a room temperature of 17 °C the pressure exerted by the vapour is approximately 380 mmHg . The gaseous mixture in the flask is composed of equal volumes of air and ether vapour.

If a saturated vapour of ether at any given temperature is cooled, condensation of some of the vapour to liquid must occur. This eventuality arises in clinical anaesthesia only in exceptional circumstances, since at room temperature the concentration of ether vapour would have to exceed 50% before condensation occurred.

In practice such a concentration is never justifiable. Analyses [1, 2] of samples taken under the mask during open ether anaesthesia gave concentrations of ether not exceeding 17%. The maximum strength of ether vapour obtainable from the 'E.M.O.' Inhaler is 20%, and it is only rarely that such a strong concentration is used.

Devices supplying ether vapour at pressures above atmospheric

There are, however, two machines which deliver 100% ether vapour. This vapour must be greatly diluted with air or gas and oxygen to prevent overdosage. Condensation at room temperature would occur only if the percentage of ether vapour in the mixture exceeded the grossly excessive figure of 50.

In both the Pinson 'bomb'[3] (figs. 78 and 79) and the Oxford Vaporiser type II[4] (fig. 80) liquid ether, in a robust metal container, is maintained at a temperature well above its boiling-point. The pressure of ether

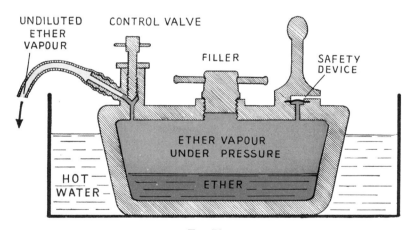

FIG. 78

vapour within the container considerably exceeds atmospheric pressure, so that when the valve is opened undiluted ether vapour is released.

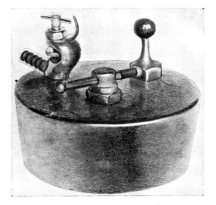

FIG. 79

In the Pinson 'bomb' the vapour is led through a narrow rubber tube to an open mask where it is freely diluted with air. At first when ether vapour from the 'bomb' is released some condenses in the rubber delivery tube. The heat of condensation derived from this process soon warms the tube above the boiling-point of ether. From now on undiluted ether vapour reaches the distal end of the narrow tube.

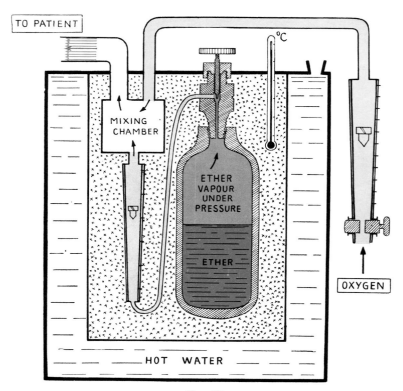

FIG. 80

In the Oxford Vaporiser type II the ether was maintained at a temperature well above its boiling point. The situation is now analogous to a cylinder of nitrous oxide. As soon as the tap is opened, vapour escapes freely. The flow rate of undiluted vapour is measured by a Rotameter in the same way as the flow of other anaesthetic gases, such as nitrous oxide and cyclopropane. For ether vapour, however, the flowmeter is kept warm, otherwise condensation would occur within it.

From the flowmeter the ether vapour is led to a warm mixing chamber in which it is mixed with oxygen with or without nitrous oxide.

In this vaporizer the ether can be maintained at any temperature between, say, 40 °C and 100 °C, depending on the melting point of the crystals used in its construction. The vapour pressure of ether between these two temperatures ranges from 1·5 to 6·5 atmospheres.

We have used this vaporizer both for semi-closed and for absorption anaesthesia. Although it is of interest to see the flow of ether vapour actually measured, we have not found any other advantages.

Respiration at High Altitudes

An understanding of some of the problems connected with high flying[5] will help the anaesthetist to appreciate the significance of the term 'partial pressure'.

Carbon dioxide is excreted from the blood stream into the alveoli and the partial pressure it exerts in the alveoli remains practically constant at 40 mmHg . Another gas inevitably present in the alveoli is water vapour. The pressure it exerts is the saturation pressure of water vapour at body temperature. Since the body temperature remains constant the partial pressure of the water vapour in the alveoli remains constant at 47 mmHg (p. 73).

These two gases, therefore, together exert a combined pressure of approximately 90 mmHg under all conditions. At sea level the pressure of the other gases (nitrogen and oxygen) in the lungs is $(760 - 90) = 670$ mmHg , whilst if air is breathed at 30000 feet, where the total atmospheric pressure is 225 mmHg , the combined pressure exerted by the nitrogen and oxygen in the lungs will be $(225 - 90) = 135$ mmHg .

The *percentage* of oxygen in atmospheric air is unaffected by altitude and remains constant at 21. Since some of the inspired oxygen has been absorbed and metabolized the percentage of oxygen in a dry and CO_2-free alveolar gas sample is only 15%.

Sea Level

Assuming air only is breathed, the partial pressure of oxygen in the alveoli at sea level is 15% of (760 − 90) mmHg = 100 mmHg .

6000 feet

At 6000 feet (1800 m) the atmospheric pressure equals 610 mmHg and the partial pressure of oxygen in the alveoli is 15% of (610 − 90) = 78 mmHg . If the tension of oxygen in venous blood is taken as 40 mmHg there is still a sufficient pressure difference, (78 − 40) mmHg, of oxygen between alveoli and venous blood to effect adequate oxygenation of the blood.

14000 feet

At 14000 feet (4200 m) the atmospheric pressure has fallen to 450 mmHg . The combined partial pressure of carbon dioxide and water vapour in the alveoli remains at 90 mmHg . The combined pressure exerted by the oxygen and nitrogen in the alveoli is therefore (450 − 90) mmHg = 360 mmHg . The pressure exerted by the oxygen in the alveoli at this height is therefore 15% of 360 = 54 mmHg . The pressure difference of oxygen between alveoli and venous blood is now reduced to 14 mmHg . Oxygenation of the blood

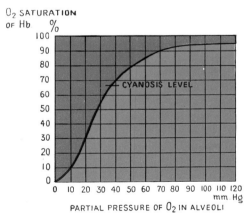

FIG. 81

resulting from this is sufficient to support life, though it leaves many of the body functions considerably impaired.

Fig. 81 shows that even when time is given for equilibrium to be reached, the blood* is only 83% saturated with oxygen when in contact with this gas at a pressure of 54 mmHg .

30 000 feet

At 30000 feet (9100 m) the total atmospheric pressure is 225 mm Hg . If air only were breathed the alveolar oxygen pressure would be 15% of (225 — 90) = 20 mmHg . This pressure is less than the tension of oxygen in venous blood.

A clinical experiment in which atmospheric conditions at 40000 feet were simulated was carried out on a colleague, E. A. P. The inspired gas mixture contained oxygen at a tension of 15 mmHg . After a few breaths the alveolar oxygenfell to 6 mm Hg . The expired gases were collected in a Douglas bag and analyses showed that oxygen had passed from the venous blood into the alveoli. Consciousness was lost quickly and the experiment had to be stopped soon owing to rapidly progressing anoxia.

Flying at 30000 feet is not possible unless the partial pressure of oxygen in the lungs is increased sufficiently to maintain an effective pressure difference between alveoli and venous blood. If instead of air oxygen from a cylinder is breathed, the partial pressure of oxygen in the alveoli is raised to 135 mmHg . The alveolar gases now consist of carbon dioxide, water vapour and oxygen.

Total atmospheric pressure   = 225 mmHg
Pressure of carbon dioxide and water
vapour   = 90 mmHg
Pressure of oxygen   = 135 mmHg

Above 30000 *feet*

From 30000 feet upwards, despite the fact that the airman breathes undiluted oxygen, the difference in pressure of the oxygen between alveoli and venous blood falls. At 42000 feet (atmospheric pressure 127 mmHg) this pressure difference is just enough to ensure adequate oxygenation. Above this height the partial pressure of oxygen in the alveoli becomes insufficient to oxygenate the venous blood and support consciousness and life. At 50000 feet (15200 m) the total atmospheric pressure is 90 mmHg . In theory the alveolar space would be entirely occupied by carbon dioxide and water vapour.

---

* The graph has been coloured in this way to make it easier for the reader to appreciate the state of saturation of haemoglobin for any partial pressure of oxygen in the alveoli. Thus at 50 mm Hg oxygen in the alveoli, haemoglobin is 80% saturated with oxygen. This is shown as though 80% were fully oxygenated (red) and 20% completely reduced (blue).

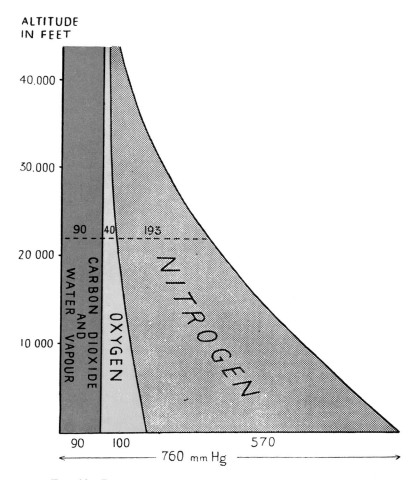

ALTITUDE
IN FEET

FIG. 82. Pressures of alveolar gases when breathing air at varying altitudes. The colours show the partial pressures exerted by the component gases. The broken line indicates the approximate height at which consciousness is lost due to anoxia.

The curve to the right of the grey field represents the atmospheric pressure as function of the altitude. Thus at the height indicated by the broken line the atmospheric pressure is 323 mmHg (= 90 + 40 + 193).

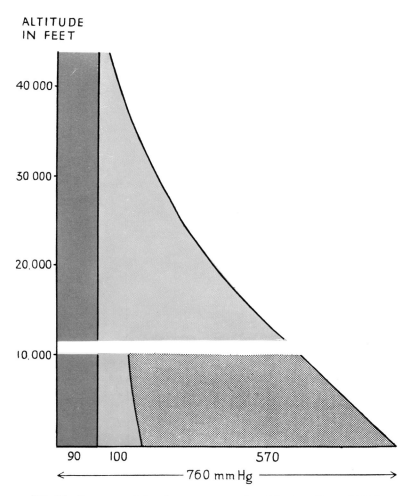

FIG. 83. Pressures of alveolar gases at varying altitudes. Up to 10 000 feet air is breathed; above this pure oxygen. Above 10 000 feet it is assumed that the nitrogen in the alveoli has been completely replaced by oxygen.

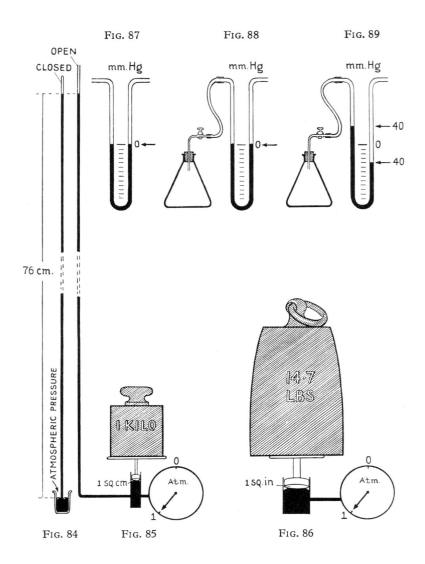

FIG. 87   FIG. 88   FIG. 89

FIG. 84   FIG. 85   FIG. 86

Normal Atmospheric Pressure

Fig. 84—In the barometer a vacuum exists above the mercury column. There is therefore no pressure on the top of the mercury column. At sea level the pressure of the atmosphere acting on the surface of the mercury in the jar supports a column of mercury 760 mm high.

Fig. 85—The top of the tube is opened. Atmospheric pressure now acts on the top of the mercury column in the tube. In order to support the weight of the column of mercury 760 mm high, counterpressure must be made by a weight of 1 kilogram* acting on the surface of 1 cm² of mercury at the base of the column.

Pressure gauges are calibrated in one of two ways. Some indicate 'absolute pressure'. These manometers when open to the atmosphere indicate a pressure of 1 atmosphere (fig. 105A, p. 106). The gauges indicating vapour pressure throughout this book register absolute pressure.

Other gauges indicate what is known as 'gauge pressure'. On these, readings indicate pressures in excess of the outer atmosphere. A gauge of this sort when open to the atmosphere indicates '0'. With such a gauge a reading of 735 lb/in² (50 atmospheres) shows that the absolute pressure within a cylinder is 750 lb/in² (51 atmospheres).

Fig. 86—Expressed in the avoirdupois system, atmospheric pressure is equivalent to 14·7 lb/in².

Fig. 87—Mercury has been poured into a U-tube. Since atmospheric pressure acts on both limbs the heights of the mercury are equal.

The total pressure of gases within a flask can be estimated by substituting the pressure within the flask for the atmospheric pressure acting on one limb of the U-tube.

Fig. 88—The levels of the mercury remain unaltered. The pressure within the flask is therefore atmospheric.

Fig. 89—Another flask is substituted. When the tap is turned on there is a shift in the mercury level and atmospheric pressure is seen to exceed the pressure within the flask by 80 mmHg . The pressure within the flask is therefore 680 mmHg .

* The precise value is 1·033 kg/cm².
As the specific weight of mercury is 13·6 g/cm³, the weight of a 76 cm high column of 1 cm² cross section is 13·6 × 76 = 1033 g. The pressure at the base of this column is 1033 g divided by 1 cm², or 1·033 kg/cm².

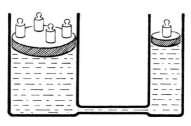

FIG. 90

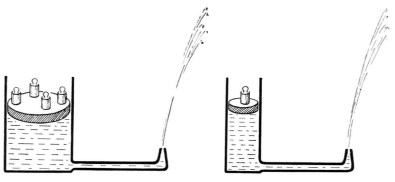

FIG. 91

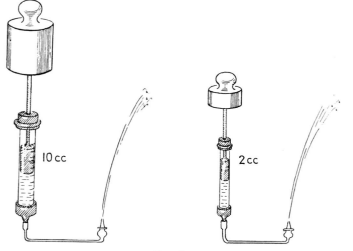

FIG. 92

Hydraulic Pressure

Fig. 90—Two cylinders containing water are connected at their bases. The diameters of the pistons are in the ratio of 2 to 1. Since the area of a circle is proportional to the square of its diameter, the surface area of the larger piston is 4 times greater than that of the smaller. 4 units of weight on the larger piston are necessary to counteract the effect of 1 unit on the smaller. The pressure of the water at the bases of the cylinders is the same.

Fig. 91—Equality of pressure is shown too by the height to which the water is forced. The pressure energy given to the liquid in the syringe is transformed into kinetic energy. The height to which the jet of liquid is forced is a measure of the kinetic energy at the nozzle and therefore of the pressure energy within the syringe.

Fig. 92—The cross-section of the piston of the 10 cm³ syringe is considerably greater than that of the 2 cm³ syringe. For the water to

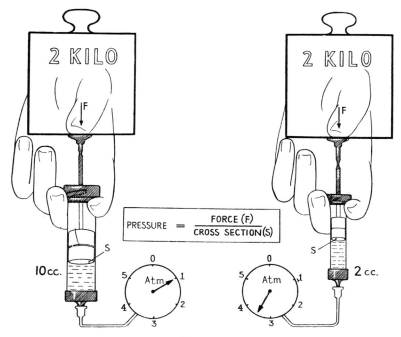

$$\text{PRESSURE} = \frac{\text{FORCE (F)}}{\text{CROSS SECTION(S)}}$$

FIG. 93

emerge from the syringes at equal pressures a correspondingly greater force must be applied to the larger piston.

Fig. 93—A 2 kg weight (equivalent to a comfortable thumb force) is applied to the pistons of a 10 cm³ and a 2 cm³ syringe. The cross-section of the former is 2·6 cm² and of the latter 0·8 cm², a ratio of 3½ to 1. Although the force applied is the same, the pressure in the smaller syringe is seen to be three and a half times greater.

Experiment

Take a 10 cm³ syringe, attach a needle, and see how far water can be squirted through it. Repeat with a 2 cm³ syringe and the same needle. *Moral*—A high pressure of liquid can be obtained without expending undue effort by using a syringe with a small diameter. This is of considerable practical importance in local anaesthesia where the resistance of long narrow needles, and of certain tissues themselves, may have to be overcome.

REFERENCES

[1] HEWITT, Sir Frederic, and SYMES, W. L. (1912). *Lancet*, i, 215–17.
[2] DRESSER, H. (1895). *Johns Hopk. Hosp. Bull.*, **6**, 7–12.
[3] WILSON, S. R., and PINSON, K. B. (1921). *Lancet*, i, 336.
[4] COWAN, S. L., *et al.* (1941). *Ibid.*, ii, 64–6.
[5] ARMSTRONG, H. G. (1952). *Principles and practice of aviation medicine*, 3rd ed. London.

CHAPTER X

COMPRESSED GASES AND GAS LAWS

PROVIDED its temperature is below a certain level, every substance in the gaseous state can be liquefied by pressure. This temperature, which varies for each gas, is known as the *critical temperature* of that gas. Above its critical temperature a substance cannot exist as a liquid however much pressure is applied.

Since the critical temperature of **oxygen** is — 116 °C, it follows that it cannot be liquefied by pressure at room temperature. At — 116 °C a pressure of 50 atmospheres is required to liquefy it. Visitors to an oxygen bottling plant are often shown liquid oxygen in open vessels, but here the temperature is much lower. If liquid oxygen is transferred to a thermos bottle open to the atmosphere it continues to boil furiously. Since the liquid oxygen is in a thermos flask, the latent heat of vaporization must come from the liquid oxygen itself, the temperature of which falls rapidly. When subsequently the temperature has fallen below — 183 °C, the liquid oxygen ceases to boil as the vapour pressure of the liquid at this temperature no longer exceeds 1 atmosphere.

If a cylinder were completely filled with liquid oxygen, the valve closed and the cylinder allowed to acquire room temperature, the previously liquid oxygen would become gaseous. Since the volume of the cylinder and the weight of the oxygen within it remain unchanged, the specific volume (p. 97) of the gaseous oxygen is the same as that of the liquid. The pressure in the cylinder would rise to the enormous height of 4000–4500 atm (over 60000 lb/in²). The storage of oxygen under this pressure is impracticable. The cylinder walls would have to be extremely thick. In addition, packing glands to withstand these pressures are difficult to construct. At these great pressures, oxygen is likely to cause spontaneous ignition of the cylinder material. Risk of fire would indeed be great if the cylinder were to crack. Cylinders capable of withstanding 5000 atmospheres have, in fact, been made, but only for experimental purposes.[1]

The cylinders in common use have comparatively thin walls. Into these cylinders gaseous oxygen is pumped until the pressure reaches 132 atmospheres (1940 lb/in²); formerly the pressure was only 120 atm (1760 lb/in²). The cylinders are now stated to be 'full',

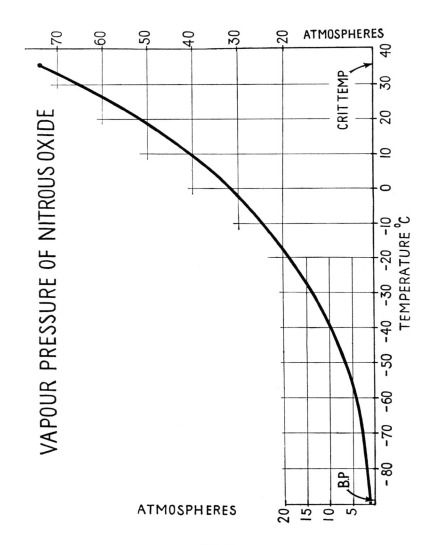

FIG. 94

although, in order to leave a wide margin of safety, they are tested[2] to withstand* a pressure of 3000 lb/in².

The critical temperature of **nitrous oxide** is 36·5 °C, and the pressure required to liquefy it at just below this temperature is 74 atmospheres. The more the gas is cooled the less the pressure required to liquefy it.

The critical temperature of **ether** is 194 °C, and just below this temperature a pressure of 36 atmospheres would be required to liquefy it.

Vapour and Gas

The terms vapour and gas are not sharply distinguishable. The former is generally employed to refer to the gaseous state of a substance which at room temperature and pressure is a liquid. Thus we refer to water vapour and to ether vapour. Expressed in more scientific terms a vapour is a gaseous substance below its critical temperature. The term 'gas' should be reserved for a substance which at room temperature exists only in the gaseous state. Liquefaction is impossible since the temperature of the room is above the critical temperature of such gases.

Pressures in Nitrous Oxide Cylinders

There is a common misconception that the pressure inside a cylinder containing liquid nitrous oxide is always 750 lb/in² (51 atmospheres). The pressure of the vapour above liquid nitrous oxide, like that above any other liquid, varies with temperature.

Fig. 94—shows that if the temperature of the liquid falls below − 89 °C the vapour pressure falls below 1 atmosphere. Above this temperature the cylinder valve must be closed to prevent the liquid nitrous oxide boiling away. At 0 °C the vapour pressure is 31 atmospheres. If the cylinder is left standing overnight at a temperature of 10 °C the vapour pressure will be 40 atmospheres. At 20 °C the vapour pressure is 51 atmospheres (750 lb/in²). See also the right hand side of fig. 110 on p. 116.

In a hot climate working conditions will often be above the critical temperature of nitrous oxide (36·5 °C), and the contents of the cylinder will therefore be wholly gaseous. Although the cylinder contents change from the liquid to the gaseous state it will be seen (fig. 110) that there is no sudden rise of pressure within the cylinder as the critical temperature is passed; the pressure at 35 °C is 72 atmospheres and at 37 °C, 76 atmospheres.

Under tropical conditions cylinders may attain a temperature as high

* The 'test pressure' of a cylinder, although it exceeds by 50% the maximum working pressure, is still only half the pressure which bursts the cylinder.

as 65 °C, at which the pressure of a 'full' cylinder (see later) would be 175 atmospheres. On this account nitrous oxide cylinders are exposed to the same pressure tests to which oxygen cylinders are submitted.

In temperate climates when the cylinder valve is opened the liquid nitrous oxide boils readily, reverting to the gaseous form, which is its natural state at room temperature and pressure. As with any other liquid, heat must be supplied to convert nitrous oxide from the liquid to the gaseous state. The latent heat of vaporization of nitrous oxide at various temperatures is shown in fig. 22 (p. 30). If the cylinder valve is opened widely and evaporation is rapid, the consumption of heat is correspondingly rapid. The temperature of the liquid nitrous oxide, of the cylinder and of the air in the immediate neighbourhood falls sufficiently for the water vapour in the surrounding air to condense and even to freeze on the cylinder wall (fig. 20, p. 28).

In the manufacture of nitrous oxide great care is taken to ensure that the gas is free from water vapour before it is compressed to the liquid state in cylinders.[3] The cooling which inevitably takes place when the cylinder valve is opened is sufficient to freeze any water vapour mixed

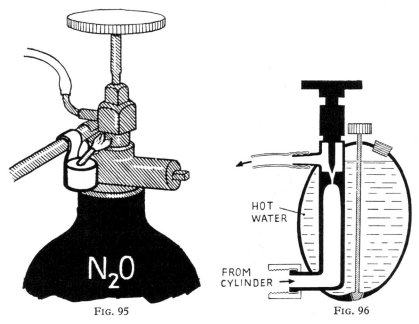

FIG. 95   FIG. 96

with the issuing gas and so block the exit valve with ice. In the early days of liquefaction of nitrous oxide, water was a common 'impurity', and blockage of the valve by ice was a frequent embarrassment. To guard against this, heat in various forms was applied locally[4]—most commonly by spirit lamps[5], warm water[6] (figs. 95, 96), or by surrounding the valve with a towel soaked in warm water. Any of these devices

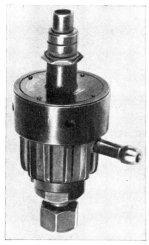

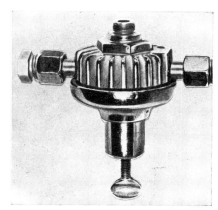

FIG. 97   FIG. 98

keeps the temperature of the exit valve above the freezing-point of water. With the same object many reducing valves (figs. 97, 98) had fins. These facilitate transfer of heat from the surrounding atmosphere and so keep the temperature within the valve above 0 °C. Owing to the meticulous care with which nitrous oxide is now dried before it is bottled, the problem of the frozen exit valve no longer arises. Fins are no longer regarded as a necessity on modern reducing valves.

Specific Volume

A gaseous substance always occupies the whole of the vessel which contains it. Gases, like other fluids, have an inherent tendency to expand. Under room conditions the restraining cohesive forces in a gas, unlike those in liquids, are negligible. Thus the molecules of gas thin out, as it were, to suit the size of the containing vessel. The volume which 1 gram of any substance, solid, liquid or gas, occupies under given conditions of temperature and pressure is known as its *Specific Volume*. The specific volume is inversely proportional to the density (see p. 6). This can be expressed by the formula:

$$\text{Specific Volume} = \frac{1}{\text{Density}}$$

When a given weight of gas is allowed to expand its specific volume increases. There are now fewer molecules per cm³, and fewer molecular impacts on each unit area of the walls. The pressure falls (p. 60). The fall is proportional to the reduction in the number of molecular impacts on each unit area of the containing vessel, and is thus inversely proportional to the increase in the specific volume. The relationship between the pressure and the volume of a given mass of gas was stated by BOYLE in 1662.

Boyle's Law can be expressed in the following ways:

(*a*) The pressure of a gas kept at constant temperature varies inversely as the specific volume.

$$\text{Pressure} \propto \frac{1}{\text{Specific Volume}}$$

Since the density of a gas is inversely proportional to its specific volume, this statement can be reworded:

The pressure of a gas kept at constant temperature is proportional to its density.

$$\text{Pressure} \propto \text{Density}$$

(*b*) The product of the pressure and the specific volume of a gas kept at constant temperature is constant.

$$\text{Pressure} \times \text{Specific Volume} = \text{K}$$

or more shortly

$$\text{P v} = \text{K}$$

If P is expressed in   atmospheres
v is expressed in   1/g
M = gram molecular weight of gas or vapour

the value of $\text{K} = \dfrac{22 \cdot 41}{\text{M}}$ at 0 °C

Examples

(*a*) Find the specific volume of oxygen under a pressure of 10 atmospheres at a temperature of 0 °C .

$$\text{M} = 32 \qquad \text{K} = 22 \cdot 4/32 = 0 \cdot 70$$
$$\text{v} = \text{K}/\text{P} = 0 \cdot 70/10 = 0 \cdot 07 \ 1/\text{g}$$

In other words: If oxygen is compressed to 10 atm at 0 °C, 0·07 litres weigh 1 gram; its density is 1/0·07 = 14·3 g/l .

(*b*) Find the pressure of hydrogen with a specific volume of 45 1/g at a temperature of 0 °C.

$$\text{M} = 2 \qquad \text{K} = 22 \cdot 4/2 = 11 \cdot 2$$
$$\text{P} = \text{K}/\text{v} = 11 \cdot 2/45 = 0 \cdot 25 \text{ atm} .$$

In other words: Hydrogen with a specific volume of 45 1/g, or a density of 1/45 = 0·022 g/l, exerts a pressure of 0·25 atm at 0 °C .

Applications

An oxygen cylinder contains oxygen under pressure. If some is allowed to escape the remainder expands and still occupies uniformly the whole of the cylinder. There are now fewer oxygen molecules per cm^3, and since there are fewer molecular impacts on each unit area of the cylinder wall the pressure falls. The relationship between the reduction in the number of molecules per cm^3 and the reduction in pressure is so exact that the pressure gauge shows what proportion of the full cylinder remains. Thus in a 'full' cylinder the pressure is 120 atmospheres. If half of the contents of the cylinder is allowed to escape, the weight of oxygen which was initially contained in 1 cm^3 is now contained in 2 cm^3 of cylinder space. The specific volume of the oxygen has doubled. Boyle's Law is confirmed since the cylinder pressure is now found to be half.

It is noticeable that pressure gauges are rarely used in conjunction with cylinders of nitrous oxide, carbon dioxide or cyclopropane. These gases are liquefied under pressure and are delivered in cylinders in this state. In a cylinder of, say, nitrous oxide, described by the manufacturers as 'full', liquid does not occupy the whole cylinder volume. A certain amount of space is taken up by nitrous oxide in the gaseous state, and the pressure exerted by this saturated vapour varies with the temperature. At room temperature the saturated vapour exerts a pressure of 51 atmospheres (p. 94). If a considerable portion of the cylinder content is allowed to escape, and the cylinder allowed to regain room temperature (there will have been a fall in cylinder temperature due to the abstraction of heat for the evaporation of the liquid nitrous oxide), it will be found that providing some liquid remains the pressure of the vapour within the cylinder is still 51 atmospheres. A pressure of 51 atmospheres at 20 °C shows that *some* liquid remains in the cylinder, but it gives no idea of *how much*.

The way to ascertain the amount of nitrous oxide within a cylinder is to weigh it. The weight of the cylinder when empty is stamped on its neck. Any difference is accounted for by nitrous oxide, 100 gallons of which at 15 °C and 1 atmosphere weigh 30 oz; converted to the metric system 455 litres weigh 850 grams. This relation will be derived in example (*c*) on p. 117.

A pressure gauge attached to a cylinder of nitrous oxide in use might give an inaccurate idea of the amount in the cylinder. At the commencement the pressure in the cylinder when 'full' is 51 atmospheres. After it has been in continuous use for some time the temperature of the liquid may fall to, say, — 20 °C. The pressure of the vapour, read on the gauge, will then be only 18 atmospheres (p. 94). If the cylinder is now turned off it will gradually reacquire the temperature of the room. If some liquid still remains the pressure will gradually rise to 51 atmospheres again. In some nitrous oxide apparatuses a pressure gauge is fitted and the above limitation to its value should be borne in mind.

During the use of a nitrous oxide cylinder a moment arrives when the last drop of liquid evaporates. Assuming the temperature to have been kept constant, a state of affairs which never obtains during clinical anaesthesia, the cylinder pressure will have remained constant at 51 atmospheres during use. From now onwards, however, the pressure within the cylinder gradually falls. If nitrous oxide vapour behaved like an 'ideal' gas and followed Boyle's Law, there would at this point still be $1 \cdot 3 \times 51 = 66$ litres of N_2O gas within a 100 gallon* cylinder (internal volume $1 \cdot 3$ litres). This would be approximately $\dfrac{66}{455} = \dfrac{1}{7}$ of the original content. In fact the cylinder contains a greater fraction. A vapour so near its saturation point is much more compressible than an 'ideal' gas. Nearly a quarter of the 'full' cylinder still remains when the last drop of liquid nitrous oxide has just evaporated.

It is commonly believed that when the last drop of liquid nitrous oxide (say at a pressure of 51 atmospheres) evaporates, the pressure within the cylinder falls quickly to zero. At this stage the cylinder is full of nitrous oxide vapour under a pressure of 51 atmospheres. The rate of fall in pressure depends on the size of the cylinder and the rate at which the gas is allowed to flow. In the case of the commonly used 200 gallon cylinder, delivering nitrous oxide at the rate of 6 l/min, the fall is spread over approximately 40 minutes. The state of affairs within a nitrous oxide cylinder when the last drop of liquid has just evaporated may be compared with a 200 gallon cylinder of oxygen at the same pressure. At 51 atmospheres the oxygen cylinder is still $\dfrac{51}{120}$ (or over $\dfrac{1}{3}$) 'full'.

* 1 gallon (British) = 4·55 litres.

Fig. 99—Nitrous oxide flows from a full 200 gallon cylinder at the constant rate of 8 l/min until the cylinder is empty. The pressure within the cylinder is recorded at frequent intervals. Room temperature 18 °C.

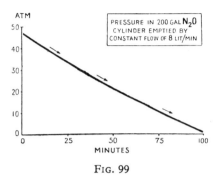

FIG. 99

The latent heat of evaporation of the liquid nitrous oxide is taken largely from the heat content of the liquid itself and from the cylinder. The temperature of the liquid nitrous oxide therefore falls and with it the vapour pressure of the liquid. It is seen that there is a continuous drop in pressure. The graph gives no indication of the moment when the last drop of liquid evaporates and the contents of the cylinder become entirely gaseous.

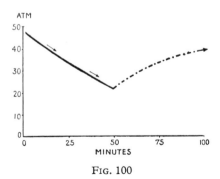

FIG. 100

Fig. 100—Here the previous experiment is repeated for the first 50 minutes. The flow of gas is now turned off. The pressure in the now cold cylinder is 22 atmospheres. The cylinder gradually warms up to room temperature. By the end of a further 50 minutes the pressure has risen to 40 atmospheres and eventually registers 47 atmospheres, showing that liquid still remains within the cylinder.

Fig. 99 might give quite a wrong impression unless the circumstances of the experiment are fully considered. At first sight it appears to demonstrate that the pressure in a nitrous oxide cylinder is a good guide to how much nitrous oxide the cylinder contains. This is in fact so if a 200 gallon cylinder is emptied in one sitting at the steady rate of 8 litres per minute. In clinical practice, however, the flow rate of gas is frequently altered and much more important still, there are almost invariably several intervals, some of very long duration, during which the cylinder is not used at all. During these pauses between operations the cylinder acquires heat from its surroundings. Provided some liquid still remains the pressure within the cylinder gradually increases until the temperature of the cylinder is again that of the room.

In the experiment in fig. 100 the pressure at the end of 25 minutes is 33 atmospheres. The flow continues for a further 25 minutes and is then stopped. At 80 minutes the cylinder has warmed sufficiently for the gauge to register 33 atmospheres. It is seen that at 25 minutes and at 80 minutes the pressures are identical, although in the first case the cylinder contains 700 litres and in the second 500 litres.

The next two experiments should be contrasted with the previous two.

Fig. 101—Oxygen is allowed to flow from a full 200 gallon cylinder at the uniform rate of 8 litres per minute. The fall in pressure is uniform.

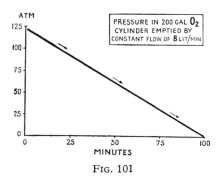

FIG. 101

Fig. 102—The above experiment is repeated but at the end of 50 minutes the flow of gas is turned off. The cylinder pressure remains constant from now on; the pressure therefore indicates at any time the content of the cylinder.

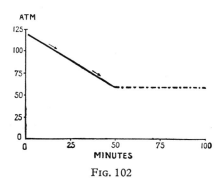

FIG. 102

The drop in temperature due to the release of the compressed oxygen is negligible. As the cylinder acquires room temperature there is a slight rise in pressure, but this is too small to be recorded on the pressure gauge used in this experiment.

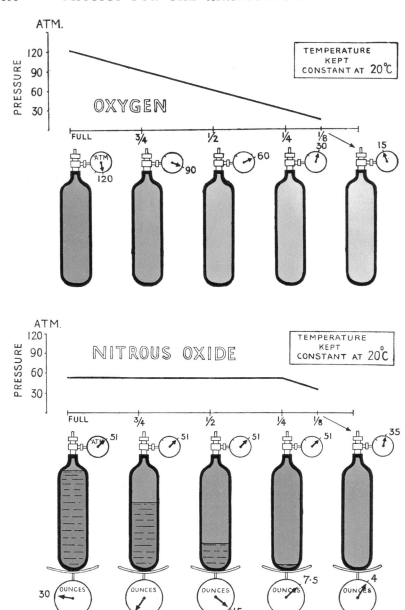

Fig. 103 and 104

Relationship between pressure in a cylinder and the amount of oxygen or nitrous oxide within it.

Fig. 103—A cylinder when 'full' contains oxygen under a pressure of 120 atmospheres. The valve is opened and the gas allowed to escape; there is a progressive fall of pressure. When the pressure has fallen to 60 atmospheres the amount of gas within the cylinder has fallen, too, to half of what it was initially. A pressure reading at any stage gives an indication of the amount of oxygen remaining in the cylinder. As the density (represented by intensity of colour) decreases there is a corresponding fall of pressure.

Fig. 104—The liquid nitrous oxide and the density of the vapour above it is represented by intensity of colour. The temperature throughout the experiment is kept constant at 20 °C, at which the pressure exerted by the saturated vapour over the liquid is 51 atmospheres. As the tap is opened gaseous nitrous oxide escapes, and is immediately replaced by further vapour from the liquid. When the cylinder is half full the density of the vapour, and therefore its pressure, are still the same. In fact these remain unaltered as long as any nitrous oxide exists in the liquid state. An accurate indication of the amount of nitrous oxide remaining in the cylinder can be obtained only by weighing the cylinder.

The horizontal line shows that the pressure of the vapour within the cylinder remains uniform until it is just less than quarter full. When the liquid is all volatilized the pressure of the gas within the cylinder begins to fall.

The relation between pressure and specific volume then gradually approximates to Boyle's Law. The Law applies only where the pressure of the nitrous oxide is considerably below its saturation pressure.

N.B.—The stamp on the neck of the 100 gallon size nitrous oxide cylinder gives 30 oz as the weight of nitrous oxide within it when full. The actual weight in a 'full' cylinder may deviate slightly from this figure in either direction.

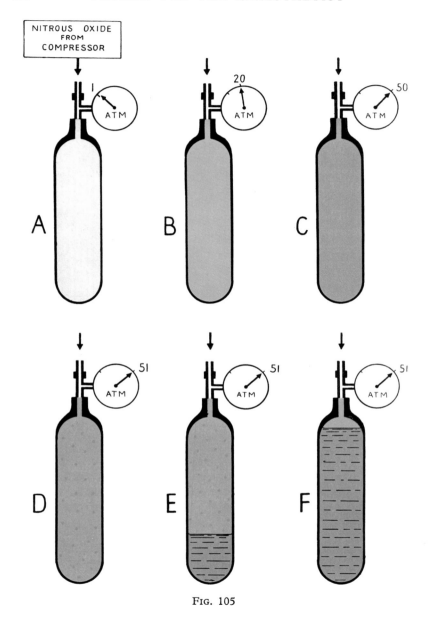

Fig. 105

Filling a Cylinder with Nitrous Oxide

Fig. 105—The temperature throughout this experiment is maintained at 20 °C.

A. The cylinder is full of nitrous oxide gas at atmospheric pressure.

B. In contrast to the ether experiment on p. 112 the capacity of the container here remains constant. Approximately 20 times the initial amount of gas has been compressed into the cylinder and the gas therefore exerts a pressure of 20 atmospheres. The specific volume of the nitrous oxide (p. 108) is now $\frac{1}{20}$ of that in A, or, expressed in another way, the density of the gas has increased 20-fold.

C. Addition of further gas from the compressor has resulted in an increase of pressure to almost the saturation pressure of nitrous oxide at 20 °C. The specific volume is still further decreased, and the increased density of the gas at this pressure is indicated by the shading.

D. Filling has continued until the vapour is saturated. The pressure gauge reads 51 atmospheres. Since at this temperature nitrous oxide in the gaseous state cannot exert a pressure greater than 51 atmospheres, further filling results in condensation of the vapour.

E. As filling continues more vapour condenses. The liquid nitrous oxide accumulates at the bottom of the cylinder.

F. Filling is continued until the cylinder is commercially 'full'.

At the factory cylinders are filled from a pipeline containing liquid nitrous oxide under a pressure well above the saturation pressure at the temperature of the filling-room.

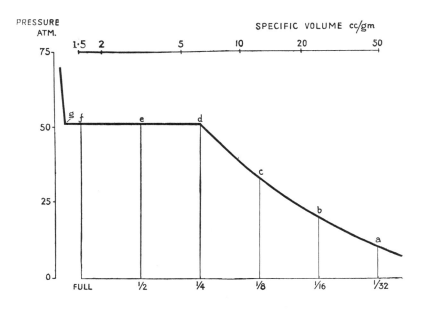

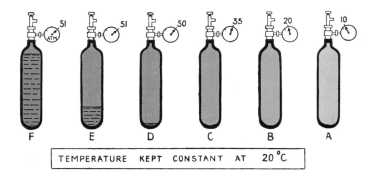

FIG. 106

Fig. 106—Pressure changes inside a nitrous oxide cylinder during filling. The temperature is kept constant at 20 °C.

The graph showing the relationship between the pressure of the nitrous oxide and its specific volume at a constant temperature is known as an 'isotherm'.

The cylinders D, E, F correspond with those in the previous figure. Between the points a and d the nitrous oxide is all in the gaseous state. The rise in pressure at the beginning is approximately inversely proportional to the specific volume (Boyle's Law, p. 98). At 20 atmospheres pressure the specific volume of nitrous oxide is 22 cm³/g, whilst at 50 atmospheres the figure has decreased to 7 cm³/g—the specific volume of the saturated vapour.

At the point d (when a pressure of 51 atmospheres is reached) liquefaction begins, and despite addition of further nitrous oxide the pressure remains constant. At f the nitrous oxide has a specific volume of 1·5 cm³/g, and the cylinder is considered to be 'full'.

Filling could be continued beyond this stage until at g the cylinder is actually full of liquid. Since a liquid is virtually incompressible the addition now of even a minute amount of nitrous oxide would result in an enormous rise in pressure.

Filling Ratio

The degree of filling of a nitrous oxide cylinder can be described by stating either the average density or the average specific volume of the contents. The specific volume of nitrous oxide in a cylinder containing liquid and vapour simultaneously is an average specific volume. This average specific volume is defined as the cylinder volume divided by the total weight of its contents, or

$$\frac{\text{cylinder volume}}{\text{weight of liquid} + \text{weight of vapour}}$$

The average density of nitrous oxide within a 'full' cylinder is easily determined. The weight of the nitrous oxide within it is found. The internal capacity of the cylinder is known (or can be found by filling a similar cylinder with water). Since the density of water is 1, the ratio

$$\frac{\text{weight of } N_2O \text{ in cylinder}}{\text{weight of water cylinder could hold}}$$

gives the average density of the contents, and the figure is known as the 'filling ratio'. Cylinders of nitrous oxide are normally filled[7] to a ratio

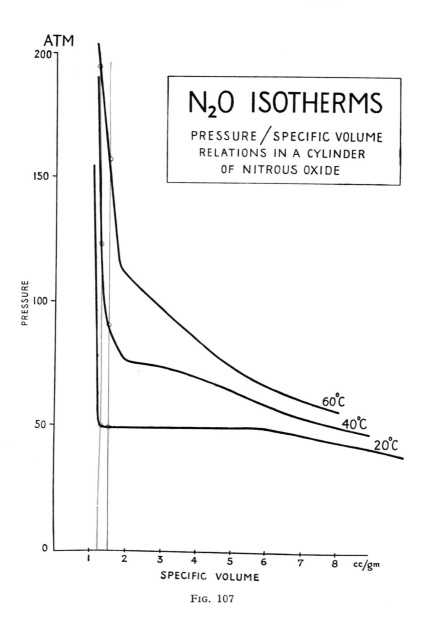

FIG. 107

of 0·67, a filling ratio which is now considered suitable for both temperate and tropical climates. A filling ratio as high as 0·75 is permissible for temperate climates. Although the higher filling ratio was formerly used in this country it has now been abandoned in favour of the 0·67 ratio.

Example

A 100 gallon (455 lit) N_2O cylinder is found to have an internal volume of 1·3 litres.

This volume of water weighs 46 oz (1300 g)

The cylinder when 'full' contains 30 oz (850 g) of nitrous oxide

$$\therefore \quad \text{the filling ratio} = \frac{30}{46} \left(\text{or } \frac{850}{1300} \right)$$
$$= 0.65$$

Fig. 107—Nitrous oxide isotherms for various temperatures, illustrating the danger which attends overfilling a cylinder.

The filling ratio of 0·65 corresponding to a specific volume of 1·5 is indicated by the vertical *blue* line. A cylinder filled to this ratio at 20 °C would have a pressure of 51 atmospheres. If the same cylinder is exposed to a temperature of 40 °C, a temperature not unknown in this country, the pressure rises to 90 atmospheres (p. 94). Should the cylinder be warmed to 60 °C—a temperature not uncommon in the tropics—the pressure would rise to 160 atmospheres, approximately the same as that of a 'full' oxygen cylinder at the same temperature (see fig. 109, p. 116).

The vertical *red* line corresponds to a filling ratio of 0·77 (specific volume of 1·3 cm³/g) for which the cylinder at 20 °C is almost completely filled with liquid. At this temperature the pressure is 51 atmospheres. At 40 °C, however, the pressure is already 125 atmospheres, and at 60 °C the high pressure of 190 atmospheres is reached, a pressure close to the testing pressure of the cylinder (p. 95).

If at 20 °C a cylinder is *completely* filled with liquid nitrous oxide (*g*, fig. 106), and a minute amount more is pumped in, there will be a sharp rise in pressure above 51 atmospheres. If such a cylinder is now warmed, as in the previous examples, the pressure will exceed the test pressure and reach dangerous values.

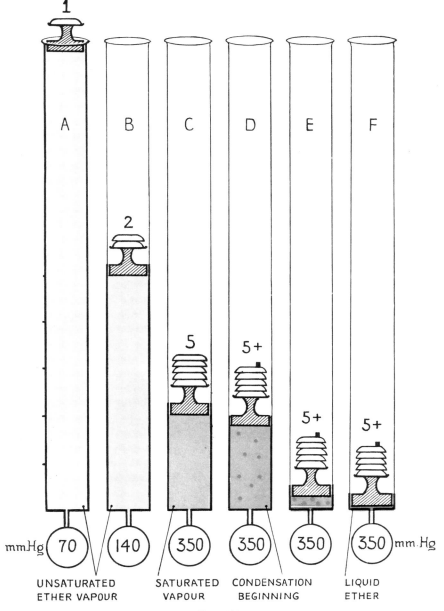

FIG. 108

The Effect of Pressure on a Vapour

Fig. 108—In this hypothetical experiment at 15 °C ether vapour is used. The cylinders are considered to be in a vacuum so that the effect of atmospheric pressure is nullified.

A. The long cylinder contains ether vapour which is compressed by a weight on the piston. The pressure exerted by the vapour is 70 mmHg .

B. The weight is doubled and the piston sinks till the volume occupied by the vapour is halved. The pressure of the vapour is found to be doubled, that is, 140 mmHg .

C. The weights are now increased to 5. The volume occupied by the vapour is ⅕ of that which it initially occupied. The pressure exerted by the vapour has correspondingly increased to 350 mmHg .

The saturated vapour pressure of ether at 15 °C is 350 mmHg (p. 80). This is the highest pressure ether vapour can exert at this temperature.

D. The small additional weight results in condensation of the vapour. Droplets of liquid form.

E. and F. Without further addition of weight the piston sinks until all the vapour is condensed as liquid ether. The pressure remains unchanged.

Compare this experiment with fig. 105 showing the liquefaction of nitrous oxide gas. In the latter the volume of the cylinder is constant, and the pressure within alters as further gas is pumped in. Here, too, when the saturation pressure of the gas at room temperature is reached (51 atmospheres) condensation begins. The pumping in of more gas results not in any increase in pressure but in further condensation.

In these two experiments the specific volume of the vapours was altered by different means. The specific volume of nitrous oxide was gradually decreased by raising the amount of N_2O within a container of fixed volume. In the experiment with ether the specific volume was decreased by diminishing the size of the container; the amount of ether was kept constant.

Charles' Law

When a gas is heated molecular movement increases, and the gas tends to expand. If this expansion is prevented, the number of molecular impacts on the walls of the container increases and the pressure rises. Charles in 1787, and after him, Gay-Lussac in 1802, found experimentally that equal volumes of all gases kept at constant pressure expand by equal increments of volume for each degree centigrade rise in temperature. For an 'ideal' gas this increment is $\dfrac{1}{273}$ of the volume of the gas at 0 °C. Conversely, when an 'ideal gas' is cooled its volume decreases by $\dfrac{1}{273}$ of its volume at 0 °C for each degree centigrade of cooling.

Charles' Law can be stated thus:

A given quantity of 'ideal' gas, kept at constant pressure, expands by $\dfrac{1}{273}$ *of its volume at 0 °C for each degree Celsius rise in temperature.*

*Examples**

(a) 1 cm³ of liquid ether when vaporized occupies 220 cm³ at 0 °C and 760 mmHg (p. 10). What will the volume be at 20 °C and 760 mmHg ?

$$\text{Increase in volume for 1 °C rise} = \frac{1}{273} \times 220 \text{ cm}^3$$

$$,, \quad ,, \quad 20 \text{ °C } ,, \quad = \frac{20}{273} \times 220 \text{ cm}^3$$

$$= 16 \text{ cm}^3$$

$$\text{Final volume} \quad = 236 \text{ cm}^3$$

(b) One mole (p. 3) of an ideal gas at 0 °C and 760 mmHg occupies 22·4 litres. What will this volume be at 20 °C ?

$$\text{Increase in volume for each 1 °C rise} = \frac{22 \cdot 4}{273} \text{ l.}$$

$$,, \quad ,, \quad 20 \text{ °C } ,, \quad = \frac{22 \cdot 4}{273} \times 20 \text{ l.}$$

$$= 1 \cdot 6 \text{ l.}$$

$$\text{Final volume} \quad = 24 \text{ l.}$$

If for each degree Celsius drop in temperature a gas at constant pressure contracts by $\dfrac{1}{273}$ of its volume at 0 °C, it would follow that by

---

* In the examples on this and subsequent pages it has been assumed that the gases under the conditions stated obey the laws for an ideal gas. This is not strictly correct but the approximation is quite adequate for our purposes.

the time the gas has been cooled to — 273 °C it would cease to occupy any space. However, at extremely low temperatures none of the laws for 'ideal' gases (for example, Boyle's Law, Charles' Law) holds good. In fact every gas liquefies before — 273 °C is reached.

In calculating the change of volume resulting from change of temperature the *Absolute scale of temperature* is used. On this 0 °Abs. is equivalent to — 273 °C, and 273 °Abs. is equivalent to 0 °C.

Temperature scales are usually named after scientists. This is obvious in the case of °F (Fahrenheit) but °C does not only signify centigrade. The latter should be pronounced as *degree Celsius*, named after a Swedish scientist.

Similarly the scale for absolute temperature is not usually described as °Abs. but is written as °**K**. This symbol refers to Lord Kelvin who made outstanding contributions to the theory of heat.

The rise of temperature of a gas from, say, 0 °C to 20 °C is expressed on the Absolute scale as a rise from 273 °K to 293 °K. The volume of a gas at constant pressure is directly proportional to its absolute temperature.

Example

(c) A gas occupies V cm^3 at 0 °C (273 °K).

What is its volume at 20 °C (293 °K) if the pressure is kept constant?

$$\text{Increase in volume for a rise of } 1° C = \frac{V}{273}$$

$$\therefore \quad ,, \quad ,, \quad ,, \quad 20 °C = \frac{20V}{273}$$

$$\therefore \text{ final volume} = V + \frac{20V}{273}$$

$$= \frac{273V + 20V}{273} = \frac{293}{273} \times V$$

Thus a gas which at 0 °C occupies 100 c.c. will at 20 °C occupy

$$\frac{293}{273} \times 100 \text{ cm}^3 = 107 \text{ cm}^3$$

and a gas which at 0 °C occupies 22·4 litres will at 20 °C occupy

$$\frac{293}{273} \times 22·4 \text{ l.} = 24 \text{ l.}$$

Gay-Lussac's Law

If the specific volume is kept constant, for each 1 degC rise in temperature the pressure of a gas rises by $\frac{1}{273}$ of its pressure at 0 °C, or

the pressure of a gas kept at constant volume is directly proportional to its absolute temperature.

OXYGEN

NITROUS OXIDE

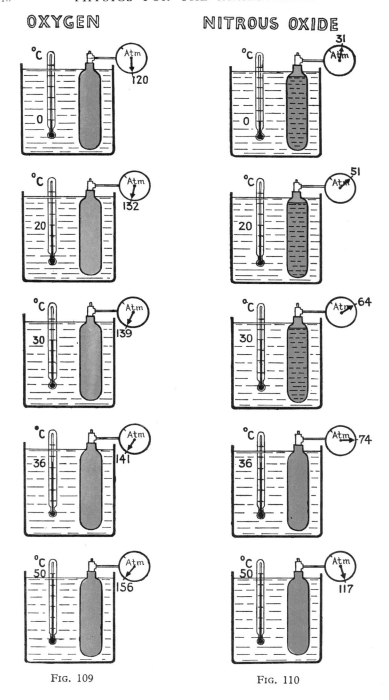

FIG. 109   FIG. 110

Examples

(a) A cylinder of oxygen showing a pressure of 132 atmospheres at 15 °C is moved to a room with a temperature of 25 °C. What pressure will the cylinder register at the higher temperature?

Initial temperature $= 288$ °K

Final temperature $= 298$ °K

∴ final pressure $= \dfrac{298}{288} \times 132$ atm

$= 136 \cdot 6$ atm

(b) The pressure inside a closed vessel containing compressed air is 12 atm at 20 °C. After immersion in a cooling bath the pressure in the vessel decreases to 10 atm. What is the final temperature?

Initial temperature $= 293$ °K

Final temperature $= T$ °K

$$\frac{T}{293} = \frac{10}{12}$$

$$T = \frac{10}{12} \times 293 \qquad = 244 \text{ °K}$$

Final temperature $= -29$ °C

(c) Confirm that 455 lit N_2O at 15 °C and 1 atm weigh 850 g (see p. 111).

From p. 98 one obtains, with $K = \dfrac{22 \cdot 41}{44}$, for the specific volume of nitrous oxide at N.T.P.

$$\frac{22 \cdot 4}{44 \times 1} = 0 \cdot 509 \ 1/g$$

From Gay-Lussac's law one obtains then the specific volume at 15 °C (288 °K)

$$0 \cdot 509 \times \frac{288}{273} = 0 \cdot 537 \ 1/g$$

The volume of 850 gm (30 oz) is therefore

$$850 \times 0 \cdot 537 = 457 \ 1.$$

Pressure increases resulting from rise of temperature in cylinders of oxygen, and of nitrous oxide 'filled' to British Standard.

Fig. 109—In this country oxygen cylinders were formerly filled till the pressure registered was 120 atmospheres. Since World War II this has been increased to 132 atmospheres.

The pressure in the oxygen cylinder rises according to Gay-Lussac's Law; it is proportional to the absolute temperature of the gas.

Fig. 110—Nitrous oxide cylinders are 'filled' till they hold a predetermined weight of nitrous oxide for a given size of cylinder. Thus 60 oz of nitrous oxide are compressed into the so-called 200 gallon cylinder. This represents a filling ratio of 0·65, at which the average specific volume of the nitrous oxide is 1·5 cm³/g . At this filling approximately $\frac{9}{10}$ of the interior of the cylinder is occupied by liquid, the remainder by gaseous nitrous oxide.

Above the critical temperature (36 °C) gas only fills the cylinder; notice, too, that there is no sudden rise in pressure as this temperature is reached and passed.

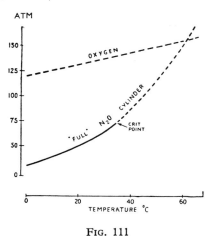

FIG. 111

Fig. 111—This graph shows the rises in pressures in 'full' cylinders of oxygen and nitrous oxide resulting from increase in temperature.

Nitrous oxide just above its critical temperature and pressure does not obey Gay-Lussac's Law. In this figure the pressure curves for nitrous oxide and oxygen cross at about 60 °C. The pressure to which cylinders are tested is given on p. 95.

REFERENCES

[1] BRIDGMAN, P. W. (1949). *The physics of high pressure*, Ch. ii. Lond.
[2] BRITISH STANDARD 1045 (1942). *Manganese steel gas cylinders for atmospheric gases.*
[3] STOVIN, G. H. T. (1952). *Gas and air analgesia in midwifery*, 2nd ed., pp. 34–5. Lond.
[4] BOOTHBY, W. M. (1912). *Boston med. Surg. J.*, 166, 86–90.
[5] HADFIELD, C. F. (1923). *Practical anaesthetics*, p. 85. Lond.
[6] CLOVER, J. T. (1876). *Brit. med. J.*, ii, 74–5.
[7] BRITISH STANDARD 1736 (1951). *Filling ratios for liquefiable gases.*

CHAPTER XI

PRESSURE REDUCING VALVES

THE importance of Pressure Reducing Valves (reduced pressure regulators) for the practising anaesthetist is based on three factors.

1. The presence of a reducing valve ensures that the bobbin or pointer of the flowmeter on the anaesthetic machine remains steady in whatever position it has been adjusted by the setting of the flow control valve; the anaesthetist has no longer to readjust the flow control every few minutes in order to keep the flow steady. This was a problem in the early days of nitrous oxide/oxygen anaesthesia. The first semi-open anaesthetic apparatus of the 'Boyle' type had no reducing valves on either oxygen or nitrous oxide cylinders. As soon as this apparatus became more popular, a demand arose for an automatic regulator which would obviate the need for continuous adjustment of the flow control.

2. The second factor is the undesirable, large change in the flowrate resulting from a small movement of the control valve spindle when the high cylinder pressure is controlled directly by a simple needle type valve. This makes the adjustment of the flow rate very difficult. With the low pressure supplied from pressure regulators, small variations in the gas flow can be made much more easily.

While originally the needle valves were placed at the outlet from the reducing valves, a further development placed these control valves on the flowmeters of the anaesthetic machine.

3. The third factor thus introduced is the limited positive pressure which can be carried by a normal flexible tube. If simple, thick-walled rubber tubing is used to connect cylinder and flowmeter, the pressure supplied through these tubes must be kept low and values down to about 6 lb/in² have become established. At this pressure a rubber tube does not blow off if it is simply pushed over a metal connector.

119

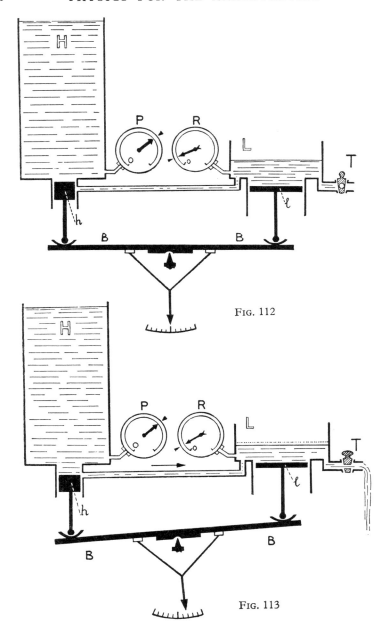

Fig. 112

Fig. 113

The Principles of the Reducing Valve

Fig. 112—A tall tank H (high pressure chamber) and a short one L (low pressure chamber) contain liquid. The hydrostatic pressures (P and R) at the bases of H and L and indicated on the manometers are proportional to the heights of the liquids.

The base of each tank opens into a short cylinder in which a piston (h and l) is free to move. The weights of the two pistons are equal. The sectional area of the piston (h) at the base of H will be referred to as 'a', and the sectional area of the other piston (l) as 'A'. The former area is much smaller than the latter.

A pipe leads from the cylinder at the base of the high pressure tank to the base of the low pressure tank: but the opening into the pipe is for the moment occluded by the piston (h).

One piston is connected by a rod to one arm of a balance, the other piston to the second arm. A state of equilibrium is illustrated, with the balance arms (B) horizontal. The forces transmitted by the pistons through the rods are therefore equal.

As the pressure at the base of H is P, the hydraulic force acting on piston (h) is:

$$F_h = P \times a$$

Since the two arms of the balance are in equilibrium, this force is equal to the force acting on piston (l) at the base of L, i.e.

$$F_l = R \times A$$

$$
\begin{aligned}
P \times a &= R \times A & . & & . & & (1) \\
R/P &= a/A & . & & . & & (2) \\
R &= (a/A)P & . & & . & & (3)
\end{aligned}
$$

The ratio of the low pressure (R) to the high pressure (P) is equal to the ratio of the sectional area of the high pressure piston to that of the low pressure piston;—see Eq. 2.

It will be noticed that tap (T), the outlet from the low pressure tank, is closed, and the pipe connecting the two tanks is occluded by the high pressure piston.

In the illustration, the piston areas are in the ratio $1/6$. The value of the reduced pressure is therefore $1/6$ of P.

Fig. 113—Here tap (T) has just been opened and liquid flows from the low pressure chamber. The level of the liquid in L falls slightly and the pressure acting on piston (*l*) is reduced. Since the pressure acting on the high pressure piston is unchanged, the balance of forces is upset; piston (*h*) sinks, freeing the opening into the connecting pipe sufficiently to allow a flowrate of liquid from H to L equal to the loss from L through T.

If, at any time, tap (T) is closed, some liquid will continue to run from H to L until the force exerted by piston (*l*) on the right balance arm comes into equilibrium with the force exerted by piston (*h*) on the left arm. As soon as the balance arms again become horizontal, the entrance to the connecting pipe is occluded by the high pressure piston, and the flow from H to L ceases. This state of affairs would be similar to that illustrated in Fig. 112, on the assumption that only a small quantity of liquid has flowed out through T during the experiment, so that the level in H is practically unaltered.

If the level in H falls noticeably while T is open, the value of R is again given by the equation

$$R = (a/A) \times P \qquad (3)$$

But P is smaller than at the beginning of the experiment, and R will have *decreased* proportionally.

Simplest type of reducing valves

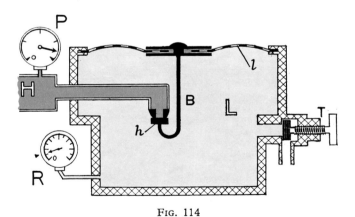

FIG. 114

Fig. 114—Here the principles described in the previous two figures are applied to the construction of a gas pressure reducing valve in its simplest form.

The tank (H) in fig. 112 is replaced by a container (H) of gas under high pressure (P), registered on the upper pressure gauge. The piston at the base of H in fig. 112 is replaced by a seating or disc (h) which occludes the nozzle through which the high pressure gas can enter the chamber (L) containing gas at low pressure (R)—indicated on the lower gauge. The effective area of the seating—the part which occludes the nozzle opening—is 'a'.

The seating (h) is connected by a rod (B) to the rigid plates which clamp the centre part of the diaphragm (l). This flexible, non-elastic diaphragm (l) of effective* area (A) is equivalent to the piston at the base of L in fig. 112.

The connecting rod (B) can be identified with the balance arms in fig. 112. The outflow tap (T) is shut and a state of equilibrium is illustrated—compare fig. 112. The force of the high pressure gas tending to push the seating (h) away from the nozzle opening is

$$F_h = P \times a$$

The force exerted by the low pressure gas on the diaphragm is

$$F_l = R \times A$$

and this is the force with which the diaphragm pulls the rod with its attached seating upward. In the position of equilibrium** the forces acting on each end of the connecting rod are equal:

$$F_h = F_l$$

$$R \times A = P \times a \qquad . \qquad . \qquad . \qquad (1)$$
$$R/P = a/A \qquad . \qquad . \qquad . \qquad (2)$$
$$R = (a/A) \times P \qquad . \qquad . \qquad (3)$$

The ratio of reduced to high pressure is equal to the ratio of the effective seating area to the effective diaphragm area (Eq. 2).

If the diameter of the high pressure nozzle is $1/17$ of the effective diaphragm diameter, the reduced pressure will be $(1/17)^2$ or approximately $1/300$ of the high pressure.

---

* If a diaphragm would behave as a piston, the force exerted by it on the connecting rod (B) would be equal to the product of diaphragm area times pressure (R). Actually the force is *smaller* and depends amongst other factors on the size of the clamping plates which keep the central region of the diaphragm flat. The effective area of the diaphragm is that area which multiplied by R gives the force exerted on the connecting rod; it is *smaller* than the actual area of the diaphragm.

** See also footnote on p. 132.

Fig. 115—When the tap (T) is opened gas flows out; the pressure in L will tend to fall slightly, and with it the force exerted on the diaphragm (l).

Since the force exerted by P on the seating (h) is unchanged, the

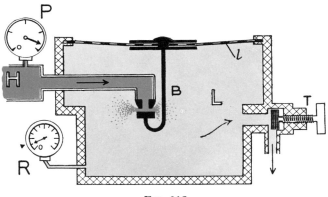

FIG. 115

balance of forces acting on connecting rod (B) is upset; the seating is pushed away from the nozzle sufficiently to allow a flow rate of high pressure gas from H to L equal to the loss from L through T.

If at any time tap (T) is closed, some gas will continue to stream from H to L. Equilibrium is soon restored when the force exerted by the gas pressure in L on the diaphragm again equals the force exerted by the high pressure gas downwards on the seating. The seating is then pulled by rod (B) against the nozzle with sufficient force to prevent any further flow from H to L. This state of affairs is similar to that in fig. 114, on the assumption that only a small quantity of gas has flowed out through T, so that the pressure in H is practically unaltered.

The pressure of gas (P) in the cylinder (H) does *not* remain *constant*, but falls gradually as the cylinder is emptied. The corresponding value of R is again given by

$$R/P = a/A \qquad . \qquad . \quad (2)$$

The diaphragm and nozzle areas are of course constant, i.e. the ratio a/A is constant.

Therefore the ratio P/R must also be constant.

If P falls, R falls proportionally.

Example

Effective radius of diaphragm $= 30$ mm

Radius of nozzle opening $= 2$ mm

As area is proportional to $(radius)^2$:

$$(a/A) = (2^2/30^2) = (1/15)^2 = 1/225$$

If the initial cylinder pressure

$$P = 1800 \text{ lb/in}^2 \ (122 \text{ atm})$$

Then (Eq. 3) reduced pressure $R = 1800 \times (1/15)^2$ lb/in²

$$= 1800/225$$
$$= 8 \text{ lb/in}^2 \ (0.54 \text{ atm})$$

When the cylinder pressure falls to $P' = 1/3\ P = 600$ lb/in² (41 atm), representing a relative decrease by $(1800-600)/1800$ or 66%, the reduced pressure will have fallen to

$$R' = 600 \times (1/15)^2 \text{ lb/in}^2 = 1/3\ R = 2.7 \text{ lb/in}^2 \ (0.18 \text{ atm}).$$

The relative decrease in R is $(8-2.7)/8$ or 66%.

Variation of reduced pressure with cylinder pressure

If P is the initial pressure in H, and P′ the pressure when the cylinder is partly empty, Eq. 3 on p. 123 gives the corresponding decrease of the reduced pressure from R to R′.

$$R = (a/A)P; \quad R' = (a/A)P'; \quad (R - R') = (a/A) \times (P - P')$$
$$(R - R')/R = (P - P')/P = (1 - P'/P) \qquad (4)$$

The left side of this equation is the *relative* change in reduced pressure which occurs when the pressure in H decreases from P to P′. For further reference it should be noted that this relative variation in R depends only on the ratio (P′/P) and is independent of R itself; this is evident because the ratio (a/A) no longer appears on the right side of the equation.

For example, if the cylinder pressure falls to $\frac{1}{3}$ of its initial value, the reduced pressure decreases by $(1 - \frac{1}{3}) = \frac{2}{3}$ or by 66%.

The simple valve scheme of figs. 114 and 115 has thus the disadvantage that the reduced pressure decreases rapidly, while the cylinder empties. Furthermore, the reduced pressure cannot be varied at will and is determined by the dimensions of the seating and diaphragm of the particular valve.

A pressure regulator of this type would fulfil the conditions (2) and (3) on p. 119; it would, however, not meet condition (1), and has the outstanding inconvenience for the anaesthetist that the control tap would need frequent readjustments while the cylinder pressure decreases.

When the pressure in an oxygen cylinder falls from $P = 1800$ lb/in² to, say, $P' = 1/10\ P = 180$ lb/in², the reduced pressure which at the beginning was set at, say $R = 6$ lb/in², will have fallen to $R' = 0.6$ lb/in².

If the flowrate through T were proportional to the pressure in L, an initial flowrate of 1000 cm³/min would fall to 100 cm³/min, if T is not adjusted while the cylinder empties.

Improved types of reducing valves

The simple valve design (p. 122) must be improved in certain respects to supply the anaesthetist with a practical reducing valve. The most important improvement must ensure that the reduced pressure does not alter appreciably while the cylinder of compressed gas empties gradually from the initial high pressure.

In addition, the reduced pressure must be adjustable at will within certain limits.

To realize these aims, a different principle of force-balance must be introduced.

In the primitive design just considered, the force exerted by R is used solely to overcome the force due to the *variable* high pressure (P) acting on the seating.

In the improved schemes which will now be discussed, the hydraulic force exerted by the reduced pressure is used principally to overcome some *constant*, mechanical force.

Such an external, mechanical force could be supplied most accurately by a weight, but this is not practicable in regulators on mobile anaesthetic equipment, on which the position of the valve is liable to change.

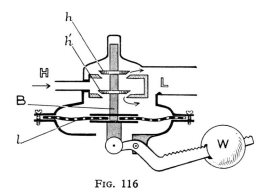

Fig. 116

Fig. 116—Technical steam pressure reducing valve, weight operated. High pressure steam enters at H and escapes past two high pressure seatings (*h* and *h'*). The weight (W) attached to a lever keeps the seatings

(h and h') open so long as the pressure in L is below the reduced pressure R which is determined by the effective area of diaphragm (l) and the force exerted by the weight (W) at the lower end of connecting rod (B). This force is determined both by the size of the weight and its position on the lever arm*.

In contrast to a weight, the force exerted by a compressed helical *spring* is uninfluenced by its position; on this account springs are used to supply the pre-determined, constant, external force. This force is constant in so far as it does not alter once the spring has been initially compressed by a regulating screw.

The force exerted by the reduced pressure in the improved valve scheme has to overcome:

1. the large constant force exerted by the compressed spring, and
2. the much smaller, variable force due to the varying high pressure acting on the seating.

If this improved valve is to supply reduced pressures of the same order as those previously considered in the primitive valve design, the dimensions of the valve diaphragm and/or nozzle must be altered because the force exerted by R on the diaphragm must *now be large compared with the force exerted by P on the seating*. Formerly, these two forces were equal at equilibrium.

For this purpose, one can use a larger diaphragm so that R exerts on it a much larger force than previously; this force would then also be considerably greater than F_h ($= P \times a$).

On the other hand, the size of the high pressure nozzle can be diminished and the high pressure force on the seating thus reduced, so that it becomes small compared with the force exerted by R on the diaphragm. In practice the diaphragm area is increased and the effective seating area decreased, but there are technical limits to these changes.

* Although two high pressure seatings (h, h') of this kind are not used in valves for medical gases, their advantage for large seating area (a) is easily understood. The high pressure (P) exerts the force $a \times P$ on the seating. If the valve should deliver high flowrates, the area a must not be too small. The force ($a \times P$) may then become fairly high and this has an adverse effect on the performance of the reducing valve (see p. 133). When using two high pressure seatings, one (h) is pushed upwards and the other (h') downwards by the high pressure. The forces on the two seatings are equal and opposite; they cancel one another and the resultant high pressure force on the seatings is nil. The operation of the valve does no longer depend on the value of P.

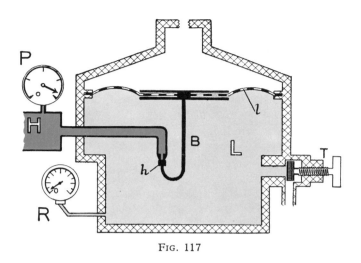

FIG. 117

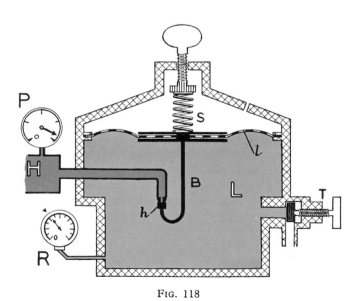

FIG. 118

Fig. 117—This shows part of the improved valve scheme and illustrates the consequences of the change in size of seating and diaphragm.

The outlet tap (T) is closed. High pressure gas has flowed from H to L until the hydraulic force exerted by the pressure in L on the diaphragm overcomes the force with which P tends to push the seating away from the nozzle.

The position of the pointer on the lower gauge shows that a very small pressure in L now exerts sufficient force on the diaphragm to pull the seating by means of the connecting rod (B) tightly against the nozzle so as to prevent further influx of high pressure gas. This small pressure in L is considerably *below the lowest reduced pressure* to which the valve can be adjusted in practice; it is also very small compared with the value of R in the primitive design shown in fig. 114.

Fig. 118—gives the complete scheme of the improved valve.

A spring (S) is placed above the central clamping plates of the diaphragm to which the connecting rod is fixed. A thumbscrew has been inserted through the casing above the diaphragm, and serves to vary the compression of the spring.

Let us consider what happens when the spring is compressed while tap (T) remains shut. A turn of the thumbscrew will push the spring against rod (B) thus forcing the seating away from the nozzle. High pressure gas flows from H to L until the pressure in L rises sufficiently to push the diaphragm upwards against the force of the compressed spring. Rod (B) is thus raised and pulls up the seating (*h*) against the nozzle. The seating must further be pressed against the nozzle strongly enough to overcome the force exerted by the high pressure gas on the seating.

The quantitative theory of the improved design will show that the least compression of the spring by the thumbscrew admissible in practice must produce a spring force which is large compared with the force necessary to occlude the nozzle against the force exerted by P on seating (*h*).

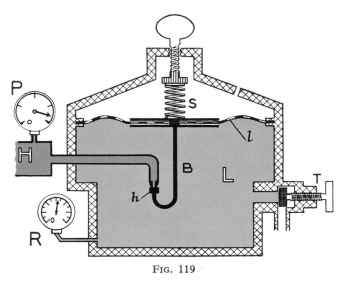

FIG. 119

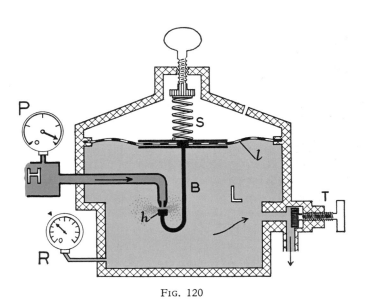

FIG. 120

Fig. 119—If the spring is further compressed by tightening of the thumbscrew, a larger pressure will build up in L before the seating again occludes the nozzle. This is indicated by the increased density of colour in L and by the movement of the pointer on the reduced pressure gauge to a higher position. The compression of spring (S) therefore regulates the reduced pressure.

Fig. 120—In this illustration the regulating spring (S) is adjusted to the same value as in fig. 118. As soon as T is opened, the pressure in L falls slightly and with it the hydraulic force on the diaphragm; the various forces acting on the connecting rod (B) are no longer balanced and the seating (h) moves away from the nozzle. The seating quickly takes up a position in which the inflow of high pressure gas through the nozzle into L equals the outflow of low pressure gas through T.

Theory*

Fig. 121—Tap T is again assumed shut as in Fig. 118.

F_S represents the force of the compressed regulating spring acting downwards on the connecting rod when the seating is just touching the nozzle.

Neglecting at first the small force ($P \times a$) exerted by the high pressure on the seating, the equilibrium condition is given approximately by the equality of F_1 with the force of the spring F_S

$$R \times A = F_S \qquad . \qquad . \qquad . \quad (5)$$

$$R \quad = F_S/A \qquad . \qquad . \qquad . \quad (6)$$

Here F_S depends only on the nature of the spring and the extent to which it has been compressed by the thumbscrew.

In this approximation R is thus *independent* of P; it remains constant for a given compression of the regulating spring. Furthermore, R can be varied at will; it is proportional to the compression of the spring by the thumbscrew.

This as well as the following, more accurate relations are valid only until the cylinder pressure (P) has fallen to the value of R. From then onwards the valve no longer regulates, R remains equal to P and both decrease together.

---

* The few existing surveys on the theory of reducing valves are highly specialized and rather inaccessible—see, for example, refs. 1 and 2.

In a more accurate theory, the small force exerted by the high pressure gas on the seating has to be taken into account.* The equilibrium equation becomes:

$$F_1 = F_S + F_h \qquad \text{or}$$
$$R \times A = F_S + P \times a \qquad . \qquad . \qquad (7)$$

R is seen to depend on P but any variation of R with falling P can be

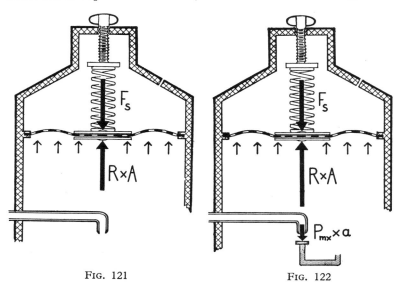

FIG. 121   FIG. 122

minimized by ensuring that the smallest value of F_S (spring compression) is always large compared with $(P \times a)$; this condition must be fulfilled even if P represents the 'full' cylinder pressure, P_{mx}. The condition that F_S is always set so as to be large compared with $(P \times a)$ was already utilized in the discussion of Fig. 118.

Fig. 122—shows the forces acting on the connecting rod (B) when T is closed and equilibrium is established. It should help to visualize both the direction and relative magnitude of the forces concerned. The high pressure cylinder is assumed to be 'full', i.e. $P = P_{mx}$.

When writing the equilibrium condition (7) in the form:

$$R = (F_S/A) + P \times (a/A) \qquad . \qquad . \qquad (8)$$

it becomes obvious that the variation of R with decreasing P can be

* The force exerted by R on seating (h) in opposition to the high pressure (P) is neglected throughout.

made insignificant by building the valve with a nozzle area which is small compared with the diaphragm; (a/A) must become sufficiently small in order to make $(a/A) \times P$ small compared with R.

Examples

Many valves used by anaesthetists, in which the reduced pressure is adjustable do not function for settings lower than approximately R = 6 lb/in² (0·41 atm). In a certain type, the diaphragm radius = 1·0 in (2·5 cm); its area A = π × (radius)² = π × (1·0)² in². The upward hydraulic force exerted by the low pressure gas on the diaphragm is

$$R \times A = 6 \text{ lb/in}^2 \times \pi (1\cdot0)^2 \text{ in}^2$$
$$= 18\cdot8 \text{ lb} \qquad (8\cdot56 \text{ kg})$$

In equilibrium, with tap T shut, this hydraulic force has to overcome the mechanical force exerted by the compressed regulating spring and also the hydraulic force exerted by the high pressure gas on the seating.

In the particular valve under consideration the opening of the nozzle has a radius of (1/50) in (= 0·05 cm); its area a = π × (1/50)² in²

The ratio of (a/A) is here   = (1/50)²/1²
$$= 1/2500$$

This is much smaller than the corresponding ratio in the primitive valve design (p. 125).

Variation of reduced pressure with cylinder pressure

The quantitative expression for the variation in R when P decreases can be found by repeating the calculation made on p. 125 for the simple valve scheme. The result for the improved type of valve is:

$$(R - R')/R = (a/A) \times (P - P')/R \qquad (9)$$

The left side is again the relative change of reduced pressure when the cylinder pressure falls from P to P'. In contrast to the result previously found for the simple type of valve, the *relative* change in reduced pressure depends now on the dimensions of the valve (a, A) and is insignificant if (a/A) is very small.

Furthermore, R appears in the denominator on the right side of the equation; the larger R, the smaller the right side. In other words, the relative decrease in R (l.h.s. of equation) with emptying cylinder gets less the larger the value of R to which the valve has been adjusted.

For: $(a/A) = 1/2500$;   P = 1800,   P' = ⅓P = 600
With S adjusted to give   R = 8 lb/in²

one obtains R' = 7·5 lb/in² and for the percentage drop of R:

$$100 \times (R - R')/R = 100 \times (1/2500) \times (1200/8) = 6\%$$

Compare this with the decrease of reduced pressure in the simple type of valve which is 10 times as great (p. 125).

The variation of the reduced pressure, — in a valve of the improved type, which occurs with falling cylinder pressure can be also derived from first principles.

1. *In a 'full' cylinder*
   of oxygen the pressure P may have a maximum value of
$$P_{mx} = 1800 \text{ lb/in}^2 \text{ (122 atm)}$$
and the corresponding reduced pressure in the valve is again $R = 6 \text{ lb/in}^2$.

The hydraulic force exerted by P_{mx} on the seating of this particular valve is:
$$F_h = 1800 \text{ lb/in}^2 \times \pi(1/50)^2 \text{ in}^2$$
$$= 2 \cdot 26 \text{ lb } (1 \cdot 03 \text{ kg})$$

Of the total force $F_l = \underline{18 \cdot 8} \text{ lb}$ exerted by the low pressure gas in L on the diaphragm, $18 \cdot 8 - \overline{2 \cdot 26} = \underline{16 \cdot 6}$ lb will be available to overcome the mechanical spring force F_s, while $\overline{F_h} = \underline{2 \cdot 26}$ lb are required to close the nozzle against the full cylinder pressure P_{mx}. The part of the reduced pressure in L which supplies this force of $2 \cdot 26$ lb is given by the expression:
$$\frac{2 \cdot 26 \text{ lb}}{\text{area of diaphragm}} = \frac{2 \cdot 26 \text{ lb}}{\pi \times (1 \cdot 0)^2 \text{ in}^2}$$
$$= 0 \cdot 72 \text{ lb/in}^2 \text{ (0·049 atm)}$$

The hydraulic force exerted by the remaining $(6 - 0 \cdot 72) \text{ lb/in}^2 = 5 \cdot 28 \text{ lb/in}^2$ overcomes the spring force, which was shown to be $F_s = 16 \cdot 6 \text{ lb}$.

2. *If the cylinder is $\frac{1}{3}$ 'full'*
   the high pressure is only
$$P' = 600 \text{ lb/in}^2 \text{ (40·8 atm)}$$
   The force exerted on the seating (*h*) by high pressure gas (P′) is only
$$F_h' = 600 \text{ lb/in}^2 \times \pi (1/50)^2 \text{ in}^2$$
$$= 0 \cdot 76 \text{ lb } (0 \cdot 34 \text{ kg})$$

The pressure component in L required to occlude the nozzle is now only:
$$\frac{0 \cdot 76 \text{ lb}}{\pi \times (1 \cdot 0)^2 \text{ in}^2} = 0 \cdot 24 \text{ lb/in}^2 \text{ (0·016 atm)}$$

As in the case of the 'full' cylinder the low pressure gas has to exert a pressure of
$$5 \cdot 28 \text{ lb/in}^2 \text{ (0·36 atm)}$$
to overcome the pre-set spring force (F_s). But the additional pressure

required to occlude the nozzle has decreased from the value of
0.72 lb/in² to the present

$$0.24 \text{ lb/in}^2$$

This decrease of $(0.72 - 0.24)$ lb/in² = $\underline{0.48 \text{ lb/in}^2}$ accounts for the
fall of the reduced pressure from

$$R = 6.0 \quad \text{to} \quad R' = 5.52 \text{ lb/in}^2$$

This variation in R with decreasing P could have been calculated
directly from the equation 9 (p. 133):

$$(R - R') = (a/A) \times (P - P') \qquad . \qquad . \qquad (10)$$

by substituting: $(a/A) = (1/2500)$ and

$$(P - P') = (1800 - 600) = 1200$$

Therefore: $(R - R') = (1/2500) \times 1200 = 0.48 \text{ lb/in}^2$

Although this type of reducing valve is not ideal in so far as the
value of R decreases while the cylinder is emptying, the variation in
R is greatly diminished compared with that in the simple valve design
calculated on p. 125 (Eq. 4).

We see that in this improved design a fall in cylinder pressure from
1800 to 600 lb/in² is accompanied by a relative decrease in reduced
pressure of

$$100 \times (6 - 5.5)/6 = 8\%$$

In comparison, the simple type of valve would show a decrease of
66% in reduced pressure (Eq. 4; p. 125).

We repeat now the experiment carried out previously for the simple
valve type (p. 125) with gas flowing from the improved valve. Tap (T)
is again set to give a flow rate of 1000 cm³/min when the gas cylinder
is 'full'.

When the cylinder pressure has fallen to $P' = (1/10) P_{mx} = 180$ lb/in²,
the reduced pressure can be found from:

$$R' = R - (a/A) \times (P - P') \qquad \text{(see Eq. 10)}$$
$$R' = 6 - (1/2500) \times (1800 - 180) \text{ lb/in}^2$$
$$= (6 - 0.65) \text{ lb/in}^2 = 5.35 \text{ lb/in}^2$$

A fall in cylinder pressure by 90% is here accompanied by a decrease
in reduced pressure of 11%.

The outflow rate through T would have decreased at the same time
only to 900 cm³/min.

Since the time taken for the cylinder pressure to fall from 1800
to 180 lb/in² is very long in clinical practice, there would obviously

be little or no need with such a reducing valve to adjust the setting of T. It would take, in fact, 15 hours at a flow rate of 1 1/min for the pressure inside an oxygen cylinder with a capacity of 40 ft³ to fall from 1800 to 180 lb/in².

If the valve is adjusted to higher values of R, its performance is still better—as predicted by the theory (p. 133, Eq. 9). We have seen (p. 135) that with the valve set to R = 6 lb/in², a fall in the high pressure of 66% is accompanied by a fall in the reduced pressure of 8%. If, however, the regulating spring is further compressed by the thumb-screw to give R = 17 lb/in², the fall in cylinder pressure from 1800 to 600 lb/in² is accompanied by a fall in reduced pressure from 17 to 16·5 lb/in². Here a fall of 66% in the cylinder pressure is accompanied by a fall of only 3% in R.

Schemes of some practical reducing valves

Even the scheme of the reducing valve shown in figs. 117 to 120 does not yet represent that of the valve types used by anaesthetists; several of these types incorporate a further refinement.

One reason for further improvements will become apparent after a closer study of the gas flow supplied by a reducing valve. So far, we have assumed implicitly that for any increased flow rate produced by opening of outlet tap (T), the seating disc (*h*) takes up a position which ensures that the reduced pressure remains unaltered. In this case we vary the flow rate of gases into the anaesthetic apparatus by varying the flow resistance of tap (T) at a pre-set 'driving' pressure (R).

Alternatively, one could vary the flow rate by substituting for tap (T) a fixed flow-resistance or constriction, and adjust the 'driving' pressure (R).

The latter method of varying the gas flow is actually used on a number of industrial reducing valves and is also still quite common on medical gas equipment in certain countries. In these valves the spring-regulating screw is designed for easy manipulation and the outflow is limited solely by the bore of the outlet pipe.

If we try to shut off the gas flow by unscrewing the regulating screw and thus relax the spring completely, the valve type discussed so far will not give satisfaction: gas will continue to flow—if slowly. This is obvious from the discussion of fig. 117 on p. 129. It was then shown that a very small pressure in L—with T closed—is sufficient to occlude the flow from H to L. But if T is kept open the pressure in L will tend to fall, gas will flow from H to L and out through T; owing to the low pressure in L the flow will be relatively small, as stated before.

To interrupt the outflow from T when the regulating spring (S) is completely relaxed, a further external force is introduced which acts on the seating disc (h) in opposition to the force of the high pressure gas. This external force is made large enough to overcome the gas pressure of a 'full' cylinder (P_{mx}) and is, of course, adequate for all other values of P.

This additional occluding force is supplied in two different ways in various valves.

(i) By the insertion of a second, short compression spring acting in opposition to the main regulating spring.

(ii) By using an elastic metal diaphragm; the force caused by its deformation exerts the desired pull on the seating disc.

(i) The functioning of valves using the first method will be apparent from the next two illustrations.

Fig. 123—The regulating spring and –screw have been removed. Tap (T) is wide open and could be replaced by a constriction in the outlet pipe. A 'shut-off' spring (s) is inserted below the connecting rod (B). When the screw valve on the 'full' cylinder is opened, gas will flow from H to L and on through the outlet.

Spring (s) is now gradually compressed by an adjusting screw underneath, until it presses the seating disc against the nozzle strongly enough to prevent any further flow from H to L. The pressure in L is zero, i.e. atmospheric. This situation is illustrated in fig. 123.

The force (G_s) exerted by the adjusted seating spring (s) is

$$G_s = a \times P_{mx} \qquad . \qquad . \qquad . \quad (11)$$

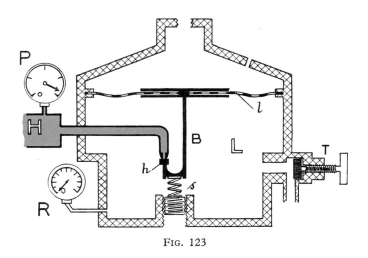

FIG. 123

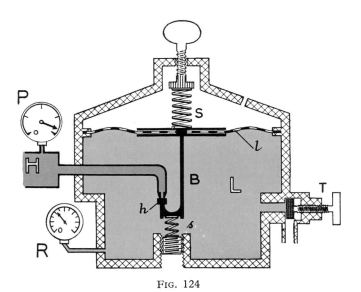

FIG. 124

Fig. 124—The regulating spring (S) is inserted and compressed by turning the regulating screw. Tap (T) is assumed closed; the turning of the regulating screw pushes h away from the nozzle and compresses S. Gas flows from H to L until R has risen to a value determined by the adjustment of the regulating screw and the characteristics of the valve.

The equilibrium of forces* is now given by

$$R \times A + G_s = F_S + P \times a \qquad . \qquad (12)$$

substituting Eq. 10 for G_s:

$$R \times A = F_S + P \times a - P_{mx} \times a \qquad .$$
$$= F_S - (P_{mx} - P) \times a \qquad . \qquad . \qquad (13)$$

Solving this for R we obtain:

$$R = (F_S/A) - (P_{mx} - P) \times (a/A) . \qquad . \qquad (14)$$

which should be compared with Eq. 8 of the previous valve scheme One can deduce from Eq. 14 that the variation of R with falling cylinder pressure is the same as for the simpler valve scheme of fig. 122.

(ii) The second method of ensuring a 'shut-off' while the regulating spring (S) is completely relaxed and with outlet (T) from L open, uses a special diaphragm.

The inelastic, slack diaphragm considered so far is here replaced by an elastic metal membrane. 'Elastic' means that the diaphragm bends from its resting position proportionally to the external force; it exerts an opposing force proportional to the displacement. In contrast, the slack, inelastic diaphragm was assumed to move within a small range without exerting any opposing force; at the limits of this range it would resist any force exerted on it without moving any further.

Fig. 125—The regulating screw of this valve has been turned back and spring (S) is completely relaxed. The outlet (T) is open and the high pressure cylinder is turned on.

Connecting rod (B) has been modified; the vertical stem passes through a short sleeve and the length of B between diaphragm and high pressure seating (h) can be fixed as required by tightening the locking screw on the sleeve at the appropriate point.

---

* In an actual reducing valve the flow of high pressure gas (P) does *not* cease completely if (h) is pulled against the nozzle with a force $= a \times P$. Owing to technical imperfections (surface irregularities of seating disc, etc.) the resultant of forces pressing the disc against the nozzle will have to be greater than $a \times P$. The actual force can be expressed as $n \times (a \times P)$, where n is a number greater than 1 depending on the degree of imperfection. Eq. 4 to 14 can be corrected for this effect by substituting $n \times a$ in place of a. The variations of R with falling cylinder pressure (Eq. 4 and 9) have to be multiplied by n.

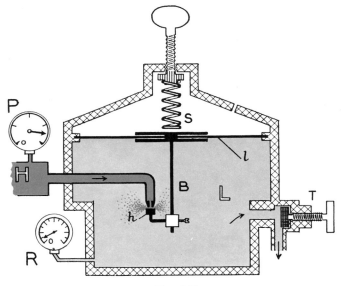

FIG. 125

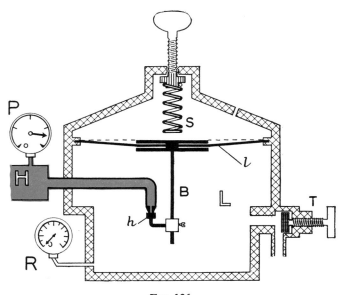

FIG. 126

When the locking screw on the sleeve is undone while h is touching the nozzle, B is free to move and the metal diaphragm will be in its undeformed position; in this situation gas would flow from H to L and out through T.

Fig. 126—The vertical stem of B is next pulled down through a small distance and the locking screw of the sleeve tightened. The diaphragm is now bent and tries to straighten out, thereby exerting an upward pull on B which is proportional to the extent to which it has been deformed.

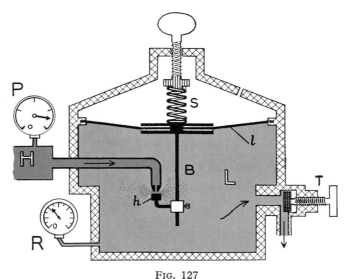

FIG. 127

This is the force which presses the seating disc against the nozzle; when the length of B has been adjusted correctly, the force exerted by the deformed diaphragm will be just adequate to prevent any flow from the 'full' cylinder.

The pressure in L is again zero as in arrangement (i) on p. 138 (fig. 123).

Fig. 127—To set this valve to the desired reduced pressure, the outlet (T) is shut and spring (S) is gradually compressed by turning the regulating screw. The downward force exerted by the compressed regulating spring deforms further the bent diaphragm and gas will flow through the nozzle until the force exerted by the pressure in L on the diaphragm overcomes F_s; l moves upwards and h is pulled tightly against the nozzle. The adjustment can also be carried out with T slightly open and while gas continues to flow from H and out through T.

If T is closed, the force exerted by the rising pressure in L will straighten the bent diaphragm against the opposing force of the regulating spring until B pulls the high pressure disc (*h*) with sufficient force against the nozzle to prevent any further outflow of gas from H. Equilibrium is again described by Eq. 14 (p. 139).

In the practical valve scheme (i) of fig. 124, a certain advance of the regulating screw will not produce an equal compression of the regulating spring (S) because seating spring (*s*) will also give way and be partly compressed (in addition to its initial compression, p. 137). In scheme (ii) of fig. 127 the elastic diaphragm will also be bent when the regulating screw is tightened.

The seating spring (*s*) is increasingly compressed when the regulating screw is adjusted to high values of R, and thus opposes the movement of seating (*h*) away from the nozzle. The practical significance of this is that the seating spring (or, in scheme ii, the elastic, bent diaphragm) acts as a 'springy' stop which limits the excursions of *h*.

Flow characteristics of reducing valves

All the preceding, quantitative discussions of the mechanism of reducing valves dealt with the equilibrium of the various forces acting in the valve when the flow of gases from the low pressure section was interrupted by closing outlet (T). The priority given to the 'no flow' situation is understandable as it is very important that the pressure in L should not gradually 'creep' above the pre-set value (R). Such excessive creep would cause particular trouble if T is not an integral part of the valve but is connected to the outlet from L by rubber tubing; this is the case on most modern anaesthetic apparatus of British manufacture, where T is the needle valve at the lower end of the flowmeter frame.

However, the performance of reducing valves when delivering gas flows at varying rates is of similar concern to the anaesthetist. In order to ensure a uniform control over all required flow rates by the adjustment of a tap (T), the ideal reducing valve should maintain the pre-set value of R independent of the flow rates.

As the theory relating pressures in L to various flow rates is not sufficiently elementary for the scope of this book, only some qualitative facts relating to this problem will be given here.

It is desirable that the reduced pressure should decrease only very little when the flow rate supplied from the valve is increased; to ensure this a slight decrease of pressure in L must then produce a considerable increase in flow from H to L. If the diaphragm moves only little for a slight drop in pressure, the seating (h) will also move only a little distance away from the high pressure nozzle. In these circumstances an appreciable increase in the flow from H to L is obtained if the bore of the nozzle is sufficiently large; this conflicts, however, with the condition that the ratio (a/A) must be kept small (p. 133). In practice a compromise solution is adopted.

To obtain large, constant flowrates the '*two-stage*' valve is indicated. In principle this consists of two valves in series; the relatively high, reduced pressure of the first supplies the input pressure to the second stage (p. 151). The variation of reduced pressure with cylinder pressure is also greatly diminished.

Commercial Reducing Valves

It is now possible to compare these schematic representations with the structure of a commercial pressure reducing valve (or 'Regulator').

Fig. 128—shows an 'exploded' view of a regulator with certain parts drawn in and positioned to assist comparison with the valve in figs. 123 and 124 on p. 138.

The rubber-covered canvas diaphragm (l) is clamped between metal plates with curved inner surfaces. Insert 128a shows a boss on the lower plate which has been engaged with 'connecting rod' B in the second insert 128b. The rod (B) consists of a hollowed, cut-out block with a screw thread in its lower part. After it has been inserted close to the high-pressure nozzle, the disc carrier (h) is screwed into B from below and touches the high-pressure nozzle. The diaphragm (l) is clamped in position on top of the valve body by the end cap (1) and threaded clamp ring (2). The seating spring (s) rests on a ledge inside tube (4). This tube is now screwed into the internally threaded, lower part of the valve body and presses thereby the seating spring (s) against the seating disc carrier (h). If all distances and the flexibility of (s) have been correctly chosen, no gas will flow from the nozzle after a compressed gas cylinder has been attached at H.

Regulating spring (S) is now inserted into 1 and comes to a rest on the upper clamping plate on l; it is compressed to set the required reduced pressure by screwing cap (3) into the threaded tube forming the upper part of 1.

The components (5) form a safety valve for the release of any

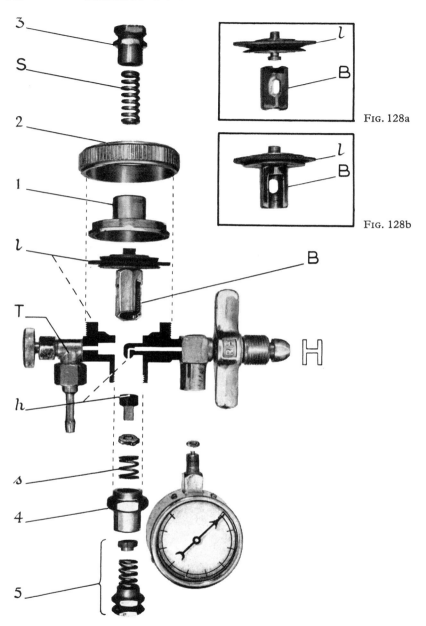

Fig. 128a

Fig. 128b

Fig. 128

excessive pressure which might build up in the reduced pressure compartment (L) should the mechanism of the regulator fail.

The foregoing will be more clearly understood by reference to the next illustration.

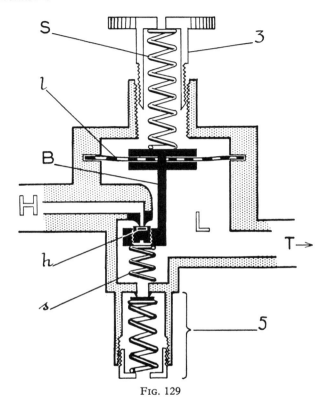

FIG. 129

Fig. 129—shows the construction of an 'Endurance' regulator drawn schematically. The mechanism of the safety valve (5) is also clearly shown.

The present-day version of the historical BEARD valve (p. 148) is the 'Adams' pressure reducing valve[3]. In contrast to the other regulators considered in this chapter, this valve is pre-set to a given, reduced pressure of about 6 lb/in² (0·4 atm.), although a small adjustment is possible. Furthermore, the movement of the diaphragm is transferred by a lever mechanism to a diminished movement of the high pressure seating.

A slight increase of pressure in L above the normal value of R will lead to a small excess hydraulic force on the diaphragm which is transferred considerably increased by the 'lazy-tongs' lever system to

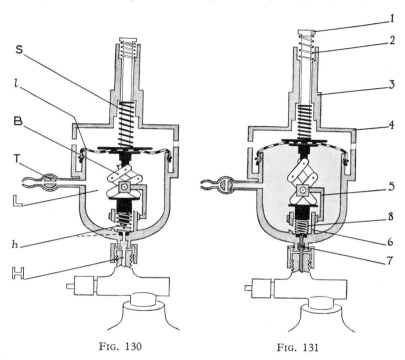

FIG. 130   FIG. 131

the conical seating (*h*); the latter will now occlude more firmly the high pressure nozzle.

The scheme of an 'Adams' valve for oxygen in which the high pressure nozzle is occluded by a steel cone is shown in figs. 130-1. In certain 'Adams' valves for nitrous oxide a small seating disc of plastic material is embedded in a holder and occludes the high pressure nozzle.

Another peculiar feature of the 'Adams' valve is that it does not shut off the outflow from the high pressure nozzle if the regulating spring (S) is un-compressed. The diaphragm is of the slack type and cannot have a shut-off function as the diaphragm in scheme ii (fig. 126). The small compression spring (8) below the conical plunger cannot possibly assist the closing of the high pressure outlet. Its function is to keep the upper part of the seating (*h*) always pressed against the lower arms of the 'lazy-tongs' so that it follows every movement of the lever system without being mechanically connected to it.

Fig. 130—shows the positions of 'lazy-tongs', diaphragm, regulating spring and cone-shaped seating if the pressure in L is atmospheric; T is open and H has been turned off. S is already compressed but the construction of the lever system prevents any further descent of the diaphragm.

Fig. 131—Here T is closed and H is open. The pressure in L has risen until it is able to push the diaphragm up against the compressed spring (S). Simultaneously, the lower lever arms are pressing the cone-shaped seating against the hydraulic force of the high pressure gas (and against the force of the small lifting spring 8) until its outflow ceases.

Fig. 132—shows an exploded view of an 'Adams' valve with the section of the valve body sketched in.

Ring (5) carries the pivot for the 'lazy-tongs' system (B) and slips over tube (6) projecting from the bottom of the valve body. Tube (6) also forms a guide for the plunger with the conical seating (*h*) at its lower end. Holes in the side of 6 allow free escape of gas from H to L as soon as *h* has moved away from the high pressure nozzle which is marked in black on the draw-

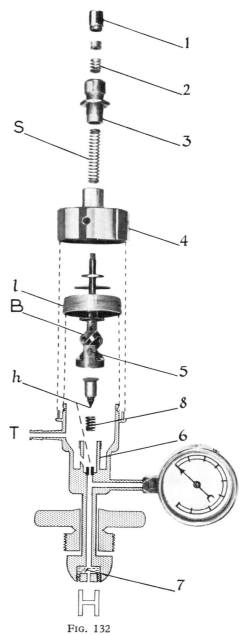

FIG. 132

ing. The slack rubber diaphragm (*l*) is cup-shaped and is pushed over the rim of the valve body when B (with 5 and *h*) are lowered into position. The externally threaded tube (3) corresponds to the regulating screw and compresses S when it is screwed down into the upper end of cap (4).

The small spring (2) rests on a shoulder inside 3; it is pushed over the extension of B above the diaphragm which ends in knob (1). If *h* is lifted from the high pressure outlet, B moves downwards and spring (2) is compressed. It thus opposes further opening of the high pressure outlet and this action steadies the valve movements: undesirable mechanical vibrations are reduced.

The small filter discs (7) form an important part of any valve; they are made from fine wire gauze and prevent dust from reaching the high pressure nozzle.

The Development of the Reducing Valve

Many features of modern pressure reducing valves were invented a long time ago. There was a spate of new designs during the last decade of the nineteenth century and within a few years most principles of our modern valves had been described and utilized.

A. Beard's Small Regulator of 1888

Fig. 133—has been re-drawn in a simplified form from the original illustration[4]; it shows that this regulator is the forerunner of the modern 'Adams' valve.

When gas enters the low pressure compartment (L), the hydraulic force on the plate (*l*) overcomes the force of the pre-set regulating spring (S), and *l* moves upwards. A 'lazy-tongs' lever system (B) couples plate (*l*) to a bar (D) at the upper end of the high pressure seating (*h*). The lower ends of the 'tongs' are round discs which can rotate about an eccentrically placed pivot. When *l* moves upwards the 'tongs' are extended and the discs at their lower end rotate about the pivot and thereby depress the bar (D). The movement of *h* is considerably less than that of *l*; according to the principles of mechanical levers, the downward force on D is correspondingly increased compared with the hydraulic force pushing upwards against *l*. Rubber bellows form the sides of the low pressure compartment and permit unimpeded movement of endplate (*l*).

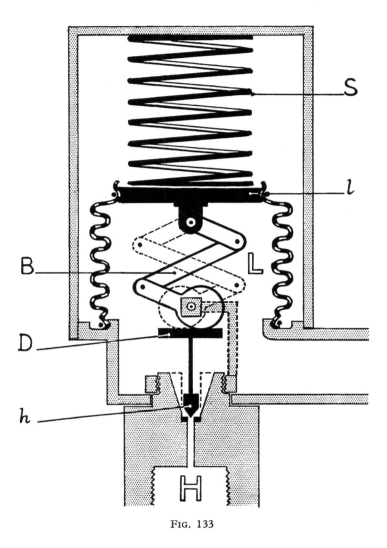

FIG. 133

The original design has a tight coupling between D and the eccentric discs at the end of the lazy tongs; seating (*h*) follows thus every movement of D.

Beard's Regulator is still in current production!

B. Suiter's Regulator of 1890

Fig. 134—is re-drawn from one of the original illustrations[5]. As in certain modern reducing valves the seating (h) is on the high pressure side of the nozzle.* A stiff, elastic metal diaphragm (l) takes over the

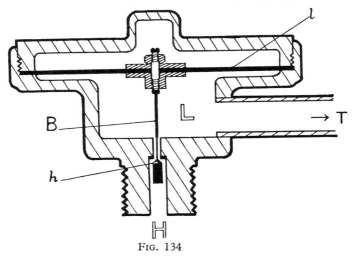

FIG. 134

function of the regulating spring; increasing gas pressure in L deflects the diaphragm upwards which opposes the bending with a force in the downward direction. The length of connecting rod (B) is initially adjusted by means of the clamping nuts at the centre of the diaphragm; this determines the extent of bending (and thereby the opposing force) before h can occlude the high pressure seat.

The original description by Suiter makes it quite clear that his 'new design' avoided deliberately any lever system or rubber diaphragm which had caused breakdown in other valve designs at that time.

C. Clarkson's Regulator of 1889

This device[6] contained two features which are incorporated in many modern reducing valves:

1. A slack, inelastic diaphragm with large, central clamping plates and a helical regulating spring.

2. A two-stage principle whereby the high gas pressure is reduced in two steps to the final low outlet pressure.

* The equilibrium condition for this type of valve is obtained from Eq. 8 (p. 132) by substituting a − instead of the + sign. If the cylinder pressure falls from the initial P_{mx}, the reduced pressure will *increase* slightly. Compare this with the slight *decrease* in R of the valve types discussed in the theoretical section of this chapter.

Fig. 135—is a simplified scheme of the original illustration. The functioning of the device is best understood by considering it as two separate reducing valves enclosed by the same container. The 'low' outlet pressure of valve (1) represents the 'high' inlet pressure of valve (2), and has been designated by 'M' (medium pressure).

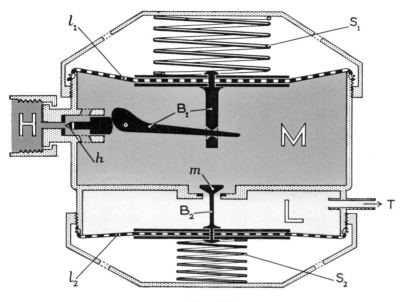

FIG. 135

The hydraulic force exerted by the medium pressure on the first diaphragm (l_1) is multiplied by a lever (B_1) before acting on the high pressure seating (h); when l_1 moves upwards through a certain distance, the lever (B_1) pushes h to the left over a much shorter distance.

The second plunger (m) regulating the entry of gas from the medium (M) to the low (L) pressure compartments is connected directly to the second diaphragm (l_2). The forces exerted by the compressed regulating springs $(S_1$ and $S_2)$ determine the medium and low reduced pressures in the valve.

The lower spring (S_2) could be adjusted to give pressures in L ranging from 24 down to only 1 inch H_2O; pressures in M were kept about six to ten times as high by suitable adjustment of S_1.

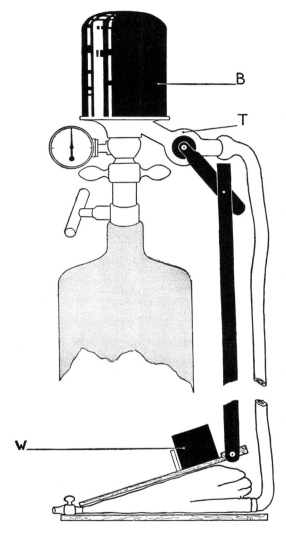

FIG. 136

Fig. 136—represents the simplified scheme of another two-stage regulator[7] which was advertised in 1891.

On top of the cylinder of compressed gas is a Beard's regulator (B). The outlet tap (T) is linked by long levers to the hinged top board of fireside bellows acting as reservoir for gas at the low, second stage pressure. The value of the second stage pressure is determined by the weight (W) placed on the hinged board.

When gas flows from the stopcock at the left end of the bellows, the upper hinged board will sink and the attached lever system gradually will open tap (T). Gas of medium pressure supplied by the Beard's valve will flow through the rubber tube into the bellows reservoir and the hinged board rises until T is completely cut off.

Early History of the Reducing Valve

The sudden activity in the design of pressure reducing valves during the last decades of the nineteenth century can be linked directly to the increasing availability of compressed oxygen in cylinders, and indirectly to the demand for improvement in public entertainment.* Lantern slide lectures enjoyed an increasing vogue and the profession of lanternist was becoming as established as that of the present cinema operator. The need for sources of bright light became more urgent.

The invention of the oxygen/hydrogen blowpipe by Newman (1816) and of the 'Limelight' by H. Davy and E. Drummond (1826) could only be fully utilized when a commercial supply of compressed gases was guaranteed. A block of lime emits brilliant light when a hot flame is played on to it. Originally the flame was produced by one of Newman's oxygen/hydrogen burners. In later years oxygen was passed over liquid ether, and the lanternist knew only too well that the resulting mixture would burn with an extremely hot flame. Two factors had to be ensured to obtain a satisfactory limelight:

(*a*) The tank and the burner should contain gas at relatively low pressure so that when the flow of gas to the burner was cut down by a stopcock near the burner, the pressure of gas within the connecting tube would not burst the tube or blow it off its connection.

(*b*) The flow should remain constant while the contents of the high pressure storage tank were gradually decreasing.

The various designs of pressure reducing regulators tried to provide

* Considerable demand for reliable pressure reducing valves was also created by the growing use of gas welding in industry. In order to obtain steady burner flames, a constant low pressure supply must be ensured.

these desirable conditions which were: a constant (regulated) supply of low (reduced) pressure gas.

It would be wrong to assume that this problem had not existed before. The development of pressure reducing regulators was also

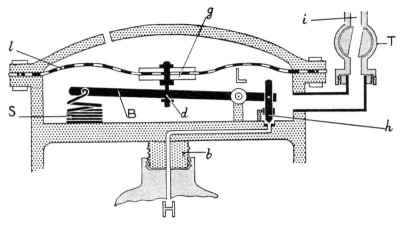

FIG. 137

closely linked with the design of containers for compressed gases and with the commercial demand for the latter.

As early as 1822 the forerunner of the modern compressed fuel gas ('Calor' gas) was supplied in portable containers at a pressure of 15 atm (220 lb/in²) by a Mr. Caslon, owner of a London gas works. Later on, filling pressures[8] were raised to 30 atm (440 lb/in²) and some of the earliest pressure reducing regulators were described in the technical literature of that time.

Fig. 137—The valve[9] is re-drawn from a patent of 1837 granted to H. Q. Tenneson, a Frenchman resident in London. The high pressure vessel is connected to 'b', the outlet (i) leads to low pressure gas burners. The connecting rod between diaphragm and high pressure plunger (h) is here a horizontal lever (B) with the hinge near its right-hand end. The high pressure plunger is attached to the right, short arm of the lever and carries at its lower end a steel cone. The centre plate (g) of the gastight diaphragm (l) is attached to the lever at (d), while a strong tension spring (S) pulls down the left end of the lever in opposition to an upward force. The reduced pressure rises until the upward force exerted by it on the diaphragm pulls up the left arm of the lever against the downward pull of the tension spring. Gas ceases to flow from the high pressure container as soon as the right arm of the lever has been lowered to a position where the steel pin occludes the high pressure orifice with sufficient force to prevent escape of gas from H to L.

REFERENCES

[1] BAILLON, A., and JURION, R. (1935). *Bull. Soc. Ing. Soud.*, **6**, 1645–73.
[2] IBERALL, A. S. (1954). *Trans. Amer. Soc. Mech. Engrs.*, **76**, 363–73.
[3] ADAMS, F. H. (1939). *Brit. Pat.* 499057.
[4] BEARD, R. R. (1888). *Brit. Pat.* 13181; also: *Optic. mag. Lant. J.* (1891), 2, 118.
[5] SUITER, A. (1890). *Brit. Pat.* 13652; also: *Optic. mag. Lant. J.* (1891), 2, 134.
[6] CLARKSON, A. T. (1889). *Brit. Pat.* 11518; also: *Optic. mag. Lant. J.* (1891), 2, 118.
[7] HUGHES, W. C. (1891). *Optic. mag. Lant. J.*, 2, 142.
[8] GORDON, D. (1823). *Repert. Arts*, 43, 275–7.
[9] TENNESON, H. Q. (1837). *Brit. Pat.* 7447; also: *Lond. J. Arts Sci.* (1839), 13, 18–22.

CHAPTER XII

LAMINAR FLOW OF FLUIDS THROUGH TUBES

Hydrostatic pressure

FIG. 138—Two containers of equal dimensions are filled with water to a height of 10 cm . The hydrostatic pressure at the outlet is due to the weight of water above this level. The pressure at any level is equal to the weight of a water column of unit cross-section area above it. Thus in the illustration the weight of such a unit column is

height (10 cm) $\times$ cross-section area (1 cm^2) $\times$ density (1 g/cm^3)

$$= 10 \text{ g} .$$

It will be seen that this weight of water is numerically the same as the height of the water column. In fact hydrostatic pressure, here 10 g/cm^2, is generally expressed in terms of *height* of a column of water, in this case 10 cm .

Hydrostatic pressure at any given depth acts equally in all directions.

Fig. 139—The tanks are connected at their bases by a tube. There is no flow of water from one tank to the other, since the pressure at each end of the connecting tube is the same.

Fig. 140—The sizes of the containers here are different. The heights of the water above the outlets remain unchanged. There is no flow from one container to the other.

Hydrostatic pressure depends solely on the head of water; it is un-influenced by the capacity of the container.

Fig. 141—The water in A stands at a higher level than in B, and is less in volume. The hydrostatic pressure at the base of A is higher than at the base of B. There is a flow from A to B until the liquid levels within the two tanks, and therefore the hydrostatic pressures at each end of the connecting tube are equal.

Conclusions

(1) Fluid flows along a tube only when there is a pressure difference between the two ends.

(2) Fluid flows along a tube from a region of high pressure to a region of low pressure.

156

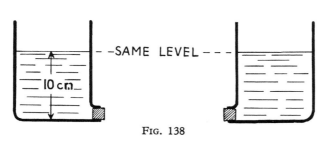

FIG. 138

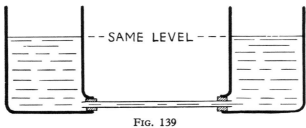

FIG. 139

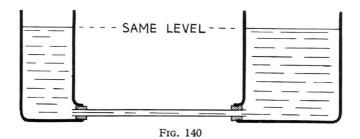

FIG. 140

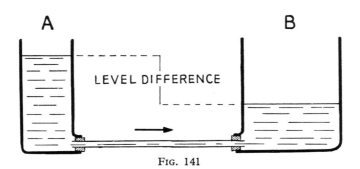

FIG. 141

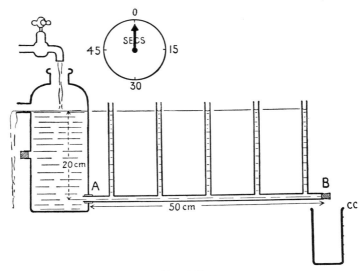

FIG. 142

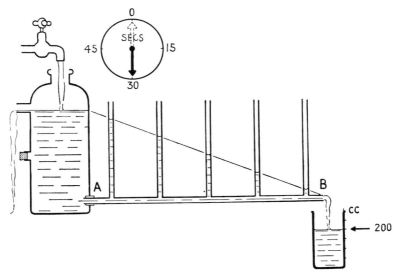

FIG. 143

Experiments on flow through tubes

Fig. 142—Water flows from a tap into a bottle, and the opening on the left ensures that the height of water, and therefore the hydrostatic pressure, above A is kept constant at 20 cm . The horizontal tube AB is 50 cm long and is closed by a cork at B.

Vertical glass tubes are attached to apertures in the horizontal tube (AB). The level to which the water is forced within them shows the hydrostatic pressure at the points in the tube AB, at which they are inserted. It is readily seen that the pressure in AB is the same (20 cm of water) throughout its length.

Although pressures are often expressed as 'cm H_2O', the official practice is to speak of 'cm water gauge' or 'cm w.g.'. The pressures expressed in these units are usually relative to the barometric pressure. Thus the absolute pressure on AB is equal to the barometric pressure plus 20 cm w.g.

The hydraulic pressure can be stated in any other units. The density of mercury (Hg) is 13·6 g/cm³. A pressure of 20 cm H_2O is therefore equivalent to one of $\dfrac{20}{13\cdot6} = 1\cdot47$ cm Hg . The absolute pressure exerted by the water on the walls of tube AB equals $760 + 14\cdot7 \simeq$ 775 mm Hg, assuming a normal air pressure of 760 mm Hg at the site of the experiment.

Fig. 143—The cork is removed and the water flows along AB. The pressure at B is now lower than at A. Pressure represents *potential energy* of the liquid. Decrease in pressure indicates that this energy has been used. In this case its loss is due to friction between the water particles as they flow along the tube (p. 175).

The pressure drop between A and B is 20 cm of water and this fall is linear throughout the length of the tube. 'Pressure gradient' is a term in frequent use to indicate the fall of pressure for each unit length of tube. In this example the pressure gradient is 0·4 cm of water for each centimetre length of tube.

In half a minute 200 ml of water pass through the tube.

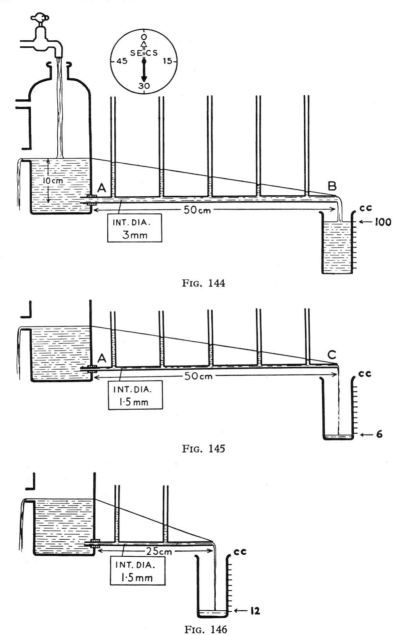

Fig. 144

Fig. 145

Fig. 146

Fig. 144—Compare with the previous experiment. The bung is removed from the lower of the two openings on the left of the bottle. The level of water above A is reduced to half (10 cm). The pressure gradient is correspondingly reduced and is now $0.4/2 = 0.2$ cm H_2O per cm length. The volume of water collected in the same time is reduced to half, i.e. 100 ml.

Fig. 145—The apparatus is the same as in the above figure except that the tube AC has a diameter half that of the tube AB. The volume of water collected in half a minute is 6 ml. This is only $\frac{1}{16}$ of the volume collected in the previous experiment. A reduction in the diameter of the tube by half has resulted in the outflow being reduced to $\frac{1}{16}$, that is, $(\frac{1}{2})^4$.

If the diameter of the tube were reduced to $\frac{1}{3}$, the volume flowing through would be reduced to $\frac{1}{81}$, that is, $(\frac{1}{3})^4$.

It was HAGEN[1] in 1839, and later POISEUILLE[2] in 1840, who discovered that the volume of fluid flowing through a tube of given length varies as the *fourth* power of the diameter of the tube.

Fig. 146—The length of the horizontal tube in fig. 145 is reduced to half. The pressure gradient along the tube is thereby doubled. The outflow is twice that in fig. 145.

Conclusions

(1) The volume flow rate through a straight tube of uniform bore is directly proportional to the pressure gradient within it.

(2) The volume flow rate is directly proportional to the fourth power of the diameter.

These relations are valid only for laminar flow (see p. 168 et seq).

N.B.—The foregoing experiments and results are idealized. In actual fact a pressure loss occurs at the entry to the horizontal tubes from the bottle. Also, the *kinetic* energy* possessed by the liquid emerging from the end of the tube is not taken into account.

* See p. 174.

Influence of Viscosity on Laminar Flow Rate*

Some fluids flow through a given tube more readily than others. The only intrinsic property of the fluid which influences its laminar flow rate is known as its viscosity.

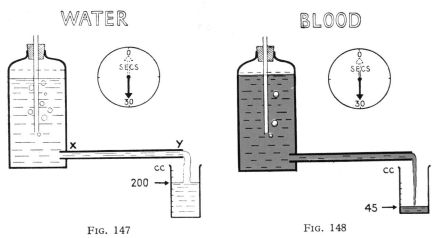

FIG. 147   FIG. 148

The coefficient of viscosity of many fluids, the measure of their rates of flow through a tube under standard conditions, is readily available** from reference books[3]. The rate of flow of a fluid is *inversely* proportional to its coefficient of viscosity.

Fig. 147—The pressure at X remains constant because the pressure in the water at the lower end of the vertical tube remains atmospheric. 200 ml of water at 37 °C flows through the tube XY in half a minute.

Fig. 148—Identical apparatus. Blood is substituted for water. A volume of 45 ml passes through the tube in the same time.

At 37 °C the (absolute) coefficient of viscosity of water = 0·007

,,   ,,   ,,   ,,   ,, blood = 0·028

∴ the flow rate of water through a tube will be $\dfrac{0·028}{0·007}$ or

4 times larger than that of blood[4] under the same conditions. The above drawings illustrate this fact (200/45 ≃ 4/1).

Viscosity has the same effect on the laminar flow rate of a *gas* as it has on that of a liquid. The laminar flow rates of different gases at the same pressure, through the same tube, are inversely proportional to their viscosities. There are considerable differences between the viscosities of the gases used in anaesthetics; their flow rates under the same

* See p. 168.   ** See also tables in Chap. XXIV, rows i, i'.

conditions vary widely. This fact is of considerable importance when measuring one gas with a Rotameter calibrated for another (see p. 205).

Figs. 149 and 150—A cylindrical vessel is filled with oxygen and an

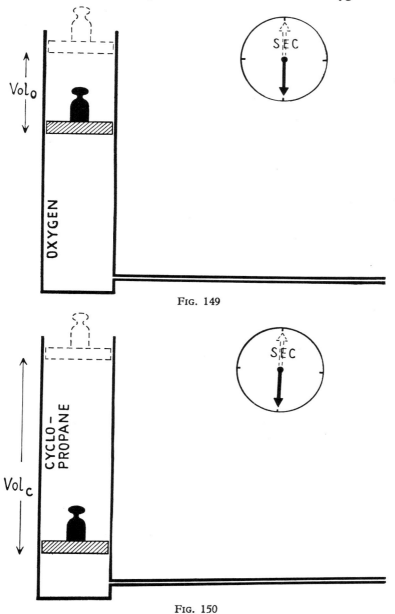

Fig. 149

Fig. 150

identical one with cyclopropane. A weighted piston keeps the gas under a constant positive pressure. Each gas flows out through a long capillary tube into the open air.

At the beginning of the experiment (ghosted clock hand) the two pistons are in the same position (ghosted pistons). The difference between the initial and the final position of each piston is a measure of the volume of gas which has flowed through the capillary tube during the interval shown on the clock. These volumes are indicated by Vol_C and Vol_O.

$$\frac{\text{viscosity of oxygen}}{\text{viscosity of cyclopropane}} = \frac{Vol_C}{Vol_O}$$

In the experiments shown

$$\frac{Vol_C}{Vol_O} = \frac{2 \cdot 3}{1}$$

The viscosity of oxygen is therefore $2 \cdot 3$ times that of cyclopropane. The viscosities of these gases relative to water at $20\ ^\circ C$ are, in fact, $0 \cdot 020$ and $0 \cdot 0087$. The absolute unit of viscosity, which will not be explained in any detail, is the *Poise* (P) named after Poiseuille. In this unit the absolute viscosity coefficient of liquid water at $20\ ^\circ C$ is nearly 10^{-2} Poise, or 1 cP. Any viscosity given relative to that of water ($= 1$) can be therefore changed into absolute viscosity by choosing 10^{-2} P as unit; a liquid with a viscosity coefficient of $0 \cdot 65$ relative to water, has an absolute viscosity of $0 \cdot 65 \times 10^{-2}$ Poise. With the help of the viscosity coefficients for certain gases and liquids listed in chapter XXIV, their flow rates under given conditions may be compared.

The negligible effect of the viscosity of a gas on flow rate through an *orifice* is discussed on p. 192.

It is worth emphasizing that the *density* of a fluid does not play a part in determining the rate of *laminar* flow through a tube. For example, benzene and olive oil have similar densities ($0 \cdot 88$ and $0 \cdot 91$) but strikingly divergent coefficients of viscosity ($0 \cdot 65$ and $84 \cdot 0$ at $20\ ^\circ C$). The flow rate of benzene through a tube is approximately 130 times that of olive oil.

On the other hand, methyl alcohol and chloroform have markedly different densities ($0 \cdot 79$ and $1 \cdot 49$) but similar coefficients of viscosity ($0 \cdot 59$ and $0 \cdot 57$). Their flow rates through a tube are approximately the same.

Similarly helium and air have markedly different densities but similar viscosities. Their laminar flow rates are the same. To the anaesthetist this point is of little interest. When helium is used to make breathing easier in cases of respiratory obstruction, the flow of gas is mainly *turbulent*; also for intermittent flow, the pressure loss due to speeding up the gas during inspiration depends on its density. For the use of helium in clinical practice see p. 195.

The coefficient of viscosity of a liquid *decreases* with rise of temperature. On the other hand the viscosity of a gas *increases* with rise of temperature, but the change is much smaller than for a liquid.

Laminar Flow Laws

The flow rate of a fluid flowing smoothly through a tube is proportional to the following:

(1) the pressure gradient, that is, $\dfrac{\text{total pressure drop}}{\text{length of tube}}$

(2) the fourth power of the diameter of the tube

(3) inversely to the viscosity of the fluid

This can be expressed by the formula:

$$\text{volume flow rate} \propto \frac{\text{total pressure drop}}{\text{length of tube}} \times (\text{diameter})^4 \times \frac{1}{\text{viscosity}}$$

This relationship may be rewritten as:

$$\text{pressure loss} \propto \frac{\text{length of tube}}{(\text{diameter})^4} \times \text{viscosity} \times \text{volume flow rate}$$

This proportional relationship may be expressed as an equation thus:

$$\text{pressure loss} = f \times \text{viscosity} \times \frac{\text{length}}{(\text{diameter})^4} \times \text{flow rate} \qquad (1)$$

These relationships which are true only for *laminar* flow in tubes, are known as the **Hagen-Poiseuille** Law.

The factor (f) depends on the units chosen.

A. In the case of *gases* it may be convenient to express the
flow rate   Q in l/min
pressure loss p in mm H_2O
length   L in cm
internal diameter   D in cm
viscosity in terms relative to that of water ($= 1$)
then $f = 6{\cdot}94 \times 10^{-2}$

AIR has a viscosity coefficient* relative to water of $1{\cdot}8 = 10^{-2}$ at 20 °C.

---

* On p. 423 (column 15, row i) the absolute viscosity coefficient is expressed in units of 10^{-4} P ($= 0{\cdot}01$ cP).

The Hagen-Poiseuille Law becomes then:*

$$p = 6.94 \times 10^{-2} \times 1.8 \times 10^{-2} \times \frac{L}{D^4} \times Q$$

$$= 1.25 \times 10^{-3} \times \frac{L}{D^4} \times Q \tag{2}$$

Example: Air is passing at a rate of 10 l/min through a cylindrical tube, 50 cm long and with an internal diameter of 1 cm. Find the pressure loss along this tube.

$$p = 1.25 \times 10^{-3} \times \frac{50}{1^4} \times 10 = 0.62 \text{ mm H}_2\text{O}$$

B. For *liquids* it may be more convenient to express the

pressure loss	P in cm H_2O
flow rate	q in ml/min
diameter	d in mm

The factor (f) becomes then:
$$f = 6.94 \times 10^{-2}.$$

For WATER at 20 °C the *relative* viscosity is 1 by definition. The equation for the laminar pressure loss becomes then:

$$P = 6.94 \times 10^{-2} \times \frac{L}{d^4} \times q \tag{3}$$

Examples:

What pressures are required to send water at a flow rate of $q = 10$ ml/min through

(*a*) a small transfusion needle, L = 3 cm, d = 1   mm and through

(*b*) a hypodermic needle,   L = 2 cm, d = 0.3 mm

Answers:

(*a*) $P = 6.94 \times 10^{-2} \times \dfrac{3}{1^4} \times 10 = 2.1 \text{ cm H}_2\text{O}$

(*b*) $P = 6.94 \times 10^{-2} \times \dfrac{2}{(0.3)^4} \times 10 = 171 \text{ cm H}_2\text{O}$

$$\text{or } 2.4 \text{ lb/in}^2$$

* Rules for the handling of powers of 10 are given in chapter XXIV on p. 429.

Practical application

Fig. 151—Identical syringes are fitted with needles of different bores. The internal diameters of the needles are in the ratio of 1 to 2. The same force is applied to the pistons. The volume of fluid ejected in unit time is 16 (that is, 2^4) times greater in the case of the larger needle.

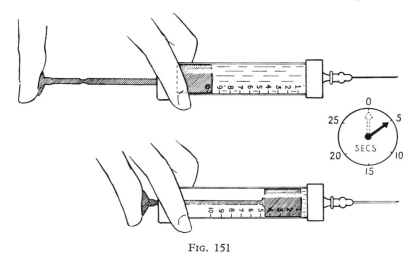

FIG. 151

If the syringes are emptied with the same thumb force, the larger needle enables this to be done in $\frac{1}{16}$ of the time required for the smaller. To empty the syringe with the small needle in the same time as with the large, 16 times as great a force would be necessary.

Moral—If a large volume of intravenous fluid is to be given rapidly, a hypodermic needle is useless (p. 191). Remember, too, that with a standard transfusion set it is more practicable to double the diameter of the needle than to increase the pressure sixteenfold.

REFERENCES

[1] HAGEN, G. (1839). *Ann. Phys., Lpz.* **46**, 423–42.
[2] POISEUILLE, J. L. M. (1840). *C. R. Acad. Sci., Paris*, **11**, 1041–8; cf. p. 1044 ff.
[3] KAYE, G. W. C., and LABY, T. H. (1956). *Tables of physical and chemical constants*, 11th ed. Lond., cf. p. 35–8.
HODGMAN, C. D. (1955). *Handbook of chemistry and physics*, 37th ed. Cleveland, cf. p. 2010–23.
[4] GREEN, H. D. (1950). In Glasser, O.: *Medical Physics*, **2**, 241. Chicago.

CHAPTER XIII

FLOW OF FLUIDS IN ANAESTHETIC APPARATUS

Laminar and Turbulent Flow

WHEN a fluid—liquid or gas, streams through a tube, the particles comprising the fluid may move along lines parallel to the walls of the tube.

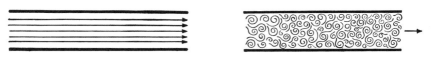

FIG. 152   FIG. 153

The flow, smooth and orderly, is referred to as *laminar* (fig. 152).

If, however, the lines of flow are not parallel to the walls of the tube but are irregular and broken up, the now disorderly flow is called *turbulent* (fig. 153).

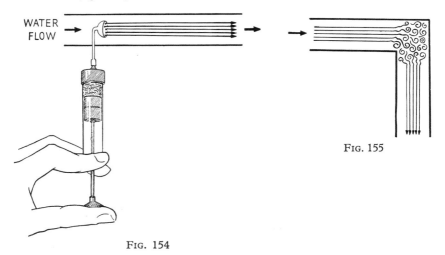

FIG. 155

FIG. 154

Fig. 154—Ink is injected through several fine jets into a stream of water. The ink flows in straight lines, parallel to the walls of the tube, showing that the flow within the tube is laminar.

Fig. 155—The previous experiment in fig. 154 is repeated, but the

168

tube has been cut and the two ends joined together at right angles so that the lumen remains unchanged. The lines of flow are no longer parallel throughout. The irregular flow is known as *local turbulence*. The stream resumes its laminar character some distance beyond the cause of the turbulence. (In an actual experiment the ink, of course, would not separate again into straight lines beyond the bend.)

For a given volume of a fluid to pass through a tube in a given time, a certain pressure difference between the ends of the tube is necessary.

Such a pressure difference is a measure of the **resistance** which has to be overcome when the fluid is forced or drawn through the tube. Whether the flow is laminar or turbulent, resistance of some degree exists.

In the case of laminar flow the pressure drop or resistance is directly proportional to the flow rate (p. 165). Where the flow is rapid enough to be turbulent, however, the resistance/flow rate graph is no longer linear; in certain conditions, such as when the inside of the tube is rough, the pressure loss rises approximately with the square of the flow rate so that the graph is no longer a straight line but approximates a parabolic curve (see also p. 195).

Critical volume flow rate

When the volume flow rate (say in litres per minute) of a given fluid in a given tube exceeds what is known as its 'critical flow rate', laminar flow is replaced by turbulent flow throughout the whole length of the tube. This critical rate of flow varies directly as the internal diameter of the tube; the larger the diameter the greater is the volume of fluid which can be made to flow through it in unit time without *general turbulence* occurring.

Table 3 lists* the *critical* volume flow rates (Q_C) of AIR at room conditions through smooth tubes of various internal diameters (D). If

TABLE 3. MAXIMUM LAMINAR FLOW RATE OF AIR

D (cm)	0·25	0·5	0·75	1·0	1·5	2·0
Q_C (l/min)	3·5	7·1	10·6	14	21	28

the actual flows are higher than these critical values, the laminar flow law is no longer valid. Thus a flow passed at the rate of 10 l/min

* The values in Tables 3 and 4 are only approximate, as the transition from laminar to turbulent flow depends on various factors. The calculations are based on the following relation:

crit. velocity (cm/s) × diam. (cm) × density (g/cm³) = 2000 × viscos. (Poise)　　(1)

through a tube of 0·5 cm diameter would be turbulent, while it would be laminar when passed through a tube of 1 cm diameter.

Table 4 gives a few critical flow rates for WATER passing through tubes of small sizes. The values can be used to assess whether the flow of water through an injection needle or a suction catheter can be laminar. The units for critical flow rate (q_C) and the internal diameter (d) are different from those used in Table 3.

TABLE 4.   MAXIMUM LAMINAR FLOW RATE OF WATER

d (mm)	0·3	0·5	1	2	5
q_C (ml/min)	28	47	94	188	470

In the case of an intravenous needle with 0·5 mm bore, the flow will be laminar unless the flow rate should exceed 47 ml/min.

Taking into account the different units chosen in Tables 3 and 4, it is apparent that the flow of *air* through a given pipe can be 15 times as large as that of *water* before the flow ceases to be laminar; thus D = 0·5 cm corresponds to d = 5 mm, and the respective flowrates Q_C = 7·1 l/min and q_C = 470 ml/min are in the ratio 7·1/0·47 $\simeq$ 15/1.

Apart from the diameter of the tube, the ratio of viscosity to density determines the value of the critical flow rate. In the case of water this ratio is 1. In the case of air the ratio is 0·018/0·0012 = 15; see p. 423 column 15, but express density (row a) in g/ml and viscosity (row i) in 10^{-2} P as units.

The laws determining the transition from laminar to turbulent flow were elucidated* by the work of REYNOLDS.[1, 2] The numerical factor in the equation relating critical velocity to pipe diameter, density and viscosity (footnote on p. 169) is known as the "critical Reynolds' number".

Resistance for laminar and turbulent flow

In anaesthetic practice the volume flow rates of inspired gases are often below that which results in *general* turbulence. However, a few comparisons between the pressure losses in laminar and in turbulent flow through tubes will illustrate the appreciable increases which may occur.

Close to the critical flow rate the pressure loss increases by about 50% if the flow is turbulent instead of laminar.

At flow rates above the critical value laminar flow no longer occurs; for the sake of comparison we shall, however, assume that laminar

* See also biographical note on HAGEN.

flow might be possible and that the corresponding pressure loss could be derived from the Hagen-Poiseuille Law.

At flow rates twice the critical value, the actual pressure loss in smooth pipes is 150% above that which would have been present for laminar flow.

If the volume flow rate is 5 times the critical value, the turbulent resistance is 400% above that for the fictitious laminar flow.

At a flow below the critical rate *local* turbulence may occur as a result of irregularities in the pathway of the gas (see pp. 169 & 175). Constrictions and sharp corners are common offenders.

During inspiration, a negative pressure is produced in the lungs (p. 184). To breathe through even an open ether mask without a reduction in respiratory minute volume, necessitates an increased intrapulmonary negative pressure of some degree. The increase in negative pressure resulting from breathing through any apparatus can be used as a measure to express the resistance of the apparatus. In order to compare the resistance of various apparatus, a continuous flow rate can be substituted for normal intermittent respiration (p. 178).

Resistance is always harmful, but a slight degree can be endured for a short time by extra effort on the part of a fit patient. An ill patient, however, may be unable to make the extra effort and his lungs will neither fill nor empty to the same extent as before the resistance was interposed.

The resistance of breathing apparatus is composed of laminar and turbulent components. Where the flow is laminar, the resistance is mainly dependent on the diameter of the tube, rising sharply as the diameter becomes smaller. The resistance due to local turbulence arises in the region of constrictions and sharp bends. Breathing tubes and connections should therefore have wide bores and be shaped to avoid local turbulence.

Velocity distribution

1. In **laminar** flow through a tube, the linear velocity at the centre (v_o) is highest, and falls to zero near the wall. The relation:

$$Q = v \times \text{area} \quad . \quad . \quad . \quad . \quad (2)$$

links the volume flowrate (Q) with the *average* linear velocity (v), which is smaller than the velocity (v_o) on the axis. It can be shown that:

$$v_o = 2 \times v \quad . \quad . \quad . \quad . \quad (3)$$

2. In **turbulent** flow the linear velocities change only little across the bore of the tube so that: $v_o \simeq v$.

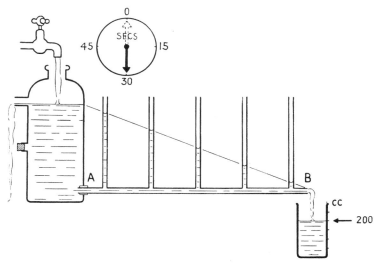

FIG. 156

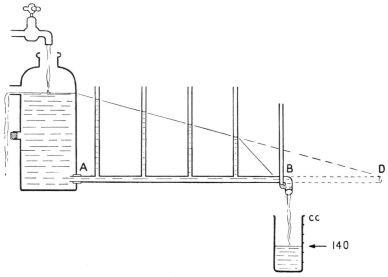

FIG. 157

Fig. 156—This is the same as fig. 143.

Fig. 157—The experiment in the previous figure is repeated, but the distal end of the flow tube is bent sharply in the horizontal plane. The abrupt pressure drop seen in the last vertical tube shows the loss of energy due to increased friction consequent on the local turbulence induced in the region of the bend.

The loss is reflected by a reduction from 200 ml to 140 ml in the volume of fluid passing through the tube in unit time.

The resistance of the bend is the same as that which would be caused by the addition of a length of straight tubing BD to the original tube AB. The end of the hypothetical tube BD is found by continuing both the flow tube, proximal to the bend, and the upper sloping line showing the pressure drop within it.

The flow rate through the bent tube AB in fig. 157 is the same as the flow would be through the straight tube AB in fig. 156, with the addition of a fictitious straight tube BD. If BD is half the length of AB, the flow rate through the bent tube in fig. 157 is $\frac{2}{3}$ that through the straight tube of the same length in fig. 156.

Pressure loss due to abrupt change in bore of tube

If the length of tube on each side of an area of local turbulence is short, there is so little laminar flow that the laws relating the size of tube, pressure loss and flow rate are altered completely.

Whenever a fluid enters a tube from a larger reservoir or another larger tube, there is an additional pressure loss which is determined by the density of the fluid, whether the flow in the tube is turbulent or laminar.

Let us consider suction applied to one end of a tube, the other end of which opens to the atmosphere. While the outer air is at rest, the air inside the tube is in motion. Energy must have been spent in speeding up the air from rest to the final velocity. The kinetic energy of this moving air is the pressure loss referred to above.

There is also a pressure loss when fluid flows from a narrow into a wide tube. If the flow passes from a tube into a large tank the kinetic energy is completely lost by friction.

If the linear velocity (v) of all the fluid particles in a tube is the same, the kinetic energy is represented by

$$H = \tfrac{1}{2} \times \text{density} \times v^2 \qquad . \qquad . \qquad . \quad (4)$$

For AIR this can be written as follows:

$$H = 2 \cdot 77 \times 10^{-3} \times \left[\frac{Q \ (l/min)}{D^2 \ (cm)} \right]^2 \ mm \ H_2O \ . \qquad . \qquad . \quad (5)$$

The expression inside the square bracket is proportional to the linear flow velocity.

The short Table 5 derived from this formula may be useful in estimating the magnitude of the kinetic energy. The actual pressure

TABLE 5

Q (l/min):	10	20	30	60
D (cm)		*H* (mm H₂O)		
0·5	4·4	17	40	160
0·75	0·9	3·5	7·8	31
1·0	0·3	1·1	2·5	10

loss is usually not equal to H; it can be obtained by multiplying H with a numerical factor of the order of 1. The latter depends on the character of the flow in the tube and on the change in diameter of the tube.

Example: Air flows from a pipe of internal bore $= 0 \cdot 75$ cm into the atmosphere. At a volume flow rate $Q = 30$ l/min the kinetic energy loss will be approximately $H = 8$ mm H_2O, if the velocity were the same at every point of the bore. In laminar flow the velocity is highest at the axis, and it can be shown that H must be multiplied by 2 to obtain the kinetic energy.

For WATER the kinetic energy is greater in the ratio of the densities of water and air. Using different units: $H(cm \ H_2O)$, $q(ml/min)$ and $d(mm)$, the kinetic energy expression for water becomes:

$$H = 2 \cdot 35 \times 10^{-3} \times \left[\frac{q \ (ml/min)}{d^2 \ (mm)} \right]^2 \ cm \ H_2O \ . \qquad . \qquad . \quad (6)$$

Example: For $d = 0 \cdot 9$ mm, $q = 70$ (ml/min) the equation yields $H = 17 \cdot 5$ cm H_2O. If water flows through a transfusion needle of $0 \cdot 9$ mm bore, the kinetic energy is equivalent to a pressure of $17 \cdot 5$ cm H_2O if the velocity were constant throughout the cross-section. If the velocity distribution is laminar, the kinetic energy would be $2 \times 17 \cdot 5 = 35$ cm H_2O. This is also the pressure *loss* when the water escapes from the needle into a wide tube or vessel. This example shows that *in addition* to the pressure necessary to overcome the laminar flow resistance of the needle, a pressure of about 35 cm H_2O must be applied at the entrance to the needle to produce the flow rate of 70 ml/min.

Pressure represents potential energy of a fluid. Any decrease indicates that some of this energy has been used. There is a fall in pressure along a uniform tube in which a fluid flows, whether the flow be laminar or turbulent, although the loss is greater in the case of the latter. In both types of flow energy is dissipated as heat in overcoming the friction between the fluid particles. During turbulence the onward flow is repeatedly interrupted by the jostling about of the fluid particles; much more kinetic energy is lost as heat and the fall in pressure is correspondingly great.

Where the flow is mainly turbulent the flow rate of a fluid is influenced much more by its density than by its viscosity.

Applications in Anaesthetic Practice

Irregularities of the inner wall of a tube, and sudden alterations in the bore of tubes and connections, particularly constrictions, are

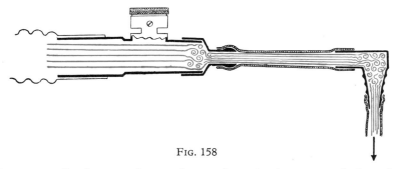

FIG. 158

frequent offenders causing a change from laminar to turbulent flow and kinetic energy losses (fig. 158).

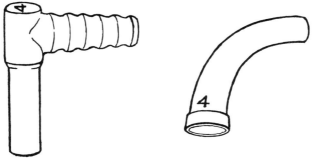

FIG. 159

Fig. 159—The curved endotracheal connection affords a smoother flow of gas and therefore offers less resistance than does one bent sharply at a right-angle.

To reduce the effort of breathing, endotracheal and other breathing tubes should be as short as possible, have a wide bore, smooth walls,

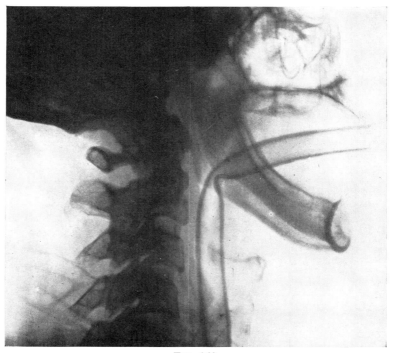

FIG. 160

gradual bends and no constrictions. Neglect of these factors increases the resistance to the passage of gases and with it the effort of breathing. Further adverse effects are discussed on p. 267.

Fig. 160—An X-ray of a patient's head. The endotracheal tube through the mouth is kinked in the pharynx causing respiratory obstruction. The risk of kinking can be avoided by the use of suitably designed tubes.[3]

Resistance

The resistance of a piece of apparatus to the flow of gases is the pressure difference, under given conditions, between the entry and exit ports of the apparatus. This resistance varies with the volume of gases flowing through it in unit time, and this flow rate must therefore be stated when resistance is described.

In the laboratory, when measuring the resistance of a piece of apparatus to breathing, a continuous stream of gas may be used (though inadequately) to take the place of the intermittent breathing of a patient. The volume flow rate of the continuous stream, however, must approximate the maximum flow rate of the air stream during normal inspiration or expiration. In an adult breathing quietly at 8 litres per minute, the maximum flow rate reaches 25 litres per minute. In a patient breathing deeply the flow rate may reach a peak of 60 litres per minute.[4]

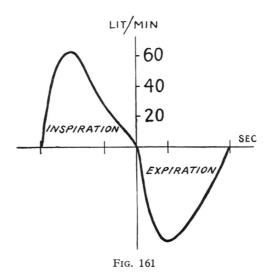

FIG. 161

Fig. 161—Rate of flow of gases during the respiratory cycle. Subject breathing deeply.

In a conscious person extremely deep breathing may cause brief periods of gas flow up to some 400 l/min.

When measuring resistance in the laboratory with a continuous flow of gas, a series of experiments is performed using a range of flow rates; the measured pressure differences are plotted against the respective flow rates (e.g. fig. 166). Such a graph enables the resistance of the apparatus to be deduced for any particular flow rate.

The following experiments illustrate the resistance to respiration due

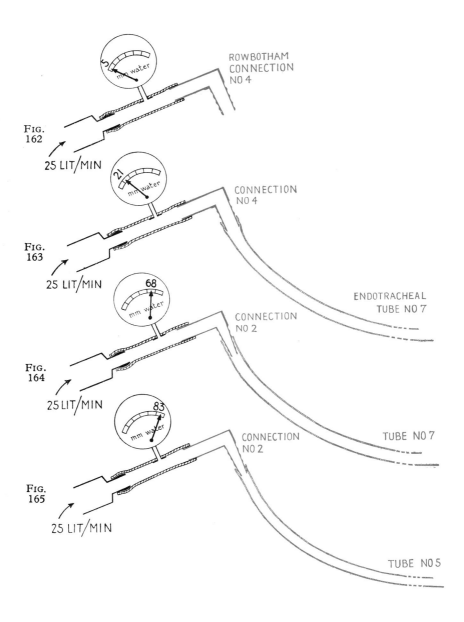

ROWBOTHAM
CONNECTION
NO 4

Fig.
162

25 LIT/MIN

CONNECTION
NO 4

Fig.
163

25 LIT/MIN

ENDOTRACHEAL
TUBE NO 7

CONNECTION
NO 2

Fig.
164

25 LIT/MIN

TUBE NO 7

CONNECTION
NO 2

Fig.
165

25 LIT/MIN

TUBE NO 5

to endotracheal connections and tubes, some of them obviously much too small for an adult. A continuous flow of 25 litres of gases per minute takes the place of adult respiration.

Rowbotham's connection No. 4

Fig. 162—A manometer, calibrated in mm H_2O, indicates the pressure at the proximal end of the Rowbotham's connection. The pressure here is above that at the distal end (that is, above atmospheric). The pressure difference, the resistance of the connection, is 5 mm H_2O.

Rowbotham's connection No. 4 and Magill's endotracheal tube No. 7

Fig. 163—The resistance of the connection and tube is 21 mm H_2O.

Rowbotham's connection No. 2 and Magill's endotracheal tube No. 7

Fig. 164—The endotracheal tube is the same as that in fig. 163. The connection is size No. 2. The resistance is 68 mm H_2O. The great increase is due to the substitution of a No. 2 connection for a No. 4.

Rowbotham connections are supplied in four sizes. They differ in the diameter of the distal end which is inserted into the endotracheal tube. The proximal end is the same for all sizes. The anaesthetist who is handed an endotracheal tube with a connection already affixed should remove the connection and inspect it to avoid the error of using one unnecessarily small.

Rowbotham's connection No. 2 and Magill's endotracheal tube No. 5

Fig. 165—When in addition to a small connection (No. 2) a small tube (No. 5) is used the resistance reaches the very high figure of 83 mm H_2O.

The experiments illustrated in figs. 162-165 are intended to give the reader only a qualitative impression of the relation between resistance and the size of tube and connector.

The combined resistance of two pieces of apparatus is not necessarily the sum of the resistances of each one measured separately. The nature of the junction between them has a great influence on the combined resistance.

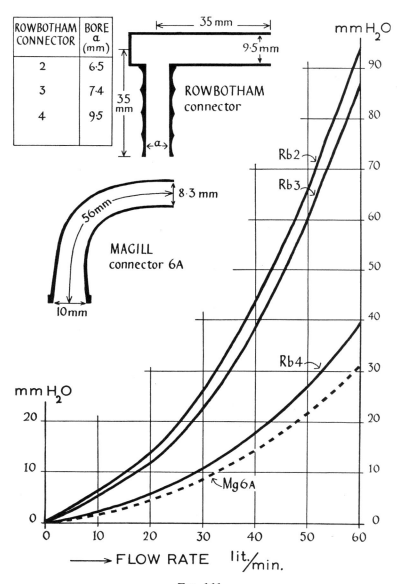

ROWBOTHAM CONNECTOR	BORE a (mm)
2	6·5
3	7·4
4	9·5

35 mm

9·5 mm

ROWBOTHAM connector

35 mm

←a→

8·3 mm

56 mm

MAGILL connector 6A

10 mm

mm H₂O

Rb 2

Rb 3

Rb 4

Mg 6A

mm H₂O

FLOW RATE   lit./min.

FIG. 166

Resistance characteristics of endotracheal connectors

Both figs. 166 and 167 show the importance of specifying the flow rate when discussing the resistance of endotracheal equipment.

Fig. 166—resistance of several endotracheal connectors as a function of the flow rate. The three curves marked 'Rb' refer to the Rowbotham connectors; their sizes are entered on the inset table.

The following features will be obvious from a study of the graphs:

(a) The resistance does not rise linearly with increasing flow rate; the resistance line curves steeply upwards. This is to be expected from ducts which are so different from an 'ideal' tube (p. 192).

(b) There is a very great rise in resistance when using a No. 3 Rowbotham connector instead of a No. 4. The increase is approximately 100%; e.g. for $Q = 40$ l/min the resistances are 38 and 17 mmH$_2$O respectively.

(c) When changing from a large size Rowbotham connector to a smoothly bent Magill connector of corresponding size, the decrease in resistance is rather insignificant at medium flow rates. At higher flow rates (60 l/min) the decrease is about 20% and may be of some importance for patients breathing deeply.

In the resistance measurements of figs. 162–165 the gauge was shown attached laterally to the supply tubing leading to the connector and endotracheal tube under investigation. Although the resistance of the supply tubing can be neglected, the lateral pressure will be influenced by the bore of the tubing: if it is made smaller, linear velocity and kinetic energy rise while the pressure (potential energy) decreases, and vice versa. Yet the volume flow rate and the resistance of the anaesthetic device have obviously remained unchanged. For that reason the experimental arrangement illustrated on figs. 162–165 is of very limited value and does not readily supply the resistance values of endotracheal equipment.

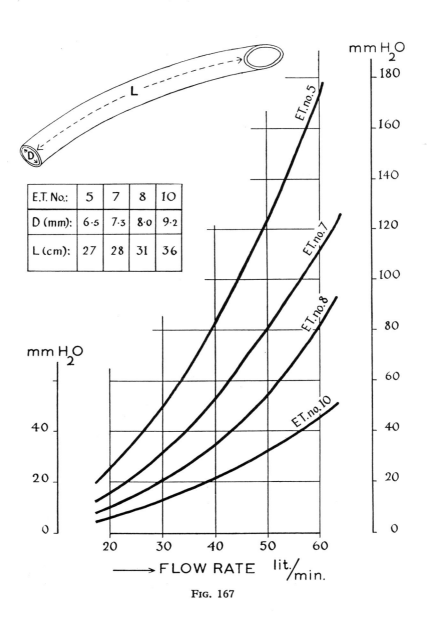

E.T. No.:	5	7	8	10
D (mm):	6·5	7·3	8·0	9·2
L (cm):	27	28	31	36

Fig. 167

In order to standardize the resistance measurement of anaesthetic devices the following procedure[5] is preferred:

One end of the device, e.g. endotracheal tube, is inserted into a large container, the other end is open to the atmosphere. A known flow rate of air is admitted to the container at another point and escapes through the anaesthetic device.

The pressure gauge is connected at a third point to a hole in the wall of the container. Owing to the large size of the container the *linear* gas velocity in it is quite small, and the kinetic effects mentioned on p. 181 are *negligible*.

The measurements illustrated in figs. 166 and 167 were carried out with this kind of apparatus.

Resistance characteristics of endotracheal tubes

Fig. 167—shows the resistance of several endotracheal tubes (Magill-type) for flow rates between 20 and 60 l/min.

(*a*) The resistance-flow rate graph is not a straight line. The resistance curve rises more steeply than linear with increasing flow rate. The reason for this is that most of the flow rates are above the 'critical' values (see p. 169) so that the flow through the tubes can no longer be laminar.

(*b*) A considerable increase in resistance results from changing an endotracheal tube to the next smaller size. In the case of the No. 7 and No. 8 tubes the difference in resistance is about 30%.

A comparison of fig. 166 and fig. 167 shows that in the case of large size endotracheal tubes, the tube resistance is of a magnitude similar to that of the metal connectors which fit them. In the case of small tubes, the tube resistance is considerably greater than that of the appropriate connector.

In using these quantitative results it has to be kept in mind that the individual resistances of an endotracheal tube and an appropriate connector are not additive. The overall resistance of a tube combined with connector is usually smaller than the sum of the individual resistances (see also p. 179).

It can also be shown that halving the length of a tube reduces its resistance by less than 50% (e.g. the decrease may be only 40%). This follows from the fact that the total resistance is the sum of viscosity and kinetic losses; the former are proportional to the length but the latter are independent of it.

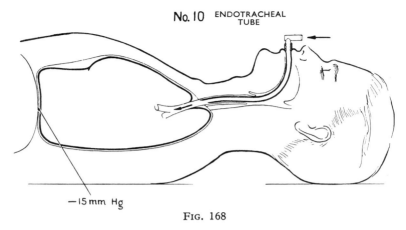

FIG. 168

Fig. 168—An adult breathes through a No. 10 endotracheal tube and the largest Rowbotham connection (No. 4). The peak intrapleural negative pressure developed during normal inspiration is estimated at — 15 mmHg .

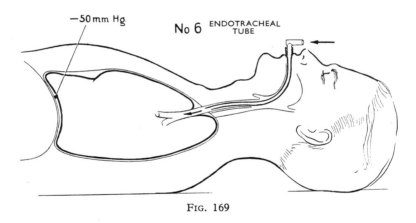

FIG. 169

Fig. 169—A No. 6 endotracheal tube is substituted. At the height of the inspiratory effort the negative intrapleural pressure may become as low as — 50 mmHg . A much greater effort on the part of the patient must be made to inspire the same volume of air in the same time through the smaller tube. In fact, the lag between the intrapleural pressure and the intrapulmonary pressure may be so great that the lungs are not filled by the inspiratory effort.

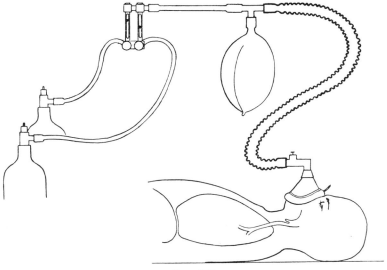

FIG. 170

Fig. 170—An anaesthetic is being administered from a continuous flow apparatus. The gases in the tube leading from the reservoir bag to the facemask travel to the patient mainly by the effort of inspiration. This tube can be regarded as an extension of the patient's respiratory

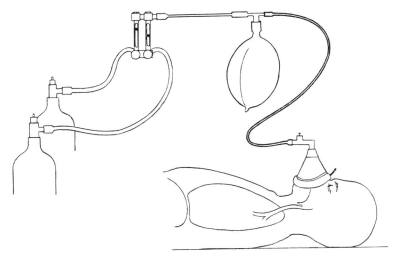

FIG. 171

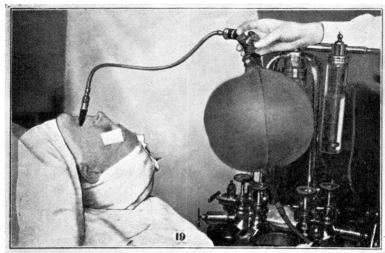

Fig. 19.—Intratracheal tube connected with the ether-vapor or gas apparatus.

FIG. 172

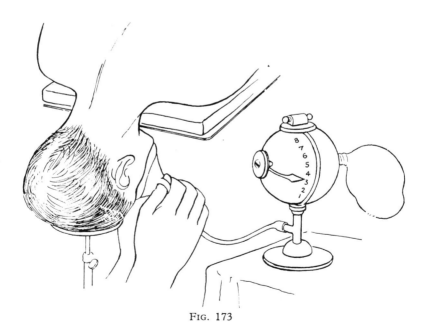

FIG. 173

tract. The diameter must be such that it causes little or no resistance to breathing. Provided the diameter is adequate, any slight difference in the lengths of the corrugated breathing tubes used in anaesthetic practice is of quite secondary importance.

Fig. 171—Should the tube between the reservoir bag and the patient be of small bore, a state of affairs is created even worse than that in fig. 169. The increased resistance to breathing means increased effort on the part of the patient, and, more important still, a great lag between intrapulmonary and atmospheric pressures with its grave potentialities (p. 268).

We ourselves have seen unconscious patients made to breathe through tubes offering a gross resistance to respiration. On the opposite page two illustrations are shown from anaesthetic literature of the thing we have in mind.

Fig. 172—From an otherwise excellent article in a 1938 anaesthetic journal.[6]

A narrow bore tube of considerable length connects reservoir bag to endotracheal tube. The expiratory valve lies between the anaesthetist's fingers. Another photograph in the same article shows that a cuff surrounds the endotracheal tube to make an airtight junction with the trachea.

The reader is advised to attempt to breathe for some time through a tube such as the one in the illustration; he will then never inflict the physiological insult on his unconscious patient.

Fig. 173—From a 1934 surgical textbook illustrating Continental procedure.

The patient is prone. An Ombrédanne's inhaler is being used. Comment on the bore of the breathing tube is superfluous.

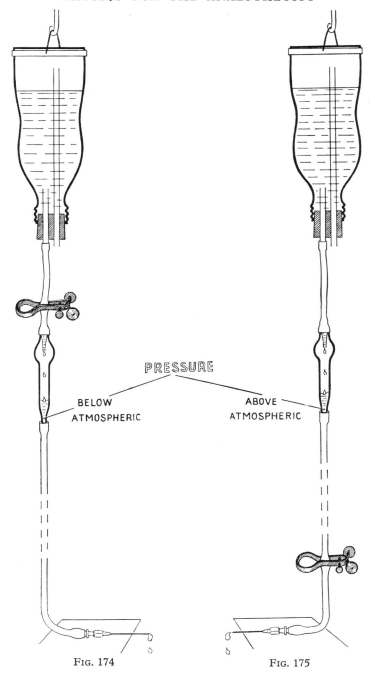

PRESSURE

BELOW
ATMOSPHERIC

ABOVE
ATMOSPHERIC

FIG. 174

FIG. 175

Intravenous Infusion

Air Embolism due to wrong position of clamp

Fig. 174—An intravenous transfusion apparatus of simple pattern is in use. The clamp controlling the flow of liquid is placed high above the level of the needle.

If the drip control clamp is closed, the weight of the liquid column in

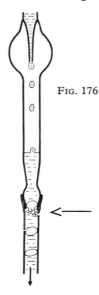

FIG. 176

the tubing below the dripper, plus the air pressure in the drip chamber, is balanced by the atmospheric pressure acting on the open end of the needle. Obviously, the pressure in the tube just below the dripper is less than atmospheric.

Fig. 176—Should there be a small hole in the tubing, as in this illustration, air will enter. When the drip control clamp is opened the small bubbles of air coalesce and are carried down with the movement of the transfusion liquid towards the needle. Fatal cases of aeroembolism from this cause have been reported.[7]

Fig. 175—The drip-control clamp here is correctly placed—almost on a level with the needle. The air in the bottle communicates with the atmosphere. The pressure at any point in the rubber tube above the clamp is equal to the atmospheric pressure plus the pressure due to the column of liquid above that point. The pressure above the clamp,

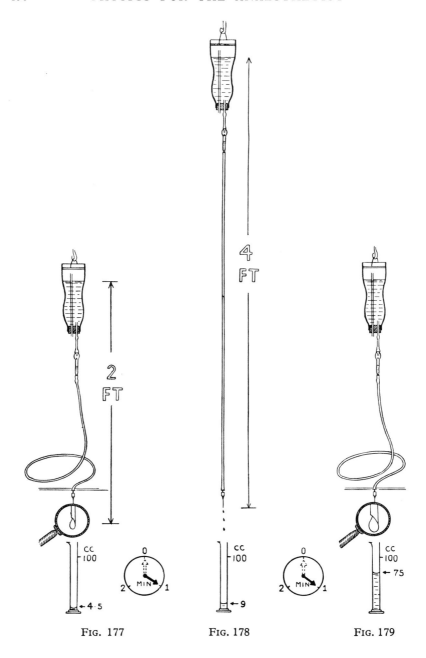

FIG. 177   FIG. 178   FIG. 179

therefore, is greater than atmospheric. Should the rubber tubing above the clamp have a hole in it, air will not be sucked in, but fluid will be forced out.

Flow rates obtainable with gravity feed

Fig. 177—A simple transfusion bottle and tubing have been set up. The level of the liquid in the bottle is 2 feet above the needle, which has an internal diameter of 0·36 mm and is 3 cm in length. In one minute 4·5 ml of liquid pass through the needle.

Fig. 178—By raising the bottle to 4 feet, the original flow of liquid is approximately doubled. The flow through the needle is directly proportional to the pressure difference.

Fig. 179—The bottle is lowered to its original height (2 feet) and a larger needle, internal diameter = 0·93 mm, substituted; its length is again 3 cm. The flow is about 17 times greater than in fig. 177.

Moral.—If a rapid flow of liquid is likely to be needed during a transfusion, use a large bore needle in preference to relying on increase of pressure.

Comparing the volume flow rates in figs. 177 and 179 it is seen that a $2\frac{1}{2}$-fold increase in bore of the needle results in a 17-fold increase in flow rate. If the pressure energy at the entrance to the needles (2 ft or 61 cm H_2O) had only to overcome the viscous resistance in laminar flow, a $(2\cdot58)^4 = 45$-fold increase would have occurred. However, the available pressure is also consumed in generating the kinetic energy which is proportional to the square of the linear flow-velocities (v) in the needles. Calculation shows that the kinetic pressure component in the large needle is 6 times greater than in the smaller one. More than 50% of the pressure at the entrance is used for kinetic energy in the large needle, while in the small needle practically the whole 2 ft H_2O pressure is available to overcome the viscous flow resistance. When checking these findings with (Eq. 3, p. 166) and (Eq. 6, p. 174), the kinetic energy obtained from the latter equation must be doubled in view of the non-uniform velocity distribution in laminar flow (p. 171).

REFERENCES

[1] REYNOLDS, O. (1883). *Phil. Trans.*, **174**, 935–82.
[2] —— Papers on mechanical and physical subjects (1901), **2**, 51–105. Cambr.
[3] ALSOP, A. F. (1955). *Anaesthesia*, **10**, 401–2.
[4] FLEISCH, A. (1925). *Pflueg. Arch. ges. Physiol.*, **209**, 713–22.
[5] GAENSLER, E. A., MALONEY, J. V., BJORK, V. O. (1952). *J. Lab. Clin. Med.*, **39**, 935–53; cf. fig. 1.
[6] THOMAS, G. J. (1938). *Curr. Res. Anesth.*, **17**, 301–11; cf. p. 308.
[7] SIMPSON, K. (1942). *Lancet*, i, 697–8.

CHAPTER XIV

FLOW OF FLUIDS THROUGH ORIFICES

Fig. 180—The term 'tube' is applied to a fluid pathway of which the length is many times greater than the diameter.

Fig. 181—In an 'orifice', on the contrary, the diameter of the fluid pathway exceeds the length. The greater the diameter compared to the

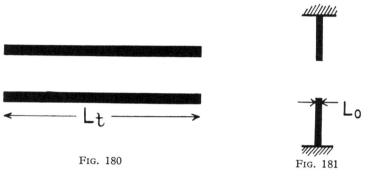

FIG. 180   FIG. 181

length the more does the opening approach the 'ideal' orifice. The flow rate of a fluid through an orifice depends on (i) the diameter, and thus on the cross-section area of the orifice, and (ii) the difference in pressures on either side of the orifice.

The flow of fluid through an orifice is always partly turbulent, and since the particles are jostled about there is inevitably a considerable loss of energy and therefore of pressure. As soon as a flow becomes turbulent the density of the fluid, rather than its viscosity, plays the important part in determining its volume flow rate. The lighter the fluid (that is, the less its density) the greater will be its volume flow rate for any given pressure difference on either side of the orifice.*

The figures on the opposite page illustrate the relative influence of density and viscosity on the rate of flow of a gas through an orifice. The densities of cyclopropane and oxygen are similar (42 : 32); their viscosities very dissimilar (8·7 : 20). The similarity in volume flow rates of the two gases through similar orifices under the same conditions indicates that the effect of viscosity is negligible.

The viscosities of oxygen and helium are similar, the ratio being 20 : 19. Their densities are very different, 32 : 4.

* This bulk flow through an orifice should not be confused with molecular diffusion through pores (see p. 251).

Experiment shows that nearly three times more helium than oxygen flows through the orifice in the same time. The ratio of flow rates derived from a simplified theory of the process is:

$$\frac{\sqrt[2]{32}}{\sqrt[2]{4}} = 2 \cdot 8$$

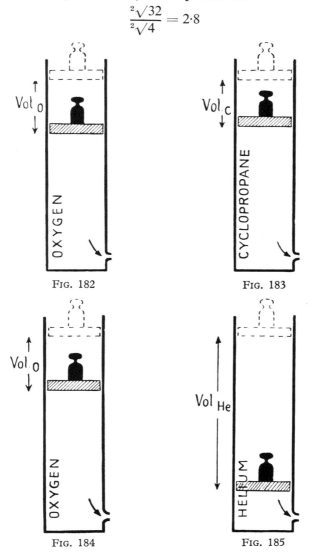

FIG. 182   FIG. 183

FIG. 184   FIG. 185

Compare these experiments with figs. 149 & 150 (p. 163) which show that viscosity plays the paramount role in determining the laminar flow rate through a 'tube'.

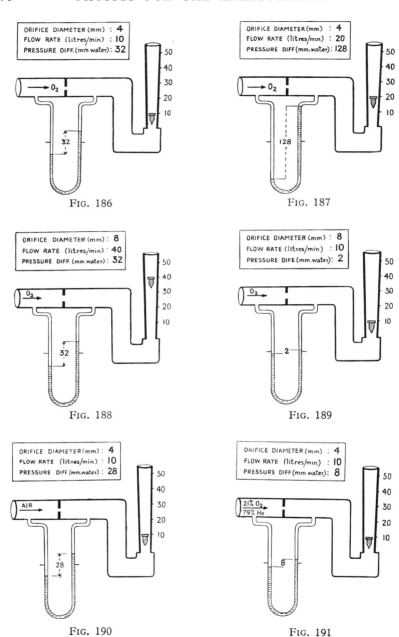

FIG. 186

FIG. 187

FIG. 188

FIG. 189

FIG. 190

FIG. 191

In the figures opposite, a series of idealized experiments demonstrate the relationship* between the diameter of an *orifice*, the flow rate of gas through it and the pressure difference on the two sides of the orifice.

Fig. 186—Initial experiment. With an orifice of 4 mm diameter, and a pressure difference of 32 mm H_2O on either side of it, oxygen flows through the orifice at the rate of 10 litres per minute.

Fig. 187—The pressure difference is now four times that of the initial experiment. The flow rate of oxygen is doubled.

CONCLUSION

The flow rate is proportional to the square root of the pressure difference.

Fig. 188—The diameter of the orifice is now double that in the initial experiment (fig. 186). With the same pressure difference (32 mm H_2O) the flow rate is four times that in fig. 186.

CONCLUSION

With a given pressure difference *the flow rate of the gas is proportional to the square of the diameter of the orifice*, or in other words is proportional to the area of the orifice.

Fig. 189—The flow rate is now reduced to 10 litres per minute, that is, to a quarter of that in fig. 188. The pressure difference is reduced to $\frac{1}{16}$. This experiment confirms the conclusion reached in experiment of fig. 187.

In the next two experiments the influence of the **density** of the gas on the flow rate is shown.

Fig. 190—Air flows through an orifice of 4 mm diameter. A difference of pressure of 28 mm H_2O on either side of the orifice is necessary for air to flow at 10 litres per minute.

Fig. 191—If a mixture of 21% oxygen, 79% helium, is substituted for air, the pressure difference necessary for the same rate of flow is now reduced to 8 mm H_2O, approximately $\frac{1}{3}$ of that required for air.

The density of a mixture of 21% oxygen and 79% nitrogen (that is, air) is 1·20 g/l. By substituting helium for nitrogen the density of the mixture is reduced to 0·41. Use is made of this fact in clinical practice. Patients who suffer from respiratory obstruction, due to such causes as growths in the larynx, scarring of the trachea or asthma, can breathe a helium/oxygen mixture with considerably less effort than air. Such a mixture may tide the patient over a stage of acute respiratory distress.

* The pressure loss caused by an orifice in a wide pipe (or in the wall of a tank) can be derived approximately from the kinetic energy expression (for air, Eq. 5, p. 174) by taking D = orifice diameter × 0·8. The factor (0·8) allows for the contraction of the stream immediately beyond the orifice before it spreads to fill the bore of the large pipe.

CHAPTER XV

FLOWMETERS

THE interdependence of flow rate, size of orifice and pressure difference on either side of an orifice or constriction is made use of in the design of the two main types of anaesthetic flowmeters. In the dry or bobbin type the pressure difference on either side of the orifice is constant and supports the weight of a bobbin. Here the size of the orifice varies for different flows. In the water depression or pressure gauge meter the size of the orifice is constant, and varying rates of flow are indicated by differences of pressure developed on either side of the orifice.

All the anaesthetic flowmeters in common use have either (a) a constant pressure difference across an orifice or annular space, the area of which varies with the flow rate of the gas, or (b) a fixed constriction with a pressure difference on either side of it which varies with the flow rate of the gas.

Variable Orifice Meters

Coxeter bobbin meter

Fig. 192—This unit consists of a glass case which encloses three flowmeters to measure the rates of flow of oxygen, carbon dioxide and nitrous oxide.

Each meter consists of a vertical glass tube of uniform bore, with a series of small holes drilled in it throughout its length. A light bobbin fits the tube closely, and as the gas enters at the lower end of the tube the bobbin is forced upwards. The bobbin rises to a certain height. At this point a number of holes have become available for the escape of gas from the interior of the tube into the outer glass cylinder on its way to the patient. The initial pressure to which the bobbin is exposed is reduced by the escape of gas through the holes to an amount just sufficient to support the weight of the bobbin. When the needle valve controlling the flow of gas to the meter is opened further, the pressure to which the bobbin is exposed increases. The bobbin rises further, permitting the gas to escape through more holes. The bobbin again comes to rest when the pressure underneath it is just sufficient to counteract its weight. The rate of flow of gas is indicated by the height to which the bobbin is raised, and can be read from the figure on the meter tube which corresponds to the top of the bobbin. Each flowmeter tube is calibrated individually for the particular gas with which it is to be used.

Very similar flowmeters were already described by JOSLIN[1] in 1879.

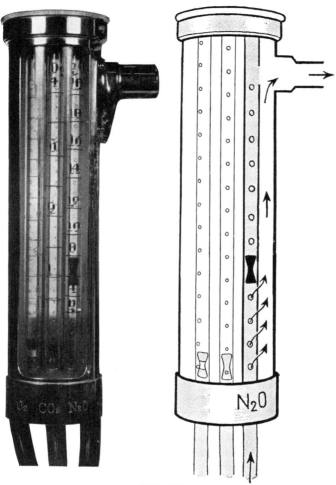

FIG. 192

The Coxeter meter is relatively inaccurate. The movement of the bobbin is impeded by friction between it and the wall of the tube, and dirt may obstruct the small exit holes, not easily cleaned. Since the bobbin moves only in steps from hole to hole the measurement of small gas flows is difficult.

The Rotameter

These meters consist of a glass tube inside which a *rotating* bobbin is free to move. The bore of the tube gradually increases from below upwards. The bobbin floats up and down the tube, allowing gas to flow around it. The higher the bobbin the wider the annular space between bobbin and tube (equivalent to a larger orifice) and the greater the gas flow through it.

Fig. 193—A bobbin is forced up the calibrated glass tube by a stream of gas in which it rotates freely without touching the walls. The internal diameter of the tube is greater at the upper end than at the lower.

Working principle

Fig. 194—Gas flows through a central opening in a horizontal tube at the rate of, say, 3 litres per minute. The constriction in this case is shaped so that an axial section through its wall resembles the section of a rotameter bobbin. The resistance offered to a flow of 3 l/min is shown on the manometer by a pressure difference of 9 mm H_2O.

Fig. 195—The opening through which the gas flows is now the annular space between an object fixed in the centre of the tube and the wall. This object is the familiar rotameter bobbin. The cross-section area of the annular space around the bobbin is the same as the cross-section area of the central opening in fig. 194. The pressure difference is again 9 mm H_2O for the same flow rate, 3 litres per minute.

Fig. 196—The tube, here placed vertically, is very similar to the previous one. The difference is that the bore increases in diameter from below upwards. The tube is, in fact, a rotameter tube. The bobbin is free to move and its weight is such that it is just counteracted by the force due to the pressure difference of 9 mm H_2O across it.

Fig. 197—A flow rate of 8 litres per minute now passes through the tube. The bobbin is forced up the conical tube by the increased flow of gas until the annular space is large enough to give rise to a pressure difference of 9 mm H_2O.

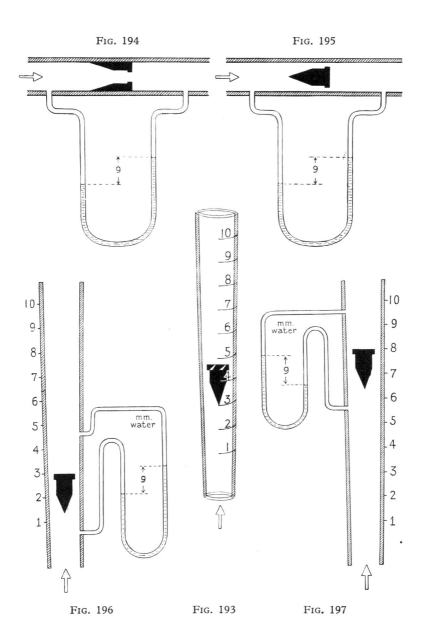

FIG. 194   FIG. 195

FIG. 196   FIG. 193   FIG. 197

History

The principle of the Rotameter was described by Kueppers in 1908. Fig. 198—is a simplified diagram of the meter. The following extract from the original patent[2] shows how little the main features have altered throughout the years.

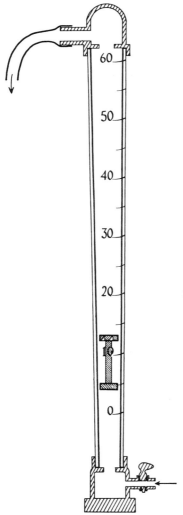

'An instantaneous flow indicator, or gas measurer, is described . . . it comprises a conical pipe . . . the float consisting of circular discs connected by a stem. In the upper disc inclined slits are provided . . . and the float is given a quick rotation . . . sticking is made impossible.'

'This flow indicator has an increasing effective cross sectional area from one end to the other.'

Shortly afterwards[3] the float was altered to its present shape.

Already in 1910 Rotameters were used in anaesthetic apparatus for measuring flow rates of N_2O and O_2; a detailed account of the early history of the Rotameter has been given by Foregger.[4]

Since then they have been used in industry on a wide scale. For many reasons, chief amongst which was the size of these meters, the industrial instruments did not arouse much interest amongst anaesthetists.

It was not until 1937, however, that, at the suggestion of R. H. Salt[5] they were modified to the now familiar form and incorporated into anaesthetic apparatus.

FIG. 198

Practical design

The gas to be measured passes upwards through a specially drawn glass tube, the axis of which must be vertical. The bore of the tube is in the form of an elongated cone with its widest diameter uppermost.

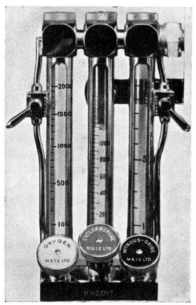

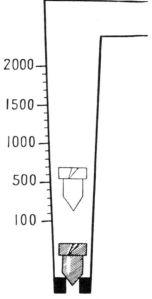

FIG. 199   FIG. 200

FIG. 199. Unit of three meters to measure rate of flow of oxygen, cyclopropane, and nitrous oxide. The oxygen and nitrous oxide meters have by-pass tubes in case large flows of these gases are needed. The provision of the former is wise since oxygen may be needed in an emergency. In the case of the nitrous oxide meter illustrated provision is already made to measure up to 10 litres per minute, and it is highly improbable that a flow in excess of this will ever be needed.

FIG. 200. The reading is taken from the top of the bobbin. The position of the 'ghosted' bobbin on the oxygen meter is that for a rate of flow of 700 cm³/min. Each meter is calibrated for a particular gas. The effect of passing through a meter a gas different from the one for which it is calibrated is discussed on p. 205.

The bobbin, usually made of aluminium, has an upper rim or head which is of a diameter slightly greater than that of the body, and in which specially shaped channels are cut. The stream of gas entering the rotameter tube at the lower end impinges on the bobbin and causes it to rise. As the gas passes between the rim and the wall of the tube the bobbin is set spinning about its vertical axis, because the rim with its channels acts like a set of vanes. The result is that the bobbin rides on a cushion of gas, and errors due to friction between the walls of the tube and the bobbin are eliminated.

Moreover, the pressure loss due to the presence of the bobbin is constant for all positions in the tube; the main loss is only determined by the weight of the bobbin. The more the control valve is opened the higher is the bobbin forced, and the greater is the area of escape for the gas between the bobbin and the meter tube.

If the tube is mounted in the truly vertical position these meters are capable of readings of an accuracy of $\pm 2\%$.

The anaesthetist may wish to measure with a rotameter a gas other than the one for which the meter is calibrated. In fact, cyclopropane is not infrequently passed through a CO_2 meter in the mistaken belief that the readings are accurate for either gas. The practice is apparently based on the assumption that since the densities of the two gases are very similar the same calibration will do for either. Another commonly held belief is that if a lighter gas (say O_2) is passed through a rotameter calibrated for a heavier gas (for example, N_2O) more gas necessarily flows than is indicated by the bobbin.

Theory

The characteristics of a gas which influence its rate of flow through a given constriction are (1) its density and (2) its viscosity.

The constriction in an anaesthetic flowmeter may be either (1) orificial or (2) tubular (p. 192).

If the constriction takes the form of an *orifice* the **density** of the gas plays a much more important part than does its viscosity in determining the rate of flow of the gas through the constriction. In fact, for an ideal orifice, across which the pressure difference is kept constant, the following formulae hold good:

(i)   volume flow rate of gas $\propto \dfrac{1}{\sqrt[2]{(\text{density of gas})}}$

and if gas A is passed through an ideal orifice in a meter calibrated for gas B,

(ii) $\dfrac{\text{actual flow of gas A}}{\text{flow indicated on B meter}} = \sqrt[2]{\left(\dfrac{\text{density of gas B}}{\text{density of gas A}}\right)}$

If the densities of the two gases are equal the right side of the equation cancels out, showing that the indicated and actual flows are equal.

On the other hand, if the constriction is a *tube*, **viscosity** plays the dominant role in determining the rate of flow of the gas; the effect of the density becomes negligible.

The nature of the constriction in a rotameter will now be considered. The clearance between the head of the float and the rotameter tube is

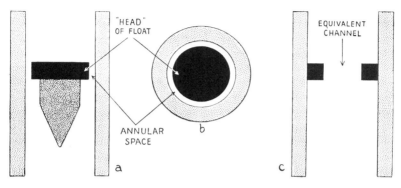

FIG. 201

annular (fig. 201 a, b) and may be considered as equivalent to a circular channel of the same cross-section area (fig. 201 c). This figure is not drawn to scale.

Figs. 202 to 205 are drawn to scale; they show the very small clearance between the head of the bobbin and the side of the rotameter tube, particularly in its lower part. The bobbin and the interior of the rotameter tube should be kept scrupulously clean, and in use the meter should always be vertical. If these details are not attended to, readings will be inaccurate.

Fig. 204—At low flows the float is near the lower end of the tube and the diameter of the equivalent channel is smaller than its length. In other words the constriction is tubular (fig. 205).

Fig. 202—As the rate of flow increases the float rises, and the diameter of the equivalent channel increases correspondingly. The length of the constriction remains, of course, constant. At high rates of flow, when the float is near the top of the meter, the diameter of the equivalent channel equals its length; the constriction approximates to an orifice (fig. 203).

Therefore, when the float spins at the lower part of the tube the viscosity of the gas plays a much more important part than does its density in determining the rate of flow through the meter. At high flow rates density plays the more important part.

Fig. 202

Fig. 203

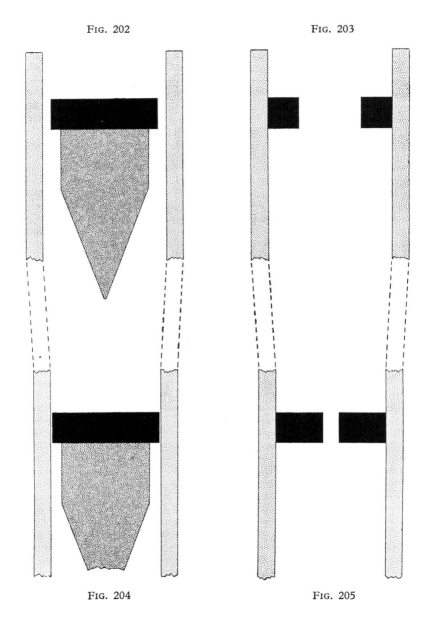

Fig. 204

Fig. 205

Experiments

These facts are well shown in the following illustrations.

The rotameters in figs. 206 (and 208) represent elongated portions of the lower part of the corresponding meters on the right in figs. 207 (and 209).

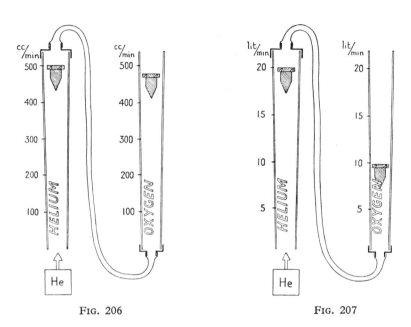

FIG. 206   FIG. 207

Helium and oxygen have similar viscosities but their densities, 0·17 and 1·33 g/l, differ markedly. At low flow rates where the influence of viscosity predominates, helium can be measured with tolerable accuracy on an oxygen rotameter (fig. 206).

At high flow rates (fig. 207) the effect of density is paramount. In this experiment the ratio of actual to indicated flow rate is 2 : 1.

If the equivalent channel through which the gases flow were an ideal orifice

$$\frac{\text{actual flow of helium}}{\text{flow indicated on oxygen rotameter}} \quad \text{would be} \quad \sqrt[2]{\frac{1\cdot33}{0\cdot17}} = \frac{2\cdot8}{1}$$

Cyclopropane and carbon dioxide have very similar densities (42 : 44), but the viscosities of the gases differ considerably (0·6 : 1). At low flow rates of cyclopropane (fig. 208) the position of the float in the CO_2 meter indicates a figure considerably below the actual flow. The true flow rate is 60% higher than that indicated on the CO_2 meter.

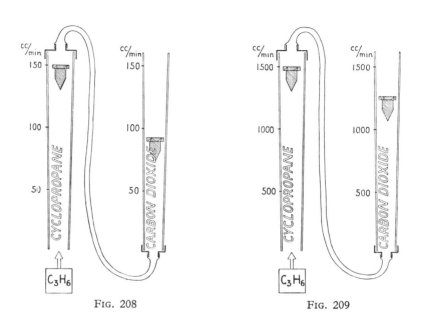

FIG. 208   FIG. 209

At high flow rates the relative discrepancy is much smaller. In fig. 209 the error is only 20%.

The succeeding TABLES on figs. 210–217 give the results of further experiments. They show the actual flow rate and the indicated flow rate when a gas is passed through a meter calibrated for a different gas. It is seen that no single factor enables the indicated flow to be converted into the actual one.

The viscosities and densities of many gases in common use are given in the tables of Chap. XXIV, p. 418-23, row i'. Reference to this will give the reader an idea as to whether the effect of viscosity or density predominates in any of the experiments tabulated on pp. 207–8.

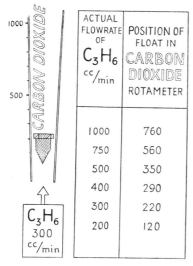

ACTUAL FLOWRATE OF C_3H_6 cc/min	POSITION OF FLOAT IN CARBON DIOXIDE ROTAMETER
1000	760
750	560
500	350
400	290
300	220
200	120

FIG. 210

ACTUAL FLOWRATE OF CO_2 cc/min	POSITION OF FLOAT IN CYCLO PROPANE ROTAMETER
1000	1180
750	900
500	620
400	520
300	400
200	320
100	200

FIG. 211

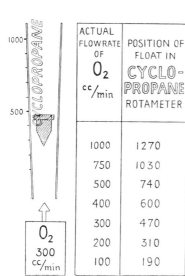

ACTUAL FLOWRATE OF O_2 cc/min	POSITION OF FLOAT IN CYCLO- PROPANE ROTAMETER
1000	1270
750	1030
500	740
400	600
300	470
200	310
100	190

FIG. 212

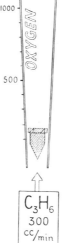

ACTUAL FLOWRATE OF C_3H_6 cc/min	POSITION OF FLOAT IN OXYGEN ROTAMETER
1000	670
750	450
500	280
400	220
300	170
200	90

FIG. 213

ACTUAL FLOWRATE OF O_2 lit/min	POSITION OF FLOAT IN NITROUS OXIDE ROTAMETER
10	9
8	7·2
6	5·5
5	4 7
4	4
3	3
2	2·2

FIG. 214

ACTUAL FLOWRATE OF N_2O lit/min	POSITION OF FLOAT IN OXYGEN ROTAMETER
10	11
8	8·8
6	6·5
5	5·2
4	4·1
3	3
2	1·9

FIG. 215

ACTUAL FLOWRATE OF CO_2 cc/min	POSITION OF FLOAT IN OXYGEN ROTAMETER
1000	890
750	640
500	400
400	300
300	240
200	150

FIG. 216

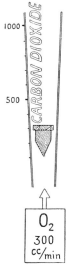

ACTUAL FLOWRATE OF O_2 cc/min	POSITION OF FLOAT IN CARBON DIOXIDE ROTAMETER
1000	1160
750	870
500	600
400	450
300	320
200	200
100	100

FIG. 217

Heidbrink meter

The conical tube (Z) is made of metal. Readings* are taken not from the base of the rod (black) but from the top which projects upwards into a glass tube. The bore of Z is not a simple cone; it is designed to give a wide range of readings. The scale illustrated is only 3 inches high yet it indicates flows from 50 to 15 000 cm³ per minute.

In principle the Heidbrink meter is similar to the flow meters described by Chameroy[6] in 1868 and to a later 'pocket' gas meter.[7]

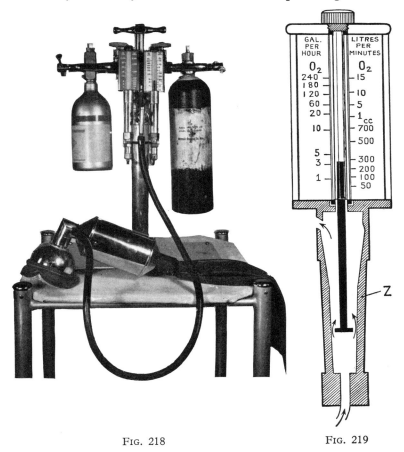

Fig. 218   Fig. 219

FIG. 218. Portable Heidbrink cyclopropane-oxygen apparatus with Waters' canister.
FIG. 219. The oxygen meter. The flow of oxygen is just under 300 cm³/min.

* The manufacturers state that 'the inherent accuracy of the Heidbrink flowmeter is as high as that of any "Thorpe Tube" flowmeter'.

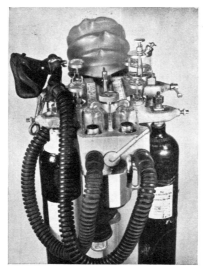

Fig. 220

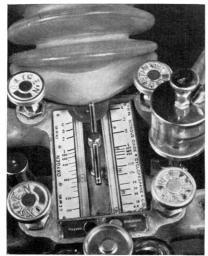

Fig. 221

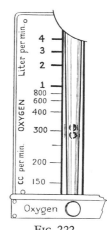

Fig. 222

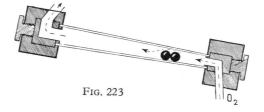

Fig. 223

Connell meter

These meters are mounted on an inclined plane. A tapered glass tube is used, but instead of a bobbin a pair of stainless steel balls is the indicator. These roll up the tube in response to the stream of gas until the difference in pressures below and above the balls counterbalances their weight component in the direction of the tube.

The pressure difference is caused by loss of pressure in the streaming gas due to local turbulence and viscosity effects in the space between the balls and the wall of the tube. Each tube is calibrated individually and the rate of flow is read from the point of contact of the balls. If a single ball is used it tends to oscillate; a pair ensures steadiness.

The inside of the hardened glass tube is not drawn out, but is ground with a high degree of accuracy. The bore does not increase uniformly as in the Rotameter, but is compound so that both large and small flows can be measured on the one meter about six inches long (cf. Heidbrink meter, p. 209). In the lower part of the tube the inner diameter increases by only 1/1000 of an inch for every inch in length.

The makers state that over the lower three inches of the meter the readings are accurate to within 10 cm³ per minute. In the upper part the taper is parabolic, opening out rapidly. This part of the tube is calibrated for large flow rates such as are used for continuous flow anaesthesia and resuscitation.

The meter illustrated was introduced in 1930.

Fig. 220—Connell 'Stratosphere' anaesthetic apparatus.

Fig. 221—Close up of head of apparatus.
Note concertina type rebreathing bag. The flowmeters are in the centre. Controls for the two cylinders of oxygen are on the left, and those for cyclopropane and nitrous oxide on the right. The ether drop bottle is between the last two.

Fig. 222—A Connell meter as seen by the anaesthetist. 300 cm³/min of oxygen are flowing.

Fig. 223—Connell meter—side elevation. The taper of the tube is not drawn true to scale.

The 'Connell'-meter uses the same principle as the 'Ball-and-tube' flowmeter invented in 1876 by Sir Alfred Ewing. This meter was devised to indicate the rate of flow of liquids. The glass tube was very slightly tapered; in one example it increased from 10 mm at the bottom

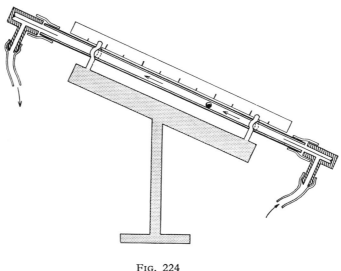

Fig. 224

to 11 mm at the top over a length of 100 cm, while the ball diameter was 9·5 mm.

This author studied the contribution of density and viscosity of the fluid to the pressure drop which keeps the ball in a certain position for a given flow rate.

Fig. 224—adapted from Ewing's article[8] shows that apart from the addition of a second ball the resemblance between the meters is quite close. The Connell meter might be appropriately described as a miniature edition of the Ewing meter incorporating two balls.

Fixed Orifice Meters

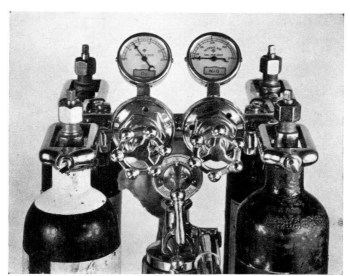

FIG. 225. Heidbrink pressure gauge flowmeter unit.

Pressure gauge meter

Fig. 226 illustrates a fixed orifice flowmeter utilizing a Bourdon pressure gauge. The gas flowing from its source passes through the small orifice (C). A pressure builds up proximal to the constriction and

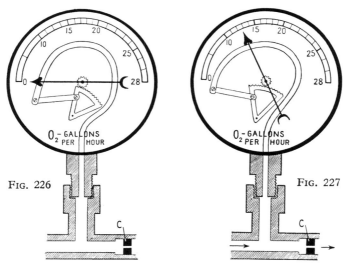

this pressure is transmitted to the flexible metal Bourdon tube of oval cross-section which tends to straighten out (compare fig. 228). The position of the needle indicator varies with the pressure within the Bourdon tube, and the scale is calibrated in terms of rate of gas flow

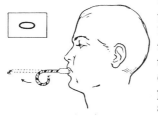

through the constriction (C). In this meter the gauge indicates the pressure difference between the proximal side of the orifice and the atmosphere. This is virtually equivalent to measuring the pressure difference on either side of the orifice, since in anaesthetic practice the pressure on the distal side approximates closely to atmospheric.

FIG. 228. *Inset*—The cross-section of the flexible tube before inflation is not circular.

This type of meter has not proved satisfactory for measuring small flows of gas.

Owing to the pressure necessary to cause the Bourdon tube to straighten out, a very small aperture (C) is used to provide the resistance to gas flow. If the orifice becomes partly blocked the meter reading increases, whereas, in fact, the actual flow is decreased; if the orifice becomes completely blocked the meter reading suggests that a flow of gas is being maintained.

Conversely, if the orifice (C) is enlarged by cleaning or scouring, the gas flow will be increased, but owing to the decreased resistance to the flow the meter reading will be decreased.

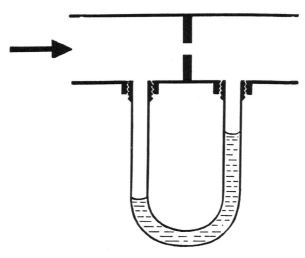

FIG. 229

Water depression meter

Fig. 229—The gas flows through a fixed orifice and the resultant pressure difference on the two sides is measured by means of a water manometer. The greater the flow rate of gas the greater the difference in pressure on either side of the orifice. In the case of an 'ideal' orifice

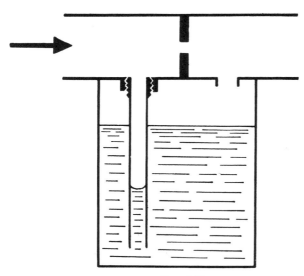

FIG. 230

the pressure difference is proportional to the square of the flow rate (see p. 195).

Fig. 230—In practice the upstream (or proximal) limb of the U-tube is immersed in an airtight glass container of water; the downstream limb is represented only by an opening. The meter is calibrated by passing a gas at known flow rates through the orifice and marking the corresponding water levels in the vertical tube on a scale.

The orifices used in anaesthetic flowmeters of this type are no larger than a small carburettor jet. They have two outstanding disadvantages:

(1) the orifice is easily obstructed by dirt. Much less gas will then be passing through the orifice than is indicated on the scale.

(2) the graduations are close together in the region where the flow rate is small, and far apart where it is big (fig. 231 left, and fig. 235). This is contrary to what is wanted in clinical practice.

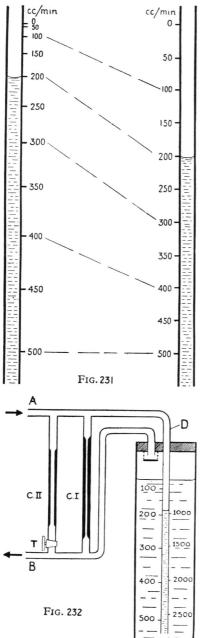

FIG. 231

FIG. 232

Meters with capillary constriction

This latter difficulty has been overcome by substituting[9, 10] a length of capillary tubing for the orifice. The resultant scale becomes nearly linear (fig. 231 right).

Fig. 232—The gas flows from A through a narrow capillary tube (C.I) on its way to B. Owing to the resistance of the capillary tube a pressure builds up in the tube D; the water within it is depressed, and the flow rate is read from the left-hand scale. This meter[10] has another advantage. A second wider capillary tube is incorporated. When the tap (T) of this is opened the gas passes through both capillary tubes and much less resistance is offered to its passage. A given depression in the tube D, now read off the right-hand scale, corresponds to a much greater flow of gas. Thus both fine and coarse rates of flow can be accurately measured on the same meter.

Foregger meter

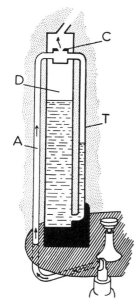

Fig. 233—After leaving the needle valve the gas enters the tube A and escapes through the constriction C into the mixing chamber D and so to the patient (see arrows). The constriction offers a resistance to the passage of the gas so that a pressure difference builds up across C, and this pressure difference bears a relation to the rate at which the gas is flowing. The more rapid the gas flow the greater will be the pressure difference—in other words more force will be required to drive the gas through C. The pressure difference is measured by the extent to which the water in the tube T is depressed below the level of the water in the main container. The lower end of the tube T enters the

FIG. 233. Foregger flowmeter, sketch.

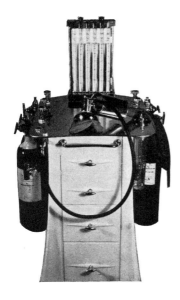

FIG. 234
Foregger anaesthetic apparatus.

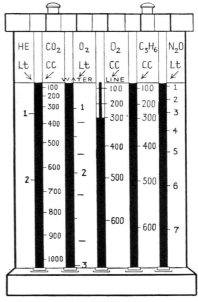

FIG. 235
Foregger flowmeters, face view.

main water container, thus forming a U-tube whose limbs are of widely differing cross-section. Any change in level in the calibrated sight tube is not accompanied by a material change of level in the main container. Tube T corresponds to the proximal side of the U-tube of fig. 229 and the main water container to the distal side of the U-tube. The main container is made of metal; the tube T, however, is transparent and a scale is provided alongside it which is graduated in terms of rate of gas flow. When looked at from the front (fig. 234) it will be seen that thin coloured strips are painted on the main container immediately behind the various tubes T and these facilitate the reading of the calibrations. Fig. 235, for instance, indicates that the only gas being used is oxygen, and this is flowing at 300 cm³/min.

The constriction in this meter is of larger bore than in the Bourdon gauge type, since a water manometer permits accurate reading of smaller pressure differences. The liability of the constriction to become obstructed with dirt is therefore less.

Water sight-feed meter

Each meter[11] consists of a metal tube. In practice two or three meters for measuring different gases are placed in the same bottle which is filled with water to the level of the horizontal metal plate which binds the tubes together. The part of the tube beneath the water is perforated by five small holes placed one below the other. As the gas flows it escapes through the holes, bubbles through the water and is led away from the top of the bottle. The greater the rate of flow of gas the greater the number of holes through which the gas will emerge into the water. A rough measure of the rate of flow of gas is thus provided by noting the number of holes from which the gas is bubbling.

Each meter is calibrated individually and to each bottle is attached a card (Table 6) giving the rate of gas flow which corresponds to the number of holes through which gas is bubbling. The rate of flow of nitrous oxide for a given number of holes is not the same as for oxygen. This is accounted for in part by the difference in density between these two gases.

Owing to the disturbance of the water which would result this method is not suitable for the measurement of large flows of gases. To prevent excessive bubbling a tap (T) is provided on the N_2O entry tube by which approximately 5 litres per minute of this gas can be by-passed without passing through the water meter. The nitrous oxide tube is on the right of the sight-feed bottle, and the by-pass tap T is situated at the top of the tube. This by-pass is closed when the tap is horizontal and open when the tap is set in the vertical position as in fig. 237. For

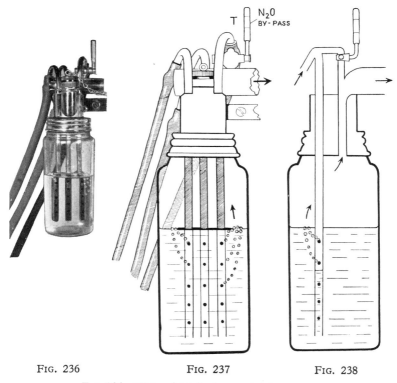

FIG. 236   FIG. 237   FIG. 238

FIG. 236. Water sight-feed meter bottle.
FIG. 237. Meter bottle enlarged.
FIG. 238. Pathway of gases from bottle to patient.

moderate flows of nitrous oxide the by-pass tap is left in the horizontal ('closed') position, but when more nitrous oxide is required than already passes through the five holes of the meter, the by-pass tap is raised to the vertical ('open') position. The gas now follows the line of least resistance and the bubbling ceases unless the needle valve is opened further.

Reference to fig. 237 and Table 6 show that 8·5 litres of nitrous oxide and 1·5 litres of oxygen are being delivered to the patient.

Though inaccurate this is the only meter in which the volume of

TABLE 6

		LITRES PER MIN.	
		N₂0	O₂
	1	·5	·5
	2	1·5	1·5
	3	2·5	3·0
	4	3·5	4·5
	5	4·5	6·0
BY-PASS OPEN	1	6·0	
	2	7·5	
	3	8·5	
	4	10·0	
	5	11·0	

gases passing to the patient is actually seen; the only other positive evidence of gas flow through a meter is the spinning of a rotameter bobbin.

REFERENCES

[1] JOSLIN, G. (1879). *Brit. Pat.* 2428; cf. fig. 6.
[2] KÜPPERS, K. (1908). *German Pat.* 215225.
[3] ANON. (1910). *Chemikerztg.* 34, 725.
[4] FOREGGER, R. (1952). *Brit. J. Anaesth.* 24, 187–95.
[5] MACINTOSH, R. R. (1941). *Lancet*, ii, 718.
[6] CHAMEROY, A. M. (1868). *French Pat.* 80129; cf. Pl. XIV, fig. 1.
[7] FRENZEL, P. (1902). *Das Gas* (in Hartleben's Chemisch Technische Bibliothek 259, 56–8; cf. fig. 26). Wien.
[8] EWING, SIR J. ALFRED (1924–5). *Proc. roy. Soc. Edinb.*, 45, 308–21.
[9] SCHOFIELD, R. K. (1937). *Proc. R. Soc. Med.* 1937–8, 31, 443–5.
[10] PASK, E. A. (1940). *Lancet*, ii, 680–1.
[11] WELLESLEY, G. (1930). *Brit. Pat.* 331050; cf. fig. 2.

CHAPTER XVI

THE INJECTOR AND ITS APPLICATIONS

Flow of fluid through constriction in pipe

Figs. 239 and 240—The experiment on p. 159 is repeated with a very long horizontal pipe so that the pressure drop per unit length is

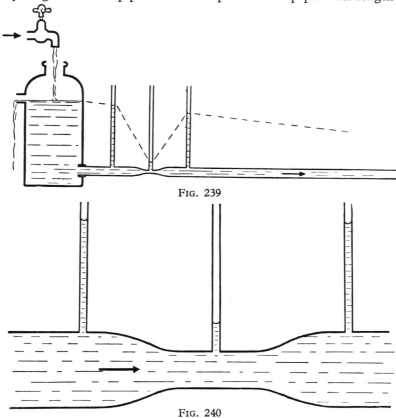

FIG. 239

FIG. 240

small. At one point the pipe is tapered *smoothly* to a constriction and then opened out again to its original bore. The heights of the water in the vertical tubes show that the pressure of the water at the site of the constriction is markedly lower than on either side. The pressure at the constriction depends on the speed of the liquid through it. In the experiment depicted the increased speed is such that the pressure is only just above atmospheric. By increasing the volume flow rate through the pipe this slight positive pressure can be further reduced. When the flow rate is large enough the pressure at the constriction

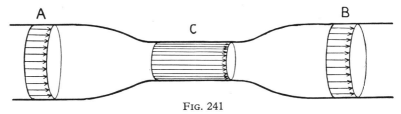

FIG. 241

becomes subatmospheric (or negative); instead of water being forced up the vertical tube air is drawn in through it (see fig. 245, p. 224).

Fig. 241—C represents a smooth constriction in a glass tube (compare fig. 240). The volume flow rate at all points along the tube is the same. The length of the arrows at A indicates the distance travelled by water in one second, that is, the linear speed of the water at that point.

The length of the arrows represents *average* speed, calculated from the formula $\dfrac{\text{volume flow rate}}{\text{cross-section}}$. The arrows would represent the actual speed only in a frictionless liquid.* In fact, with laminar flow the speed, greatest in the centre of the tube, decreases to zero at the walls (p. 171).

The volume of water contained in the shaded area, therefore, represents the volume flow rate of water in the tube. Since the volume flow rate is the same throughout the whole length of the tube, the length of the arrows in the constricted part C is such that the volume of the shaded area C is equal to that of A. It is seen that the speed of the water is greatest at the narrowest part of a tube.

The relationship between the speeds of the water and the cross-section areas (at A and C) is given by the ratio

$$\frac{\text{speed of water at A}}{\text{,, \quad ,, \quad C}} = \frac{\text{cross-section area of C}}{\text{,, \quad ,, \quad A}}$$

If the diameter at C is half that at A, the cross-section area at C is quarter that of A. The speed at C is therefore four times that at A.

The relationship between the speeds and the pressures at C and A is such that the pressure is least where the speed is greatest. This fact can be utilized to measure the flow rate by observing the pressure difference between A and C. Doubling the flow rate causes fourfold increase of pressure difference.

* Also in fully developed turbulent flow.

The Venturi Tube

As the liquid passes beyond the constriction to the wider part of the tube its speed gradually decreases. This is accompanied by a gradual increase in pressure as is well shown by fig. 242 taken from Venturi's original paper published in 1797 (see 'Biographical Notes', p. 436).

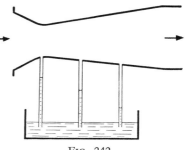

FIG. 242

Daniel BERNOULLI in 1738 formulated the laws for the flow of fluids through pipes of varying diameters. He demonstrated that the pressure of a fluid is least where its speed is greatest (fig. 240). Some sixty years later VENTURI showed that in order for a streaming fluid to regain a pressure much higher than that at the constriction (fig. 242) it was necessary for the tube immediately distal to the constriction to open out *very gradually*. He found his tube ceased to fulfil the above function if the angle of the cone exceeded 15°.

In a suitably designed tube a marked negative pressure can be created in the region of the constriction. Venturi describes an experiment in which 10 ft³ of water flowed per minute through a tube (entry $1\frac{1}{2}$ in. diameter). At the constriction ($1\frac{1}{3}$ in. diameter) a negative pressure of $4\frac{1}{2}$ in.Hg was created. Two inches beyond this point the negative pressure was only $1\frac{1}{2}$ in.Hg.

In the Venturi tube speed and pressure are closely related. The pressure drop (H) between A and C is approximately given by Eq. 6 on p. 174, if the area at C is appreciably smaller than that at A. The volume flow rate can thus be determined by measuring this pressure drop. Eighty years after Venturi's publication an American engineer, Herschel, inserted a Venturi tube in a pipe to measure flow rates through it. This principle has since become standard in engineering practice for measuring large flow rates of water.

The design of a Venturi tube is such that the pressure downstream almost regains the value it had on the upstream side of the constriction. This shows that local turbulence is small. The pressure drop seen near the constriction is due to the temporary conversion of pressure energy into increased kinetic energy (speed). There is a gradual reconversion of kinetic into pressure energy on the downstream side of the constriction.

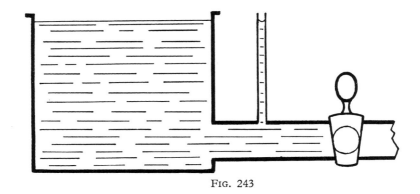

Fig. 243

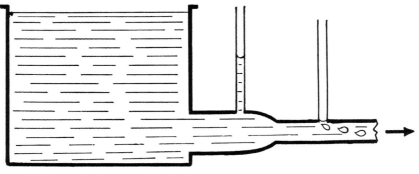

Fig. 244

Fig. 245

A simple physical explanation of why the pressure in a pipe is least where the speed of the liquid is greatest.

Fig. 243—A pipe leads from the bottom of a large vessel containing fluid. Flow through the pipe is prevented by the closed tap; the liquid is at rest. The total energy of the liquid in the pipe is in the form of pressure energy supplied by the hydrostatic pressure of the liquid in the large vessel. The height to which the liquid rises in the vertical tube, open to the atmosphere, indicates the pressure in the pipe and is a measure of the total energy possessed by the resting liquid.

Fig. 244—Throughout this experiment the level in the large supply vessel, and consequently the hydrostatic pressure at the entrance to the pipe, is kept constant. The tap has been opened and the liquid flows through the pipe. The flow rate soon becomes constant. In addition to pressure energy the liquid now possesses kinetic energy by virtue of its movement. Since the total energy per unit volume necessarily remains unchanged, the kinetic energy is produced at the expense of pressure energy. The diminution of pressure energy is shown by a fall in liquid level in the vertical tube.

Fig. 245—The pipe is modified as shown. There are two vertical tubes to indicate pressure. The position of the first is unchanged; it is inserted into the original wide bore segment. The second is inserted into the narrow segment.

Since the volume flow rate throughout the length of the composite pipe is the same, the linear speed of the liquid in the narrow segment must be greater than in the wider (p. 222). The liquid obviously possesses more kinetic energy in the narrower segment.

Any increase in kinetic energy in the narrow segment is again accompanied by a decrease in pressure energy in that segment.

If the speed in the narrow segment is great enough the pressure falls below that of the atmosphere. If this occurs air is forced by atmospheric pressure into the pipe through the vertical tube.

In this discussion the effect of the viscosity of the liquid has been neglected. The effect of viscosity is to cause a loss of energy as frictional heat for the flow along straight pipes as well as for any abrupt alteration in the pipe diameter. In a fictitious, non-viscous liquid there is no loss of energy but a conversion of pressure into kinetic energy and vice versa.

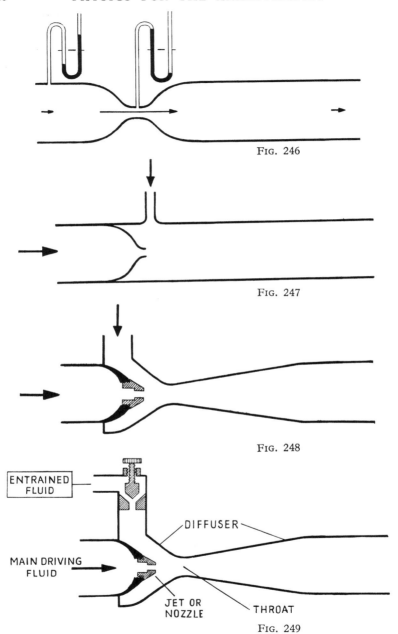

FIG. 246

FIG. 247

FIG. 248

ENTRAINED
FLUID

DIFFUSER

MAIN DRIVING
FLUID

JET OR
NOZZLE

THROAT

FIG. 249

The evolution of the injector with entrainment duct

Fig. 246—A gas flows through a constriction in a tube. The manometers show that the pressure which is positive (that is, above atmospheric) at the first manometer is negative at the site of constriction. The lengths of the arrows indicate the average linear velocities of the gas at various points along the tube.

Fig. 247—The tube is slightly modified. The principle remains unchanged. A side entry tube (or entrainment duct) replaces the manometer opposite the constriction. Since here the pressure is below atmospheric, air is sucked in (or entrained) to swell the stream of gas in the tube.

Fig. 248—A jet replaces the constriction and the tube has been modified further. The specially shaped part downstream from the jet is known as the *diffuser*.

Fig. 249—An injector device. Its development from fig. 247 is easily traced.

In a suitably designed injector the final composition of the mixture is not dependent on the volume flow rate of the driving gas: it is determined only by the size of entrainment port. Here this is controlled by the screw tap.

The function of the conical diffuser is to reduce turbulence as the gas stream slows down in the widening tube and to transform as much as possible the kinetic into pressure energy, to entrain a larger volume of gas, and to make this volume independent of fluctuations in resistance or in pressure distal to the diffuser. Such conditions arise when the gas mixture from an injector passes into a reservoir bag.

The entrainment is the result not only of the suction effect of the fast stream of driving gas,* but also of its propulsive effect on the resting gas surrounding the jet.

* The fact that gases are compressible has been neglected, although it is of vital importance for the design of injectors if the gas is supplied to the jet at a high pressure.

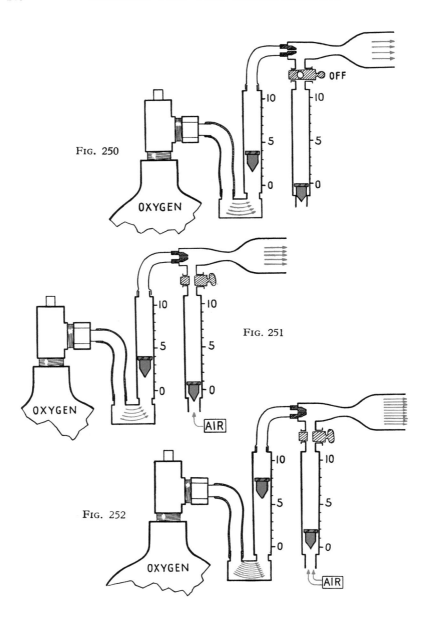

FIG. 250

OXYGEN

FIG. 251

OXYGEN

AIR

FIG. 252

OXYGEN

AIR

History of the Injector

An early application (1827) of the entraining properties of a fast stream through a jet was the blast pipe in the chimney of a locomotive. The exhaust steam was discharged through a nozzle in the chimney with the object of sucking air through the furnace to speed up combustion. The device was only moderately successful but became highly effective when, about 1850, the interior of the chimney was shaped like a Venturi tube.

James Thomson, brother of Lord Kelvin, should be considered the father of the injector. In 1852 he designed his water jet pump in which a fast stream of water is discharged through a nozzle into an appropriately shaped Venturi tube, now termed a diffuser. By this simple yet efficient combination he was able to drain large volumes of water from low-lying land.

Use of injector for supplying gas mixtures of constant composition

Fig. 250—Oxygen from a cylinder flows through the jet of an injector at the rate of 4 litres per minute (red bobbin). The air entrainment duct is shut by a tap marked 'OFF'.

Fig. 251—The tap is opened fully. The blue bobbin of this flowmeter indicates that 1 litre per minute of air is being entrained. The mixture issuing from the diffuser consists of 4 vol. oxygen and 1 vol. air; its oxygen concentration is $100 \times (4 + 0.2)/5 = 84\%$.

Fig. 252—The flow of oxygen is increased to 8 litres per minute. This results in 2 litres per minute of air being entrained. Despite the fact that the flow rate of the driving gas has been altered, the percentage *composition* of the mixture issuing from the diffuser remains unchanged, $100 \times (8 + 0.4)/10 = 84\%$.

In the injector units considered here the final mixture depends on the degree to which the air entrainment tap is opened, and on the design of the unit. With the tap closed a negative pressure is still produced in the vicinity of the jet, but there is obviously no entrainment, and the driving gas emerges undiluted. As the tap is gradually opened more and more air is entrained.*

* With a suitably designed injector the driving gas may entrain as much as twenty times its own volume.

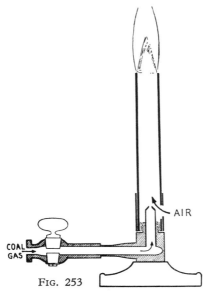

A homely example is the Bunsen burner. The coal gas flows through the jet situated in the base of the burner. When the side hole is closed air is not entrained. The coal gas burns with a yellow flame. When the side hole is open (fig. 253) air is drawn in and the mixture burns with the typical hot blue flame. The composition of the final coal gas/air mixture depends on the degree to which the hole is open and is little influenced by the setting of the gas tap.

FIG. 253

Anaesthetic Mixtures

The first reference we can find in the anaesthetic literature[1] to the use for the injector is the machine patented[2] by Marston in 1898 (fig. 254).

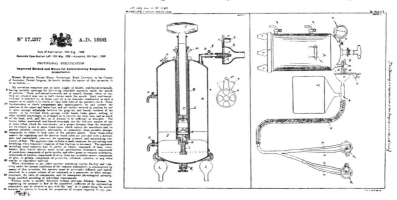

This apparatus, simplified in fig. 255, incorporated other ingenious features based on a sound knowledge of physics. The reservoir bag, sometimes misnamed 'rebreathing' bag, was even then no new feature, and the metal pressure chamber was but a compact modification of

Clover's clumsy container (fig. 9) in which the contents, being at atmospheric pressure, were soon exhausted.

The novelty of the apparatus lay in the incorporation of an injector and a tap which regulated the amount of air entrained, so that the

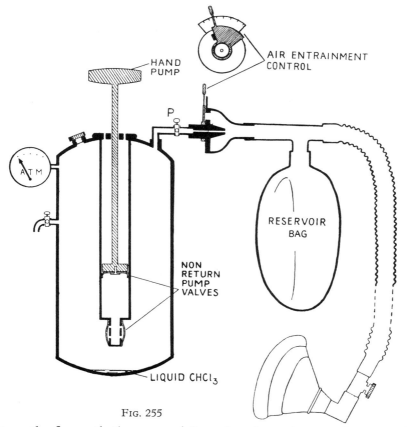

FIG. 255

strength of anaesthetic vapour delivered to the patient was known and could be varied at will.

The apparatus was designed primarily for chloroform, but of course could be used to deliver the vapour of any other liquid anaesthetic.

The metal cylinder has a capacity of 15 litres. Reference to fig. 67 shows that when the temperature of the room is 19 °C the maximum partial pressure of chloroform vapour in air is 150 mmHg . To saturate the 15 litres of air in the cylinder with chloroform vapour, 10 ml of liquid chloroform is introduced and vaporized. At this stage the pressure within the cylinder is 1 atmosphere and the percentage of chloroform vapour* is $\frac{150}{760} \times 100 = 20\%$. When further air is pumped into the cylinder the air pressure within it rises; the partial pressure of the chloroform vapour remains unchanged. When the gauge indicates 2 atmospheres (absolute pressure) the percentage of chloroform vapour is $\frac{150}{2 \times 760} \times 100 = 10\%$. If by further pumping the pressure is raised to 5 atmospheres, the percentage of chloroform vapour is $\frac{150}{5 \times 760} \times 100 = 4\%$. At this stage the cylinder contains 5 times the amount of air (75 litres) which it had at atmospheric pressure.

If the tap P is now opened 4% chloroform vapour issues from the jet. Marston's air entrainment control is simple and is calibrated so that the vapour from the cylinder can be diluted with air in known proportions. When the control is fully open 9 volumes of air are entrained for every volume issuing through the jet. Thus any mixture of chloroform vapour and air between 4% and 0·4% can be delivered by suitable adjustment of the control.

Distal to the injector unit of Marston's apparatus the essential features of any continuous flow machine—reservoir bag and wide bore tubing leading from it to the patient—are readily recognized. Compare with fig. 301, p. 274.

Oxygen therapy

Fig. 256—Oxygen from a cylinder flows through the jet of an injector.[3] The air entrainment duct is covered by a rotating disc which has holes of varying size drilled in it. As the disc is rotated any one hole can be made to coincide with the air entrainment duct.

In this illustration the disc is rotated until the indicator points to 40. Here the largest hole coincides with the entrainment duct so that the maximum amount of air is entrained. At this setting 1 volume of oxygen entrains 3 volumes of air, and the issuing mixture contains 40% of oxygen. The disc can be rotated and any smaller hole made to coincide with the entrainment duct, when the amount of air entrained will be correspondingly smaller. If the disc is rotated so that the indicator points to 100, the entrainment duct is completely blocked and undiluted oxygen issues from the diffuser. Once the disc is set, the number to which the indicator points gives the percentage of oxygen in the

---

* To simplify the calculation it is assumed that a volume of air equivalent to that of chloroform vapour has escaped from the cylinder.

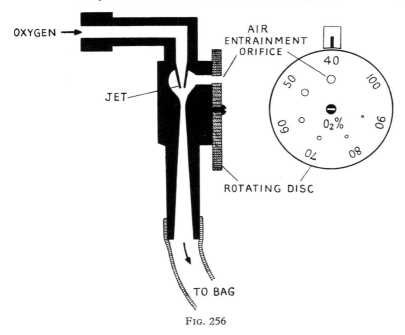

FIG. 256

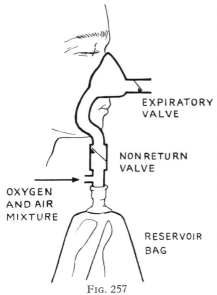

FIG. 257

mixture issuing from the injector unit. This is uninfluenced by any alteration in the oxygen flow rate from the cylinder.

When this method of administering oxygen is chosen a reservoir bag with non-return valves is used (fig. 257). A flowmeter is unnecessary: the flow rate is adjusted so that it is adequate to keep the reservoir bag moderately full. If the oxygen supply fails, the fact becomes apparent immediately since the bag remains deflated.

The method has other advantages. Any desired percentage of oxygen can be given, and if desired the patient can gradually be 'weaned' from high to lesser concentrations. There is no rebreathing.

Nitrous oxide/Air analgesia apparatus[4]

Nitrous oxide from a cylinder issues intermittently through a jet, entraining air through an orifice the size of which is such that the final mixture of nitrous oxide and air contains 50% of air. The mixture passes into a rubber bag from which it is breathed by the patient. Inside the bag are two levers which tend to move outwards through the action of a spring, thereby occluding the nitrous oxide jet. To overcome the action of this spring a negative pressure of a few mm H_2O must be produced in the bag. This negative pressure is produced by the inspiratory effort of the patient.

Fig. 258—When the patient inspires, the bag empties, pushing the levers towards each other against the force of the spring. The seating to which the levers are attached moves away from the jet allowing gas to flow. Air is entrained and the mixture passes to the patient.

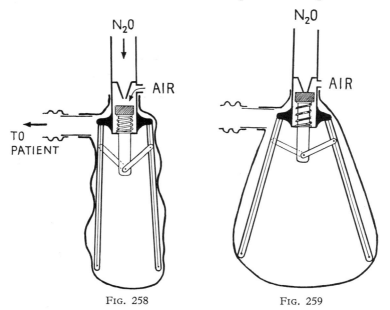

FIG. 258   FIG. 259

Fig. 259—When inspiration stops the bag fills with gas mixture. The spring can now force the levers apart; the seating rises and occludes the jet. Gas flows only on inspiration; if the mask is removed from the face the nitrous oxide is automatically cut off.

Portable suction apparatus

The injector principle has been used to provide suction for nearly a hundred years, the driving fluid being either steam or water.

Saher and Salt[5] have applied this principle, using compressed gas, to a suction apparatus for anaesthetic purposes. Suction is thus made available whenever a cylinder of oxygen or other compressed gas is to hand. The writers have found this portable suction apparatus a life-saving measure when suction was wanted urgently in wards where suction by other means was not available.

Fig. 260—The complete unit. The foot control is seen immediately below the cylinder. Sections of the device are shown in the following two illustrations.

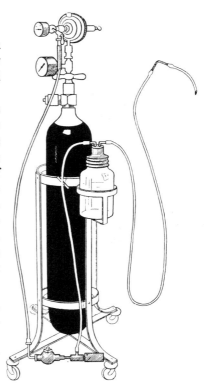

FIG. 260

Fig. 261—Foot control of the injector unit. Oxygen flows only when the spring is depressed by the foot. Immediately the foot is raised suction ceases.

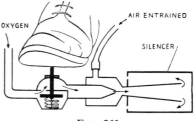

FIG. 261

Fig. 262—The working principle is illustrated. As oxygen is made to flow through the injector nozzle, air is entrained. A vacuum is created in the bottle. The tube leading into the bottle is used for suction and the aspirated fluid collects in the bottle.

Negative pressures of -400 mmHg below atmospheric can be obtained for an oxygen pressure of 45 lb/in² (3 atm) supplied to the jet; the oxygen consumption is in the region of 20 l/min.

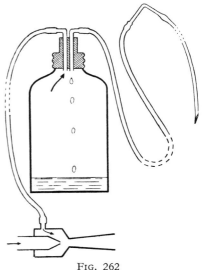

FIG. 262

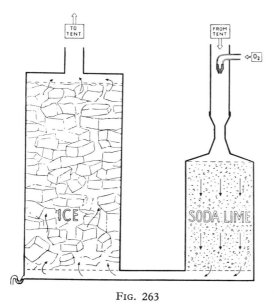

FIG. 263

The Heidbrink oxygen tent

Fig. 263—The oxygen supply enters through a jet. The negative pressure so created sucks air and other gases out of the tent. Carbon dioxide is absorbed by the soda lime and the water vapour condenses in the ice container. Cooled and dry oxygen and air re-enter the tent. The efficiency of the injector in circulating the air of the tent is stated by the manufacturers to be high. According to their figures a flow rate of only 3 l/min oxygen passing through the jet circulates 40 times as much air from the tent. If the flow of oxygen is increased to 5 l/min, the circulation rate becomes 50 times the oxygen flow.

The various examples of the application of the injector discussed so far represent only a small selection of the many uses to which this device has been put in anaesthetic and related equipment. In present-day anaesthetic apparatus, for example, the injector is incorporated in many mechanical respirators which provide both a positive and a negative pressure phase.[6]

REFERENCES

[1] MARSTON, R. (1899). *The anaesthetist's pocket companion*, p. 48 ff. Leicester.
[2] —— (1898). *Brit. Pat.* 17237.
[3] COWAN, S. L., and MITCHELL, J. V. (1942). *Brit. med. J.*, i, 118–9.
[4] TALLEY, H. A. E. (1942). *Brit. J. Anaesth.* 1942–3, **18**, 81–7; cf. p. 82.
[5] SAHER, N. F., and SALT, R. (1943). *Brit. med. J.*, i, 790.
[6] MUSHIN, W. W., RENDELL-BAKER, L., and THOMPSON, PETER W. (1959). *Automatic Ventilation of the Lungs*. Oxford.

CHAPTER XVII

SOLUTION OF GASES

GASES dissolve in liquids. This is evident from such everyday phenomena (fig. 264) as:

(a) the liberation in the form of bubbles of air dissolved in water when the latter is heated to say 60 °C;

(b) the ability of fish to live in water;

(c) the liberation of dissolved carbon dioxide in a soda water siphon when the lever is depressed, soda water forced out and the tension in the bottle lowered.

When a gas is in contact with a liquid the molecules of the former in their ceaseless motion impinge on the surface of the liquid. Some intermingle with the molecules of the liquid and are said to be in solution.

Fig. 265—Oxygen at a pressure of 1 atmosphere (absolute) is introduced to a vessel $\frac{9}{10}$ full of recently boiled (and therefore air-free) water at 20 °C. Some of the gas dissolves in the water and when equilibrium is reached the pressure of the oxygen has fallen from 1 to $\frac{3}{4}$ of an atmosphere.

Fig. 266—Here the initial pressure of the oxygen in contact with the water is 2 atmospheres—double that in fig. 265. The fall in pressure is twice that in the previous experiment, showing that double the amount of oxygen has dissolved.

Fig. 267—The experiment in fig. 265 is repeated but the temperature of the water is now 40 °C instead of 20 °C. Less oxygen passes into solution.

The gauges are assumed to indicate absolute pressures.

Conclusions

The amount of a given gas which dissolves in a given liquid is directly proportional to the pressure of the gas (Henry's Law). The amount varies with the temperature of the liquid; the higher the temperature the less the amount of gas which goes into solution.

Saturated Solutions of Gases

At any given temperature and pressure a gas dissolves in a given liquid only to a certain extent. When no further gas dissolves in the liquid a state of equilibrium exists between the gas over the liquid and

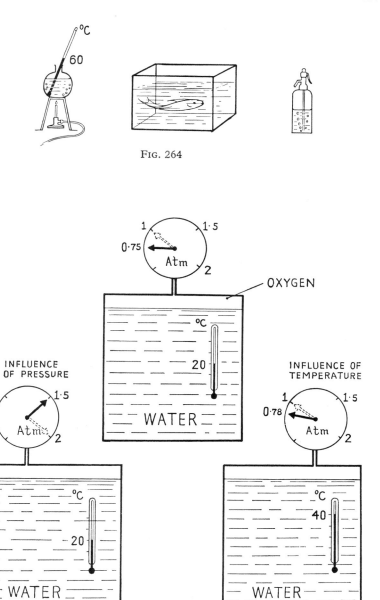

FIG. 264

OXYGEN

INFLUENCE
OF PRESSURE

INFLUENCE OF
TEMPERATURE

FIG. 266   FIG. 265   FIG. 267

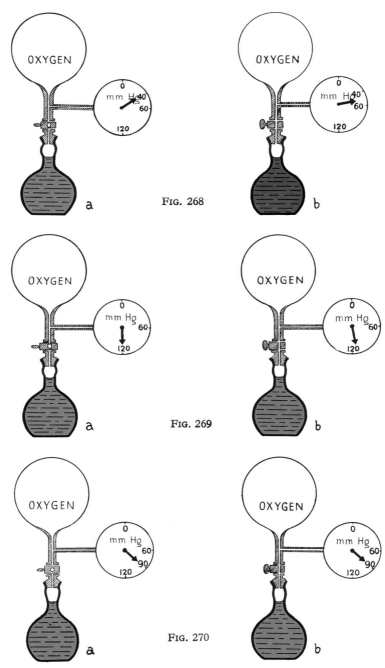

FIG. 268

FIG. 269

FIG. 270

the gas dissolved in it. The liquid is said to be fully saturated with the gas at that temperature and pressure. It is a convention to state that the gas in solution exerts the same *'tension'* as the partial pressure of the gas over the liquid in equilibrium with it.

Example: The partial pressure of oxygen in the alveoli is 100 mmHg If the oxygen in the blood after passage through the lungs is assumed* to be in equilibrium with the alveolar gases, its tension equals 100 mmHg .

This definition of 'tension' of a dissolved gas gives the clue to a method whereby the tension of a gas (say oxygen) in a liquid (say blood) can be determined. Small amounts of the blood are brought into contact with samples of oxygen at varying known pressures, till one is found where oxygen neither enters nor leaves the blood. The oxygen in solution in the blood is here in equilibrium with the oxygen sample. The tension of the oxygen in the blood is then the same as the partial pressure of the sample of oxygen with which it is in contact.

To determine the tension of oxygen in a given sample of blood

Fig. 268a—A fraction of the blood sample is placed in a flask and is connected to a closed bulb containing oxygen at a pressure of 40 mmHg .

Fig. 268b—The tap is now opened and the gaseous oxygen comes into contact with the blood. The pressure of the oxygen rises to 50 mmHg and the blood becomes darker in colour. Oxygen has passed from the blood into the bulb.

Fig. 269a—Another fraction of the blood sample is used with oxygen at a pressure of 120 mmHg .

Fig. 269b—When the tap is turned on the pressure in the oxygen chamber drops to 110 mmHg . Oxygen has passed from the gas flask into the blood.

Fig. 270a and b—Here the blood sample is brought into contact with oxygen at a pressure of 90 mmHg . When the tap is opened no change in pressure occurs. The blood oxygen is in equilibrium with the oxygen in the flask. The tension of the oxygen in the blood, therefore, is 90 mmHg .

* Complete equilibrium may not be established owing to uneven ventilation of the lungs and other causes.[1]

Under the same conditions of temperature and pressure, different gases dissolve to different extents in any given liquid.

TABLE 7. SOLUBILITY IN WATER

Gas (dissolved in water)	Coefficient of solubility at	
	0 °C	40 °C
Oxygen	4·9	2·3
Nitrogen	2·4	1·2
Carbon dioxide*	170	53

A measure of the amount of a gas which dissolves in a given liquid is the 'coefficient of solubility' of the gas in that liquid; the value of this for different gases in water is given on p. 419.

There are many *coefficients of solubility*. A coefficient in common

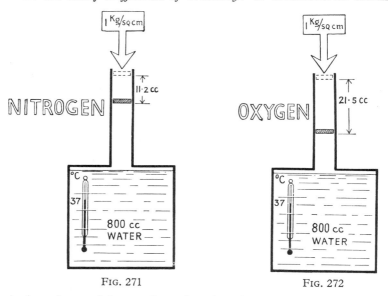

FIG. 271   FIG. 272

use is the volume of the gas (in cm³, reduced to N.T.P.) which dissolves in 100 cm³ of the solvent when the partial pressure of the gas is 1 atmosphere.

* This large coefficient is due to the chemical reaction of CO_2 with water forming carbonic acid.

The coefficient of solubility decreases with rise of temperature and the latter must, therefore, always be stated.

Fig. 271—800 cm³ of water at body temperature exposed to nitrogen under a pressure of 1 kilogram per square centimetre (approximately 1 atmosphere) dissolve 11·2 cm³ of nitrogen.

Fig. 272—Under the same conditions of temperature and pressure 21·5 cm³ of oxygen are dissolved.

At 37 °C the coefficients of solubility of nitrogen and oxygen in water are as 11·2 to 21·5.

It is of interest to compare the *weight* of a gas, say oxygen, dissolved in water, with that of a solid.

Oxygen in the alveoli has a partial pressure of 100 mmHg . At this pressure 0·3 cm³ of oxygen dissolve in 100 cm³ of water. Since the density of oxygen is 1·3 g/l, the weight of oxygen which dissolves in 100 cm³ water is $0·3 \times (1·3/1000) = 0·0004$ g. Barium sulphate is considered 'insoluble'. Actually 0·0003 g dissolve in 100 cm³ water.

Oxygen dissolves to the same extent in plasma or water. It is striking that a permanent concentration of 0·0004 g of oxygen per 100 cm³ plasma is sufficient to supply all the oxygen necessary for the metabolism of the body. This is made possible by (1) the inexhaustible reservoir of oxygen in the haemoglobin, (2) the intimate contact between plasma and tissue cells, and the short distances the oxygen has to diffuse to reach the cells.

APPLICATIONS

1. Oxygen Therapy.

The partial pressure of oxygen in the alveoli, when air is breathed at sea level, is 100 mmHg . Arterial blood in these circumstances contains 20 cm³ of oxygen per 100 cm³ of blood. Of this 19·7 cm³ are combined with haemoglobin in the red cells, the remaining 0·3 cm³ being in solution in the plasma. Reference to fig. 81 shows that when the oxygen in the alveoli exerts a partial pressure of 100 mmHg the haemoglobin in the blood leaving the lungs is practically saturated with oxygen, assuming again equilibrium to be established (p. 241). Any increase in the partial pressure of the oxygen in the alveoli, therefore, can result only in a very small increase in the amount of oxygen *carried by haemoglobin*.

The amount of oxygen *dissolved in the plasma*, however, is directly proportional to the partial pressure of the oxygen in contact with the plasma, that is, in the alveoli. When pure oxygen is breathed the partial pressure of oxygen in the alveoli can be raised from 100 to almost 700 mmHg . This results in a sevenfold increase in the amount of oxygen dissolved in the plasma,—from 0·3 to 2·1 cm³ of oxygen per 100 cm³ of blood. The total *percentage* increase in the oxygen carried by the blood is only 10%. Nevertheless, the increase of the *dissolved* oxygen is of great importance since the transfer of oxygen from the blood to the tissues is by diffusion, and the rate of this process is proportional to the difference in oxygen tension between plasma and tissues.

2. Oxygen inhalation to relieve abdominal distension

A valuable application of the fact that gases in the body tend to come into equilibrium with the gases in the blood stream was made by Fine.[2]

Post-operative abdominal distension is distressing, and may become a serious complication. As a result of abdominal discomfort air is swallowed, and because of intestinal atony accumulates in the bowel. This still further increases the patient's discomfort, leading to further aerophagy so that a vicious circle is established. The gases in the bowel and blood tend to come into equilibrium. Oxygen passes from the bowel to venous blood in which the tension is lower. The tension of the nitrogen in the blood, however, is substantially the same as that of the nitrogen now in the bowel, so that transfer does not take place. The distension may assume grave proportions.

Normally the only exits for the imprisoned nitrogen are the two ends of the alimentary canal. However, if the patient is given pure oxygen to breathe the partial pressure of nitrogen in the alveoli falls rapidly. The tension of nitrogen in the blood stream falls. Nitrogen now passes from the gut into the blood stream, thence to the alveoli, and the abdominal distension subsides. Within a few hours the result may be dramatic.

In the same way the inhalation of oxygen often relieves the headache which may follow aero-encephalography. Here air has been injected into the ventricles to outline them for radiography. Residual nitrogen is alleged to be the cause of headache and its absorption is hastened by the inhalation of oxygen.[3]

3. Aeroembolism[4]

Nitrogen is in solution in the tissues and in the blood. Its tension there is in equilibrium with the partial pressure of nitrogen in the alveoli which at sea level is approximately 570 mmHg .

As an airman ascends he is exposed to a progressive fall in atmospheric pressure. With this there is a corresponding fall in the partial pressure of nitrogen in his alveoli. Even at low rates of climb there is no time for the nitrogen dissolved in the body to come into equilibrium with the nitrogen in the alveoli. Owing to slow diffusion and the greater solubility of nitrogen in fatty tissues, the tissue nitrogen, especially that of fats, lags behind that of the blood nitrogen and still more behind the alveolar nitrogen. The tissues become supersaturated with the gas. From about 18 000 feet upwards bubbles of nitrogen form in the tissues, particularly those of high fat content and poor blood supply. Above 30 000 feet nitrogen bubbles may form in the blood stream.

The presence of bubbles in the tissues and the vessels gives rise to symptoms which vary with their place of location. A rapid descent quickly relieves the symptoms since the nitrogen is forced into solution again.

The same phenomenon, here referred to as compressed air illness or caisson disease, may be a sequel to working in a caisson or to deep-sea diving. Here air is breathed at anything up to 10 atmospheres of pressure (corresponding to a depth of 300 feet). Breathing air at very high pressures, during which the partial pressure of the alveolar nitrogen may rise to several thousand mmHg, results in a great increase in the amount of nitrogen taken into solution in the tissues.

On decompression there is a fall in alveolar nitrogen, but there is a lag in the fall of tissue and blood nitrogen. When the pressure is reduced by more than half, bubbles of nitrogen may appear in the tissues and blood. In practice, therefore, decompression is carried out in stages. In the intervals the diver is kept at a fixed pressure till his tissues and alveolar air approach equilibrium. At no one time should the reduction of pressure exceed half. Should symptoms of compressed air illness develop, the treatment, of course, is immediate recompression.

4. Inhalation of anaesthetic gases at positive pressures

The oxygenation of a patient cannot be materially improved by increasing the *pressure* at which the anaesthetic mixture is breathed.* It has been stated that during gas and oxygen anaesthesia an increase of pressure by, say, 20 mmHg may be enough to make adequate the

---

* The following discussion should not be confused with the conclusions reached by BERT[5] in his experiments of 1879. In his arrangement the whole body of the patient was enclosed in a chamber in which the pressure was considerably above atmospheric. The partial pressures of all the components of the inhaled mixture were increased. Oxygenation could therefore be considerably improved. However, the pressure *difference* between the alveolar gases and the ambient air was no greater than normal; and the circulation remained unimpaired.

previously inadequate oxygen in the mixture. This belief is borne out neither in practice nor by a consideration of the relevant physical facts.

Let us consider a mixture of 12% oxygen and 88% nitrous oxide. Breathed at atmospheric pressure the partial pressure of oxygen

in the mixture $= \dfrac{12}{100} \times 760 = 91$ mmHg

The partial pressure of oxygen in the alveoli[6] is now $\underline{35 \text{ mmHg}}$

Breathed at 20 mmHg above atmospheric pressure (780 mmHg), the partial pressure of oxygen

$$= \dfrac{12}{100} \times 780 = 94 \text{ mmHg}$$

Assuming a linear relation between inspired and alveolar oxygen pressures over this narrow range, the partial pressure of oxygen in the

alveoli becomes $\dfrac{94}{91} \times 35 = \underline{36 \text{ mmHg}}$

The increase of the partial pressure of oxygen in the alveoli is from 35 to 36 mmHg .

The partial pressure of oxygen rises by $1/35$th.

$\therefore$ oxygen increase in *solution* $= \dfrac{1}{35} \times 0\cdot3$ cm^3 $= 0\cdot009$ cm^3 per 100 cm^3
of blood.

Reference to fig. 81 shows that the increase in the oxygen taken up by *the haemoglobin* for a rise of oxygen tension from 35 to 36 mmHg is also negligible.

Under ordinary clinical conditions it is inadvisable to administer anaesthetic gases at positive pressures exceeding 30 mmHg . Undesirable physiological effects on the circulation result from excessive positive pressures in the lungs.[7]

In current clinical practice improved oxygenation is not to be obtained by increasing the pressure of the gas mixture, but by increasing the proportion of oxygen in the inspired mixture.

REFERENCES

[1] RILEY, R. L. *et al.* (1951). *J. appl. Physiol.*, 4, 102–20.
[2] FINE, J. *et al.* (1936). *Ann. Surg.*, 103, 375–87.
[3] SCHWAB, R. S. *et al.* (1936). *J. nerv. ment. Dis.*, 84, 316–20.
[4] ARMSTRONG, H. G. (1943). *Principles and practice of aviation medicine*, 2nd ed., p. 356 ff. Lond.
[5] DUNCUM, B. M. (1947). *The development of inhalation anaesthesia*, p. 360 ff. Lond.
[6] MACINTOSH, R. R., and BANNISTER, F. B. (1952). *Essentials of general anaesthesia*, 5th ed., p. 55. Oxford.
[7] HUBAY, C. A. *et al.* (1954). *Anesthesiology*, 15, 445–61.

CHAPTER XVIII

DIFFUSION AND OSMOSIS

Molecular Movement

UNLIKE the molecules in a solid, the molecules in a fluid (that is, liquid or gas) wander freely and their range of movement extends to every

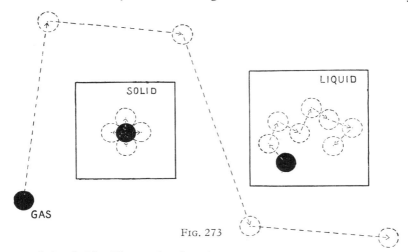

FIG. 273

part of the fluid. The path of each molecule (fig. 273) is necessarily zigzag because of frequent molecular collisions, but movement takes place in all directions and is scarcely influenced by gravity. The time taken by a molecule to cover a certain distance in its zigzag path depends on the proximity of its neighbours. The closer the molecules are packed the greater is the number of molecular impacts, and the longer a molecule takes to travel a certain distance in a given direction. A sprinter may cover 100 yards in 10 seconds on a sports field. The same distance along a crowded pavement takes longer to traverse, and the time taken is largely determined by the buffeting en route.

In gases at room conditions the intermolecular spaces are relatively big, and the molecules move considerable distances in a short time, since the number of collisions is comparatively few. The large size of the intermolecular spaces in a gas, compared to those of a liquid, can be appreciated from the following facts.

We have seen (p. 10) that 1 cm³ of liquid ether is converted into 220 cm³ of ether vapour at N.T.P.; 1 cm³ of ethyl chloride is transformed into 340 cm³ of vapour at room conditions. The molecules which initially occupied 1 cm³ are now dispersed into 340 cm³.

In the case of WATER the difference between the volumes of liquid

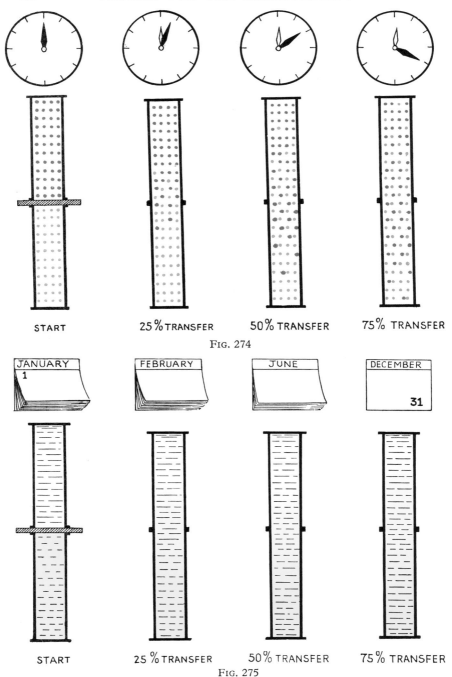

START   25% TRANSFER   50% TRANSFER   75% TRANSFER

FIG. 274

START   25% TRANSFER   50% TRANSFER   75% TRANSFER

FIG. 275

and vapour is even more marked. 1 cm³ of water is converted into 1600 cm³ of water vapour at its boiling-point. Only $\frac{1}{1600}$ of the space of the vapour is occupied by molecules; the rest is intermolecular space. The intermolecular distance in this vapour is $\sqrt[3]{1600}$ or approximately 12 times that in the liquid from which it was formed.

In a gas a molecule does not necessarily collide with its nearest neighbour. The average distance ('mean *free path*') travelled between two collisions is many times greater than the intermolecular distance. At N.T.P. the Loschmidt number $L = 2·68 \times 10^{19}$ molecules/cm³ (see p. 4). The *average distance* between two adjacent molecules is therefore given by $1/\sqrt[3]{L}$ cm which equals* 33 Å. The mean *free path* of a nitrogen molecule under these conditions was given (footnote on p. 2) as about 1000 Å, i.e. 30 times the average distance between molecules.

Diffusion in Gases and Liquids[1]

Fig. 274—(*a*) A jar containing oxygen (red) is inverted over a jar containing carbon dioxide (blue). Both gases are at the same pressure. A plate separates the two jars. The jar containing the lighter of the two gases is placed on top so that gravity will tend to keep the gases apart when the plate is removed.

(*b*) The plate is removed and within four minutes 25% of each gas has travelled into the other by diffusion.

(*c*) By the end of nine minutes a 50% transfer has occurred.

(*d*) At the end of twenty minutes transfer is 75% complete.

This molecular mixing or diffusion has taken place despite the opposing influence of gravity.

Fig. 275—The experiment is repeated using liquids instead of gases.

(*a*) The upper jar contains water and the lower a 5% solution of glucose in water (specific weight** $= 1·024$).

(*b*) The glass plate is removed and a 25% transfer of molecules takes one month to be accomplished.

(*c*) Six months elapse before a 50% transfer takes place.

(*d*) One year passes before 75% mixing is effected.

This process of molecular intermingling is called *diffusion*. Figs. 274 and 275 show that in gases at normal pressures diffusion takes place rapidly, while in liquids the process is extremely slow.

In the alveoli the inspired air diffuses readily into the residual air.

---

* Å = Angstrom unit, 1 Å = 10^{-8} cm; see also Ch. XXIV.
** The specific weight of this solution is often given as 1024, i.e. 1000 times greater. This value is based on the MKS (Meter-Kilogram-Second) system of units in which the specific weight of pure water becomes 1000 (kilogram per cubic metre).

In spinal anaesthesia the diffusion of the molecules of the injected anaesthetic drug in the cerebro-spinal fluid is so slow that it can be ignored as a factor affecting the spread up and down the spinal canal. In fact, the spread of a spinal anaesthetic solution in the cerebro-spinal fluid (c.s.f.) is accounted for by convection currents resulting in movement in bulk. These currents are set up by gravity, by the mechanical mixing of injection or of barbotage,[2] and by arterial pulsation.

Laws governing diffusion

The greater the difference in concentration of a dissolved substance between two neighbouring layers of a solution, the greater the amount of the substance which diffuses, from the more to the less concentrated region in unit time.

Fick's Law states that *the rate of diffusion is proportional to the gradient of concentration,* that is, the change of concentration per unit length in the direction of diffusion. Diffusion from regions of high to lower concentration also occurs in gases, but here the process can be better described by saying that the diffusion rate of a gas in a mixture is proportional to the difference in partial pressure of the gas between two neighbouring regions of the mixture. The same consideration applies to a gas diffusing through a liquid. The concentration of the gas in the liquid is expressed by its tension (p. 241).

Inspiration draws air as far as the terminal bronchioles. From here, where the oxygen partial pressure is high, this gas diffuses into the alveoli and then across the membrane into the venous blood where the tension of oxygen is low. Diffusion of nitrogen does not take place since the partial pressure of this gas in the alveoli is the same as its tension in the blood.*

The kinetic theory of gases states that the molecular speed in a gas is inversely proportional to the square root of the molecular weight. Diffusion depends on molecular movement and in fact the rates of diffusion of gases at identical partial pressures through a porous earthenware partition or through certain membranes *are inversely proportional to the square roots of their molecular weights* (**Graham's Law**).

Example

$$\text{Molecular weight of oxygen} = 32$$
$$\text{,,   ,,   carbon dioxide} = 44$$
$$\frac{\text{Diffusion rate of oxygen}}{\text{Diffusion rate of carbon dioxide}} = \frac{^2\sqrt{44}}{^2\sqrt{32}} = \frac{6\cdot63}{5\cdot65} \backsim \frac{1\cdot2}{1}$$

* Molecular intermingling still proceeds even if the concentration gradient is nil. However, equal numbers of molecules diffuse then in either direction through any imagined area so that the *net transport* through it will be *nil*.

Thus oxygen diffuses 20% faster than carbon dioxide through a dry, porous partition.

Comparison of diffusion with bulk flow

The laws governing *bulk* flow of fluids through orifices must not be confused with those concerning the *diffusion* of a fluid through fine pores. The fundamental difference between these two processes is that bulk flow through orifices is determined by *density* and that diffusion through pores is determined by the *molecular weight* of the fluid.

A spurious analogy between these two processes can be drawn in the case of GASES at atmospheric pressure because the density is then proportional to the molecular weight; the proportional relation for the bulk flow:

$$\text{Volume Flowrate} \propto \frac{1}{\sqrt{\text{Density}}} \quad \text{can be written:}$$

$$\text{Volume Flowrate} \propto \frac{1}{\sqrt{\text{Molecular Weight}}}$$

A specific example for LIQUIDS might make the situation still clearer.

If water and liquid ether pass through identical orifices under the same driving pressure, ether will *flow faster* than water because the volume flowrate through an orifice is inversely proportional to the square root of the density of the fluid. The density of ether is 0·74 compared with that of water $= 1$. But the molecular weight of ether is much greater than that of water (74 : 18) and ether would *diffuse slower* than water through a porous partition according to Graham's law.

Diffusion through partitions and membranes

Gases do not only diffuse freely within a container as in fig. 274, but may pass through partitions such as membranes. The rates of diffusion of gases may be affected by the nature of the membrane. In some cases the difference is striking. Thus nitrogen and carbon dioxide diffuse through an earthenware partition at comparable rates. On the other hand a rubber bag is almost impervious to nitrogen yet allows carbon dioxide to diffuse through with measurable speed.

When a gas diffuses through a water film there is another factor to be taken into consideration—the solubility of the gas in water. The rate of diffusion of the gas is not only inversely proportional to the square root of the molecular weight, but is also directly proportional to the solubility of the gas in the liquid.

The alveolar membrane, always moist, can be regarded as a water film. Owing to the marked solubility of CO_2 in water the diffusion rate of this gas is high. The small pressure difference across the alveolar membrane is sufficient to effect satisfactory excretion.

Semi-Permeable Membranes

If the molecules of any fluid pass through a thin sheet of a substance this latter is referred to as a membrane. The membrane is said to be permeable to the particular molecules it lets through. Thus parchment is permeable to water, rubber to carbon dioxide, while a filter paper is permeable to gases and to most liquids and substances dissolved in them.

Diffusion, or intermolecular mingling, can take place through a permeable membrane on both sides of which the total pressures are equal. This process should be distinguished from transfer in bulk of the fluid, caused by a difference of hydrostatic pressure on either side of the membrane. The two processes can go on simultaneously.

In fig. 286, p. 258, a membrane permeable to water only, separates two solutions of salt of differing concentration. Molecules of water pass through the membrane in both directions but more pass from the side of the weaker solution to that of the stronger, so that finally the concentrations on both sides of the membrane are equal.

The membrane illustrated in fig. 59 is permeable to all the substances used in the experiment.

It should be clearly understood that diffusion is a molecular movement and should not be confused with movement in bulk, for which some external force such as gravity must be applied. Filtration is an example of bulk transfer.

Membranes vary in their permeability to dissolved molecules and their solvents. Some (for example, filter paper) are completely permeable to all dissolved substances and their solvents. Others allow the passage through them of molecules of certain substances only—hence the name semi-permeable membrane. Some of these bar the passage of all dissolved molecules and allow the transfer of solvents only.

Parchment of a certain kind is a semi-permeable membrane. It is permeable to water but not to cane sugar in solution. Salt in solution, however, passes through. The selectivity here is probably accounted for by the smaller size of the salt ions. Other membranes, like the envelope surrounding a red blood corpuscle, are permeable to sodium ions but not to potassium ions. Here some other factor plays a part, since the sizes of these ions are similar.

A rubber bag[3] can be regarded as a semi-permeable membrane, in that it allows diffusion through it of CO_2 but is practically impermeable to, say, oxygen or nitrous oxide.

Osmosis

Fig. 276—1% glucose solution is placed in a container, the bottom of which is formed by a semi-permeable membrane, permeable to water molecules but impermeable to glucose molecules. The container is

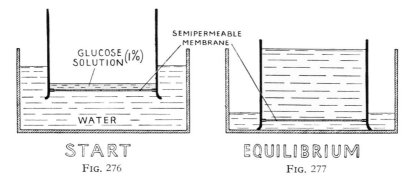

GLUCOSE SOLUTION (1%)

SEMIPERMEABLE MEMBRANE

WATER

START

Fig. 276

EQUILIBRIUM

Fig. 277

placed inside a large vessel containing water. Water molecules pass through the semi-permeable membrane and the glucose solution becomes diluted. As the quantity of liquid in it increases the glucose container gradually sinks. The transfer of water from the outer vessel into the inner glucose container ceases when the glucose solution reaches a certain height.

Fig. 277—Equilibrium is established. The difference between the hydrostatic pressures on each side of the membrane is sufficient to prevent more water entering the now very dilute glucose solution.

In the next experiment, too, a 1% glucose solution is separated by a semi-permeable membrane from water in an outer container. The tendency of the water to pass through the membrane and dilute the glucose solution is countered by the pressure exerted by the column of mercury pushed up into the capillary tube. Early in the experiment there is a transfer of water into the already full glucose container. This slight volume increase causes the mercury to be forced up the distal limb of the U-tube.

Fig. 278—*Start of the experiment.* The glucose container is full and communicates with a U-tube containing mercury. The proximal limb of the U-tube is dilated at one point to act as a mercury reservoir. A slight displacement of mercury from the reservoir is reflected by a large rise of the column in the distal limb of the calibrated capillary tube.

The pressure exerted by the glucose solution is atmospheric, as is shown by the levels of the mercury being equal.

Fig. 279—*End of the experiment.* When equilibrium is established no more water passes through the membrane into the glucose solution,

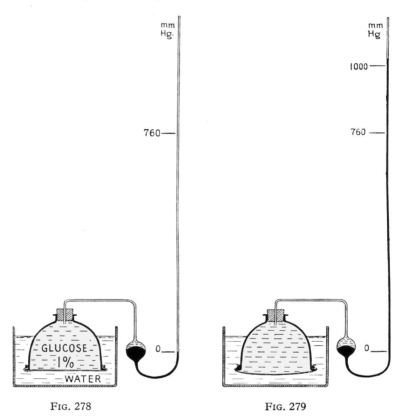

FIG. 278   FIG. 279

and the pressure inside the glucose chamber does not rise further. At this stage it will be seen that the mercury column is 1000 mmHg high. In other words a pressure of 1000 mm of mercury is necessary to counter the tendency of the water to pass through the semi-permeable membrane into the glucose solution.

Fig. 280—Diagram of a *semi-permeable membrane* with molecules of pure solvent, say water, on one side, and molecules of both water and a dissolved substance, such as glucose, on the other. Both liquids exert the same hydrostatic pressure. The semi-permeable membrane

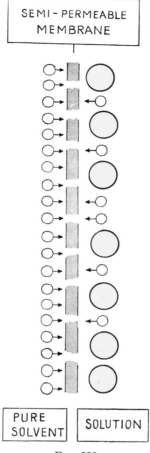

FIG. 280

allows molecules of water to pass freely through it but does not allow the passage of glucose molecules. Over a unit cross-section of membrane, more water molecules reach the membrane from the side of the pure water than from the side of the solution. Water passes freely through the membrane in both directions, but owing to the larger number of water molecules reaching the membrane on the water side, more water molecules pass through the membrane into the solution than in the reverse direction. The process continues until the solution becomes infinitely dilute. This migration of molecules of *solvent* across a membrane is called **osmosis.** Figs. 277 and 279 show that this transfer

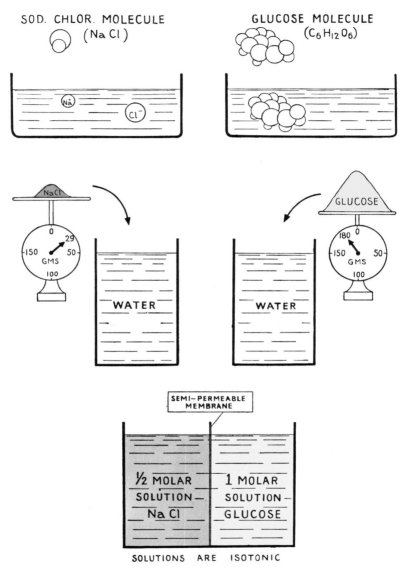

SOD. CHLOR. MOLECULE
(Na Cl)

GLUCOSE MOLECULE
($C_6 H_{12} O_6$)

WATER

WATER

SEMI-PERMEABLE
MEMBRANE

½ MOLAR SOLUTION— Na Cl

1 MOLAR SOLUTION— GLUCOSE

SOLUTIONS ARE ISOTONIC

Fig. 281

Fig. 282

Fig. 283

Fig. 284

Fig. 285

of pure solvent into the solution can be prevented by pressure applied to the solution. The pressure which just stops the transfer is known as the *osmotic pressure* of the solution.

Isotonic Solutions

Fig. 281—When in solution the molecules of many substances 'dissociate' into ions, and each ion behaves as a separate particle. For example, NaCl splits into Na^+ and Cl^- ions.

Fig. 282—Other substances do not ionize, and molecules remain the smallest particles of the substance in solution. Glucose, and many other organic compounds, fall into this latter group.

A *molar* solution of a substance (solute) is one which contains one mole of the substance dissolved in 1 litre of the final solution.* It can be prepared by placing 1 gram-molecular weight of solute into a measuring cylinder, and filling up with water (solvent) until the 1-litre mark is reached.

Fig. 283—A quantity of 29 grams of salt (NaCl—molecular weight 58) dissolved in the right amount of water to give 1 litre is a ½-molar solution of salt.

Fig. 284—Since the molecular weight of anhydrous glucose ($C_6H_{12}O_6$) is 180, a molar solution of glucose is one which contains 180 grams of glucose per litre.

Fig. 285—The osmotic pressure of a solution depends only on the number of dissolved particles per litre, and not on the nature of the substance dissolved.** A molar solution of glucose and a ½-molar solution of salt contain the same number of particles. The osmotic pressures exerted by the two solutions, therefore, are the same.

At 0 °C one mole of a substance which does not ionize, e.g. glucose, when dissolved in 22·4 litres of water, exerts an **osmotic pressure** of 1 atmosphere. In such dilutions the osmotic pressure of any given substance is directly proportional to its concentration, and the equation linking pressure and concentration is the same as for an ideal gas. Nevertheless, the phenomena of gas pressure and osmotic pressure are not strictly comparable.

Fig. 286—A bag made of semi-permeable membrane contains 500 cm³ of 0·5-molar solution of SODIUM CHLORIDE. It is immersed in the same quantity of 1-molar concentration of the same salt. Water passes from

---

* The *molarity* thus defined varies with temperature owing to the expansion of the given solution when heated. A slightly different expression known as *molality* does not alter with temperature and is often preferred. A *molal* solution contains 1 mole of solute per 1000 grams of solvent.
** This statement applies strictly only to very dilute solutions.

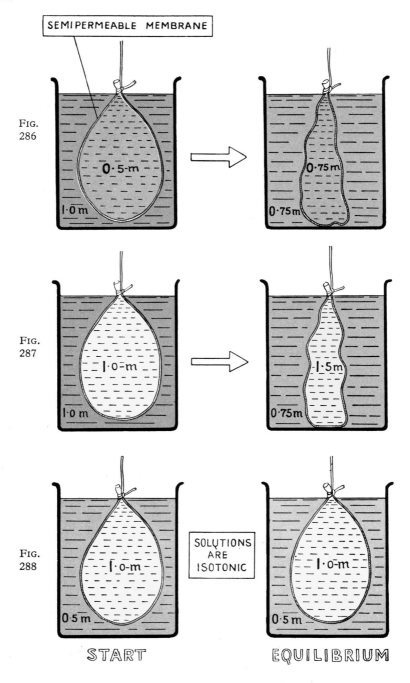

SEMIPERMEABLE MEMBRANE

FIG. 286

0·5·m

1·0 m

0·75 m

0·75 m

FIG. 287

1·0·m

1·0 m

1·5 m

0·75 m

FIG. 288

1·0·m

0·5 m

SOLUTIONS
ARE
ISOTONIC

1·0·m

0·5 m

START

EQUILIBRIUM

the interior of the bag to the surrounding solution. The bag shrinks and ultimately the concentration of salt outside and inside it becomes the same, that is, 0·75-molar concentration.

Fig. 287—Here a 1-molar solution of GLUCOSE within the bag (yellow) is immersed in the 1-molar SODIUM CHLORIDE solution (green). Water passes from the glucose solution to the salt solution; neither glucose nor salt can pass through the semi-permeable membrane. Osmotic equilibrium is reached when the bag contains a 1·5-molar concentration of glucose, and the surrounding sodium chloride a 0·75-molar concentration.

Fig. 288—A 1-molar solution of GLUCOSE in the bag is surrounded by a 0·5-molar solution of SODIUM CHLORIDE. Transfer of water does not occur since the osmotic pressure of the solutions is the same.

Haemolysis

If distilled water is added to a drop of blood the blood lakes; the red blood corpuscles swell, the membranes burst and the contained pigment is discharged. In clinical practice the red blood corpuscle is the standard of osmotic pressure, and relative to this distilled water and even 0·3% saline are *hypotonic*. If a 10% solution of saline is added to red blood corpuscles, water is drawn out from them and the cells shrink. Such a solution is *hypertonic*.

Experimentally it is found that solutions of 0·9% saline, or of 5% glucose, are isotonic.

That these solutions exert the same osmotic pressure is seen from the following calculations*:

0·9% NaCl solution = 9 grams NaCl in 1 litre saline
58 grams NaCl in 1 litre form a 1-molar solution

$\therefore$ 9 grams form a $\dfrac{9}{58}$ = 0·15-molar solution.

5% glucose solution = 50 grams glucose in 1 litre solution
180 grams glucose in 1 litre form a 1-molar solution

$\therefore$ 50 grams form a $\dfrac{50}{180}$ = 0·28 $\backsimeq$ 0·3-molar solution.

An isotonic saline or glucose solution injected subcutaneously is painless, whereas the reader can readily verify that an injection of distilled water causes sharp pain.

Circulatory Volume

In life, membranes such as the capillary walls and the lining of the tissue cells, are permeable to most of the substances dissolved in blood. Chlorine ions (Cl·), for example, pass through the membrane of an

* See also fig. 285.

erythrocyte in either direction (diffusion), and the final result is a transfer from the side of high concentration to the side of low. These living membranes, however, are at the same time impermeable to particles of other substances (for instance, the erythrocyte wall is impermeable to potassium ions) and the phenomena of osmotic pressure develop when such particles are present on one or both sides of the membrane. In the body this process of osmosis goes on simultaneously with diffusion, since absolute impermeability does not occur.

The capillary wall is relatively impermeable to sodium sulphate. On this account this salt is used intravenously to produce hydraemia. The first effect of introducing sodium sulphate is to raise the osmotic pressure of the blood; water streams in from the tissues and diuresis follows. Sodium sulphate does, however, diffuse slowly through the capillary wall, and eventually its concentration outside and inside the vessels is the same.

'Osmotic diffusion' is the hybrid term which describes the joint processes of osmosis and diffusion which go on simultaneously whenever a salt is introduced into the body.

Transfusion

An adequate intravascular volume is essential for the maintenance of an efficient circulation. The capillary walls are permeable to all substances normally dissolved in blood, except the proteins (serum globulin and albumen). The mechanism by which substances inside and outside the blood stream are maintained in equilibrium is delicately balanced. The filtration pressure in the capillaries (that is, the difference between blood pressure and tissue pressure) forces water and crystalloids out of the capillaries by filtration, while the osmotic pressure (25-30 mmHg) exerted by the colloids (serum globulin and albumen) tends to draw liquid inwards. A rise in blood pressure may cause an increase in extravascular liquid.

Salt and glucose pass through the capillary walls easily, so that equilibrium of these crystalloids on either side of the walls is soon established. Infusion of these plays little part in maintaining the circulatory volume. The integrity of the vessels carrying the blood is obviously essential. The mechanism by which the fluid balance of the body is controlled is easily disturbed by trauma, injudicious transfusion, prolonged anoxia and disease. The permeability of the capillary walls is increased by all these, even to the extent of allowing the passage of blood proteins.

Increased capillary permeability and diminished circulatory volume are essential features of 'shock', but whether they are the cause or the result of the shock is still undecided.

Transfusion of blood or plasma should be carried out early to break the vicious circle. Any improvement in circulation and of oxygenation may initiate recovery of capillary function. Delay may result in the damage to the capillary walls becoming irreparable so that they continue to be permeable to protein. An adequate blood volume and circulation cannot then be maintained. In these dire circumstances transfusion, even of blood, is not followed by the retention of fluid within the vessels; oedema of the tissues including the lungs follows.

Filtration

Many membranes (for example, the common filter paper) allow all dissolved substances to pass through unchanged, offering merely a resistance to their passage, so that only a pressure difference is required for the transfer to take place. This process of filtration is independent of the concentration of the substances on either side of the membrane.

Just as osmosis and diffusion often go on simultaneously (p. 260) so also do osmosis and filtration. A particular membrane may be freely permeable to certain substances and impermeable to others. If there is a hydrostatic pressure difference between the two sides of the membrane, both solvent and the molecules for which the membrane is permeable pass through by filtration. The passage of water by this process is opposed by the osmotic pressure of any substances left behind (which cannot pass through the membrane), and which tends to draw water in the reverse direction. The filtration pressure is the difference in hydrostatic pressure between the two sides of the membrane, and must be greater than the osmotic pressure before filtration commences.

Kidney Function

In health the glomerulus of the kidney is both a semi-permeable membrane and a filtering membrane. It bars the passage of colloids but allows salts and many other substances in the blood stream to filter through. The rate of filtration depends on the pressure difference between the two sides of the membrane and thus on the blood pressure.

The osmotic pressure of the blood colloids is 30 mmHg, and it is known that a pressure of 30–40 mmHg is required to overcome the resistance of the kidney tubules and the rest of the urinary tract. A blood pressure of above 70 mmHg is therefore required for kidney function.

The danger of a prolonged fall in blood pressure is obvious.

FIG. 289

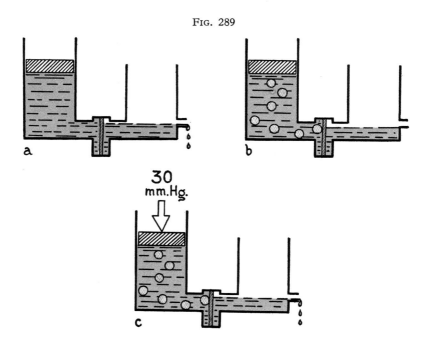

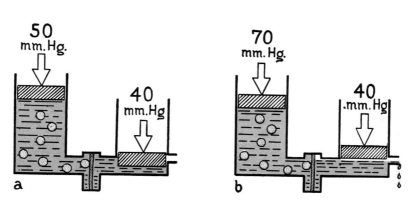

FIG. 290

Fig. 289—(*a*) Two chambers are separated by a membrane. The left-hand chamber contains a solution of salts (NaCl, urea, etc.) to all of which the membrane is permeable. The weight of the piston and the hydrostatic pressure of the liquid supply a filtration pressure which causes the solution to flow through the membrane unchanged into the right-hand chamber, and to escape through the outlet at a certain rate.

(*b*) A colloid, globulin, to which the membrane is impermeable, has been added to the solution until the concentration of globulin is equivalent to that of the total blood colloids.

The osmotic pressure due to the colloid opposes the filtration pressure. The absence of flow through the membrane shows that the osmotic pressure is the greater.

(*c*) A force is applied to the piston resulting in a pressure rise of 30 mmHg in the left-hand chamber. Solution, containing the salts to which the membrane is permeable but not the colloid, flows through the membrane at the same rate as in (*a*). The osmotic pressure of the colloid has been overcome by the added pressure of 30 mmHg .

Fig. 290—(*a*) A piston is inserted into the right-hand chamber and a force applied to it, resulting in a pressure of 40 mmHg . Even though the pressure in the left chamber is raised some 20 mmHg above that in the previous figure, flow through the membrane ceases.

(*b*) To counteract the pressure of 40 mmHg in the right-hand chamber and to ensure a flow of liquid, the pressure in the left-hand chamber must be raised by 40 mmHg over that shown in fig. 289 (*c*). The liquid again flows through the membrane at the same rate as in fig. 289 (*c*).

This illustration is meant to represent kidney function. The membrane is the glomerular membrane, the left-hand chamber the arterial blood, the right-hand chamber the urinary tract with a constant back pressure of about 40 mmHg . In order for urine to begin trickling down the urinary tract a minimum blood pressure of about 70 mmHg is required. In this diagram the pressure acting on the membrane is above 70 mmHg and the flow of liquid is more than a trickle.

Pulmonary Oedema

During inspiration the pressure in the lungs is subatmospheric and is exerted in all directions. This negative pressure tends to draw into the alveoli both air via the trachea and fluid out of the capillaries. Normally the air-route is clear; air flows freely and a high negative pressure does not develop. The difference between the capillary blood pressure and the subatmospheric pressure in the alveoli is less than the

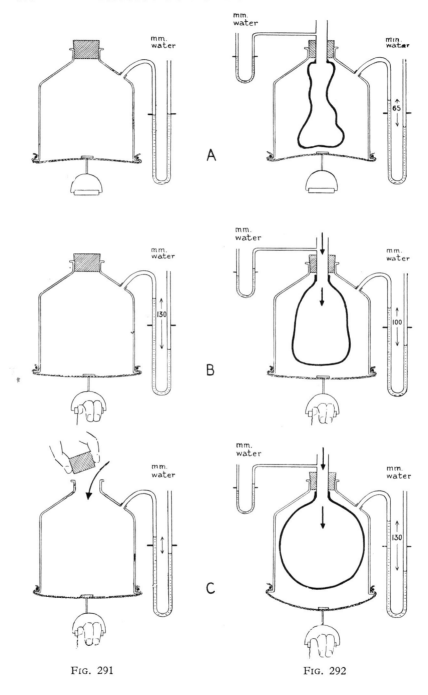

FIG. 291   FIG. 292

osmotic pressure exerted by the colloids in the capillaries, hence no liquid can exude into the alveoli. If, however, the airway is obstructed from any cause an increased negative pressure may develop in the lungs during the inspiratory effort. This negative pressure may be large enough to result in a filtration pressure sufficiently great to draw fluid out of the pulmonary capillaries into the alveoli. Pulmonary oedema results if the obstruction is long continued.

A patient with left-sided heart failure already has a raised pulmonary capillary pressure (cf. filtration pressure, p. 261). In such a case respiratory obstruction, even of short duration, may be disastrous.

The results of respiratory obstruction in the shocked patient are known to be particularly noxious. Here the capillary walls are damaged and permeable to substances to which they are normally impermeable. Pulmonary oedema soon follows.

Fig. 291—(A) A large bell jar with a well-fitting cork has its base formed by a rubber diaphragm. The water manometer shows that the pressure inside the jar is atmospheric.

(B) The diaphragm is pulled down until a negative pressure of — 130 mmH$_2$O develops.

(C) When the cork is removed air rushes in and the pressure inside the jar reverts to atmospheric.

Fig. 292—An experiment simulating normal inspiration. The bell jar now represents the thoracic cage, while the tube and an elastic bag take the place of the trachea and lungs.

(A) The pressure within the bag, measured by the manometer on the left, is atmospheric. Some air has already been sucked out from the space between the jar and the bag, producing a subatmospheric pressure of — 65 mmH$_2$O inside the jar. This represents the negative intrapleural pressure which always exists at the start of normal inspiration. This negative pressure is just enough to overcome the elastic recoil of the lungs, here represented by the elastic bag,* which would otherwise collapse completely.

(B) Inspiration—the diaphragm descends. The negative intrapleural pressure increases and soon reaches — 100 mmH$_2$O. Since air is able to pass freely into the lungs the *intrapulmonary* negative pressure, however, never rises above a few millimetres of water.

(C) Height of inspiratory flow. The intrapleural pressure reaches — 130 mmH$_2$O while the intrapulmonary pressure soon reverts to

* If the bag were sufficiently big and inelastic it would expand until the pressure outside it became equal to that inside it, that is, atmospheric.

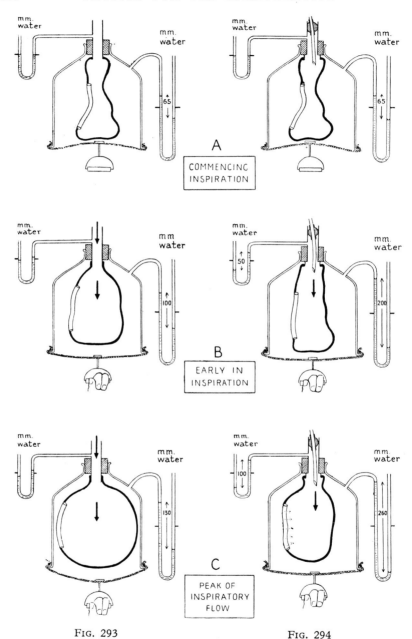

A
COMMENCING
INSPIRATION

B
EARLY IN
INSPIRATION

C
PEAK OF
INSPIRATORY
FLOW

FIG. 293   FIG. 294

atmospheric. The increased intrapleural negative pressure is necessary to overcome the increased tension of the elastic tissue in the lungs as they are made to expand.

On expiration the diaphragm relaxes. The elastic tissue in the lung recoils; the situation again reverts to A.

The effect of breathing through an endotracheal tube of inadequate bore

Fig. 293—The three figures on the left-hand side of the page, the same as those in fig. 292, represent inspiration through a normal *unobstructed* airway.

Fig. 294—In the figures on the right-hand side the inspired air has to pass through an endotracheal tube of inadequate bore. Entry of air round the tube is prevented by an inflated cuff. A capillary on the alveolar wall is indicated.

(A) *Commencing inspiration.*

(B) *Early in inspiration.*

The left figure 293 (unobstructed respiration) shows that when the intrapleural negative pressure reaches $- 100$ mmH$_2$O the intrapulmonary pressure deviates but little from that of the external atmosphere (left manometer). This is accounted for by the fact that air passes freely into the lungs.

In the right figure 294 the diaphragm descends, but owing to the resistance offered by the small bore endotracheal tube air cannot enter the lungs freely. In this experiment the negative intrapleural pressure at this stage reaches $- 200$ mmH$_2$O, and the intrapulmonary pressure $- 50$ mmH$_2$O .

(C) *Maximum of inspiratory flow.*

The negative intrapleural pressure is found to be $- 260$ mmH$_2$O, and the negative intrapulmonary pressure $- 100$ mmH$_2$O if the airway is obstructed. As a result of the inadequate tube, considerable further effort must be made for the lungs to expand more fully during the time normally taken for inspiration.

Sequelae to Respiratory Obstruction

The extra muscular work to expand the thorax is not the only evil the patient has to contend with. The increased negative intrapulmonary pressure may be sufficient to upset the delicate balance by which fluid is retained within the pulmonary capillaries. This tendency is shown by the ghosted arrows in fig. 294 C. Pulmonary oedema from this cause is discussed on p. 263.

The ultimate result to the patient depends on whether he is shocked

or not, on the degree of obstruction and on how long this undesirable
state of affairs is allowed to continue. Thus we have seen a healthy
young man exposed to moderate obstruction for twenty minutes without obvious ill effects, but we have heard of deaths from pulmonary

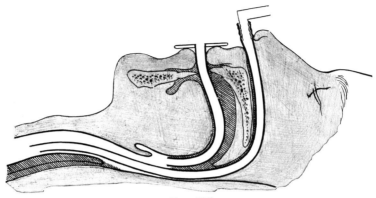

FIG. 295

oedema following prolonged operations in which the adequacy of the
airway was suspect.

If an endotracheal tube is to be used it should be of the largest
reasonable bore. If there is any doubt about the adequacy of the bore
a mouth airway should be inserted in addition, so that further air can
be inspired through the space between the outside of the tube and the
vocal cords (fig. 295). As a corollary, an anaesthetist should not use an
inflatable cuff on an endotracheal tube the bore of which is too small.

After the endotracheal tube has been passed a good idea of whether
the airpath is adequate is afforded by watching the movement of the
chest wall during respiration. With an inadequate tube the inspiratory
movements are similar to those due to obstruction from any other cause.
The diaphragm descends, and since air cannot be drawn in freely the
anomalous situation arises that on inspiration the chest wall does not
expand but is sucked in.

The paradox is explained by the fact that since air cannot be drawn
in freely a strong intrathoracic negative pressure develops, and the chest
wall collapses under the influence of the pressure of the outside
atmosphere.

Obstruction in an adult may be recognized as an indrawing of the
intercostal and supraclavicular spaces, whilst in a child, with a pliable
thoracic cage, the whole chest wall may be sucked in. If the anaesthetist

is careless, *paradoxical respiration* from respiratory obstruction may be mistaken for that which results from paralysis of the intercostal muscles —a sign of deep anaesthesia, rediscovered by successive generations of anaesthetists since the time of Snow.[4]

Endotracheal tubes can be a great boon, but they are often used quite unnecessarily, and to the detriment of the patient. Their value in certain cases, including head and neck and thoracic operations, is unquestioned. In many others they are used only because the anaesthetist is too lazy to maintain an airway by other means, or thinks that nothing can go wrong since an endotracheal tube has been passed. The passage of an endotracheal tube is not synonymous with adequate oxygenation. We have known an anaesthetist called back from a neighbouring room because the oxygen cylinder had emptied unexpectedly. The endotracheal tube itself can kink (fig. 160) and we have known it to become blocked with blood clot. The manoeuvre of passing an endotracheal tube does not relieve the anaesthetist of his obvious obligation of giving the patient his undivided attention.

The ease of respiration through an endotracheal tube rarely equals that through the normal airpath. Certainly the use of tubes of inadequate size is far too frequent an occurrence. In such cases respiratory obstruction can be relieved by the simple expedient of withdrawing the tube and giving the patient a chance to breathe normally!

REFERENCES

[1] SMITH, A. S. (1934). *Ind. Eng. Chem.*, **26,** 1167.
[2] MACINTOSH, SIR ROBERT (1957). *Lumbar puncture and spinal analgesia*, 2nd ed., p. 124. Edinb.
[3] AMERONGEN, G. J. VAN (1946). *J. appl. Physics*, **17,** cf. p. 976, Table I.
[4] SNOW, J. (1858). *On chloroform and other anaesthetics*, p. 42. Lond.

Chapter XIX

PRINCIPLES OF CERTAIN ANAESTHETIC APPARATUS

The Development of Nitrous Oxide Apparatus

Until about 1870 nitrous oxide had to be made on the spot since no commercial supply was available. The gas was made by heating ammonium nitrate in a glass retort and removing the grosser impurities by washing the gas in various reagents. The gas was collected under slight positive pressure in a large gas holder from which it could be later inhaled by the patient.

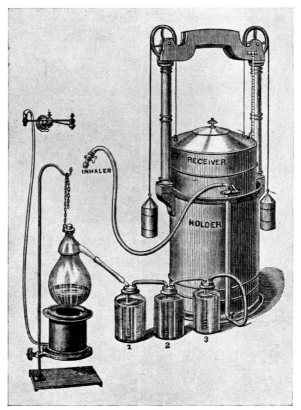

Fig. 296

Fig. 296—Old nitrous oxide apparatus designed by Sprague,[1] *circa* 1863. The nitrous oxide gas is generated in the retort on the left, passes through the wash bottles and is subsequently inhaled through the mouthpiece labelled 'inhaler'.

Wash bottles number 1 and 2 contain a solution of ferrous oxide to remove the toxic nitric oxides. Bottle number 3 contains sticks of potassium hydroxide to remove chlorine derived from impurities in the ammonium nitrate. The gas is finally stored in the 'receiver' or reservoir from which it is subsequently inhaled.

In 1868, the gas was liquefied on a commercial scale and supplied in cylinders both by Coxeter and Barth in Great Britain. The popularity of this anaesthetic at once increased. Its purity was assured, and as the size of the cylinder now containing liquid nitrous oxide was only 1/400 of the volume of gas it liberated, transport presented no problems.

The liquefaction of nitrous oxide did not at once make the apparatus for its administration less cumbersome. As will be seen later, a reservoir

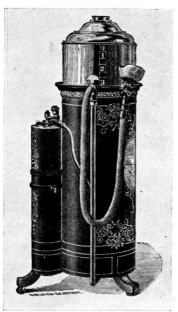
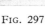
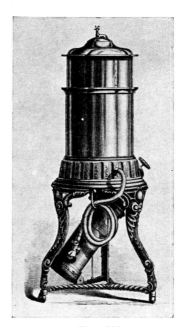

FIG. 297   FIG. 298

of some sort is an essential feature of all anaesthetic machines past and present. For some time the ornate and cumbersome gasholders continued to fulfil this function, and these were filled as required from a cylinder of compressed nitrous oxide (fig. 297). In this way a reservoir of gaseous nitrous oxide was available from which the patient could fill his lungs with ease.

Fig. 297—The gasometer is filled as required from the cylinder of liquid nitrous oxide on the left. The patient inhales from this reservoir. The facemask and wide-bore breathing tube are seen looped in front of the reservoir.

Fig. 298—The cylinder of compressed nitrous oxide is suspended beneath the reservoir. The wide-bore breathing tube is coiled in front of the cylinder.

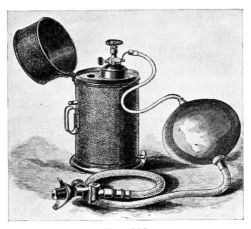

FIG. 299

In the same year that saw the introduction of compressed nitrous oxide in cylinders, a more convenient reservoir in the form of a rubber bag was introduced by CATTLIN. It took some time, however, before this bag displaced the cumbersome and immobile gasholder.

Fig. 299—Shows an early, transportable nitrous oxide apparatus[2] with reservoir bag: "for convenience in carrying to the house of a patient, or to a distance, a metal case, covered with morocco, made large enough to contain not only the cylinder, but also the bag, inhaler and tubing, is preferred". The cumbersome gasholder has given place to the more mobile rubber bag reservoir which is kept filled from the cylinder throughout anaesthesia, and from which the patient inhales. Notice the narrow bore pressure tubing between cylinder and bag, and the wide-bore tube through which the patient inhales.

The identity of Cattlin's reservoir bag and the once commonly

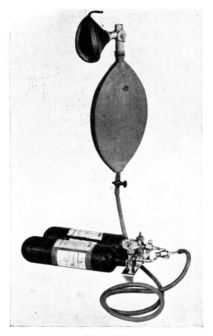

FIG. 300

misnamed 'rebreathing' bag* on modern apparatus is apparent from fig. 301.

Fig. 300—Nitrous oxide apparatus, 1912.

Here the reservoir bag happens to be near the facemask. It would function equally well if it were placed near the cylinders, *provided the breathing tube leading from it to the patient is wide enough to offer only negligible resistance to breathing.*

In skilled hands the apparatus gives satisfactory results in minor surgery. The rate of flow of gas is controlled by the foot key and, if the administration is prolonged, the requisite oxygen is derived from the air inspired as the mask is raised from the face from time to time.

Improvement of primitive apparatus is desirable, but technical elaboration can never dispense with the necessity of the anaesthetist being trained in basic principles. Better this simple apparatus in the hands of the expert than the most elaborate of gas/oxygen machines in charge of someone inexperienced.

* Although it was possible to set the stopcock next to the facemask (figs. 299 and 300) so that rebreathing occurred, the main function of the bag was as a reservoir.

The Principle of the Semi-open Anaesthetic Apparatus

Fig. 301—The 'gas and oxygen apparatus' in its simplest form consists of a cylinder of nitrous oxide and another of oxygen connected by rubber tubing to a reservoir bag. From this a length of *wide-bore* rubber

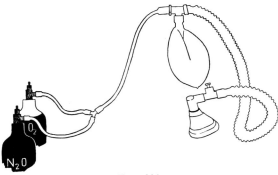

FIG. 301

tubing leads to the facemask, close to which is an expiratory valve. The gases are drawn from the reservoir bag through the breathing tube principally by the force of the patient's inspiration. The breathing tube must, therefore, have a lumen large enough to ensure that undue resistance to inspiration is not produced. The internal diameter of a breathing tube of standard length should not be less than 2 cm ($\frac{3}{4}$ in).

The Function of the Reservoir Bag

If an adult with a tidal volume of 500 ml breathes 14 times a minute, his respiratory minute volume is 7 litres. During respiration the patient inhales intermittently and the significant part of inspiration commonly occupies only about $\frac{1}{3}$ of the respiratory cycle.* During inspiration, therefore, the flow rate of gases into this patient's lungs averages about 21 litres per minute. During anaesthesia this rapid but intermittent inrush of air into the patient's lungs must be provided for either by a continuous flow of gases to the facemask of at least 21 l/min or, as is done in actual practice, by incorporating in the anaesthetic assembly a reservoir which is replenished by a continuous stream of gases from the cylinders at the slower rate of 7 l/min.

* The duration of the flow of gases in and out of the lungs during inspiration and expiration is almost equal (p. 177). The effective part of inspiration occupies about $\frac{1}{3}$ of the cycle; during this time the major part of inspiration takes place.

A certain minimum volume[3,4] of fresh gases per minute must be supplied if all the patient's carbon dioxide is to be carried away to the outside air.

The average adult patient under basal conditions consumes approximately 250 ml of oxygen per minute. Assuming a respiratory quotient of 0·9, the corresponding CO_2 output is 225 ml. If the CO_2 content of the expired air is known to be 4%, the total volume of gases exhaled is $\frac{100}{4} \times 225$ ml,—say 6 litres. This, therefore, is the minimum volume of fresh gases which must be inspired to ensure that all the expired CO_2 is carried away, thus keeping constant the CO_2 tension in the alveoli.

During anaesthesia administered with a Boyle's machine, expirations pass through the expiratory valve. To ensure that at least 6 litres of expired gases pass through the valve every minute it is obvious that not less than 6 litres per minute of fresh gases must be supplied to the patient from the cylinders. If the supply falls below this, some rebreathing into the breathing tube takes place, and there is thus inevitably some CO_2 mixed with the inspired gases. In practice the supply of fresh gases should always exceed the respiratory minute volume of the patient. For an adult the combined volumes of nitrous oxide and oxygen added each minute should not be less than 7 litres. In the case of a child this volume can be cut down but should always generously exceed the child's respiratory minute volume. It is never advisable, even in the case of an infant, to reduce the total volume below 4 litres a minute.

Pressure Reducing Valves

Fig 302—The addition of pressure reducing valves to the cylinders

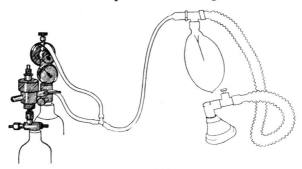

FIG. 302

of compressed gases was a considerable advance. Not only was the control of the high pressure gas made easier, but for any given setting of the tap on the flow meter, a constant flow rate was maintained independent of the fluctuation of pressure inside the cylinder. The need for cumbersome high pressure tubing between cylinder and flow meter was also obviated.

Details of the working principles of these reducing valves are given in Chapter XI.

Flowmeters

Flowmeters were incorporated to deliver with accuracy the desired flow rates of known mixtures of gases from cylinder to patient.

Fig. 303—The control tap at the bottom of the flowmeters (x) is

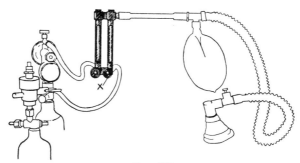

FIG. 303

usually a simple needle valve. With this arrangement reducing valves are essential. The pressure to which these are adjusted should not exceed 10 lb/in² (0·7 atm) if simple slip-on rubber connections are used. Otherwise, when the needle valve on the flowmeter is turned down, the tubing might be blown off. This arrangement is cheap compared with the high pressure tubing and unions necessary to withstand the pressure of 60 lb/in² (4 atm) at which the McKesson reducing valve is usually set.

Like a speedometer on a motor car a flowmeter is a useful refinement; neither is absolutely essential, but both contribute to safety. Both these instruments may give inaccurate readings. Just as the good motorist is guided more by his sensation of speed than by the speedometer, so the good anaesthetist is guided by the condition of his patient and not by the readings on the flowmeter. Taking for granted the airway is clear a blue patient needs more oxygen, no matter the reading on the flowmeters.

Liquid anaesthetics

Fig. 304—Bottles are incorporated to vaporize liquid anaesthetics, for example, ether, vinesthene, chloroform, trichlorethylene ('Trilene') or halothane ('Fluothane'). Each bottle is fitted with a control tap by which the gases leaving the flowmeters can be made to by-pass or to pass through the bottle. The mechanism by which this is done is illustrated on p. 278.

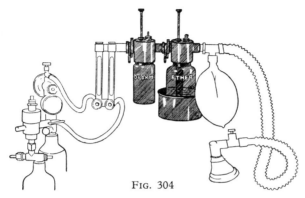

FIG. 304

The Complete Boyle's Apparatus

The addition of spare cylinders of oxygen and nitrous oxide to the apparatus in fig. 304 completes this series of illustrations.

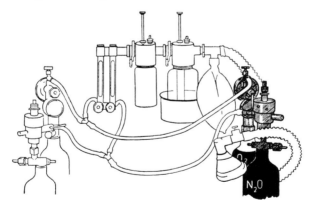

Figs. 305 and 306 will be familiar to our British readers as the ubiquitous Boyle's apparatus. The way it has been built up is now apparent. Many other continuous flow anaesthetic apparatuses incorporate individual refinements but function on the same general principles.

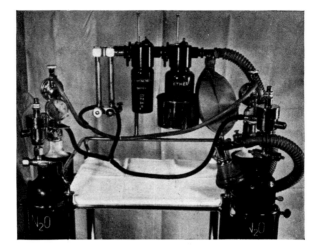

FIG. 306

Bottles for vaporizing liquid anaesthetics

The method of varying the concentration of anaesthetic vapour delivered from bottles on Boyle's apparatus is as follows.

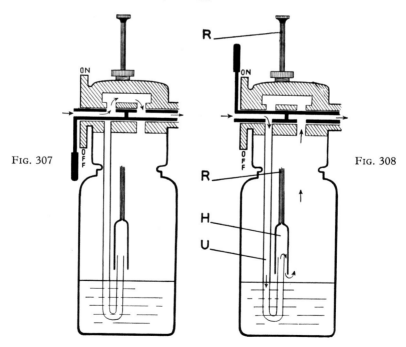

FIG. 307   FIG. 308

Fig. 307—Direct passage of the gases from the flowmeters to the patient is prevented by a permanent partition in the horizontal rotor tube. When the handle of the tap is in the OFF position (fig. 307), the gases are diverted completely from the bottle.

Fig. 308—With the tap in the ON position the gases all pass through the bottle containing the liquid anaesthetic.

The control tap can be placed in any intermediate position, and this determines how much of the total volume of gases passes through the ether bottle. This is one way of controlling the concentration of ether vapour to the patient.

A further means of controlling the ether vapour concentration is provided. Any gases which pass through the ether bottle (fig. 309) must go through the U-shaped metal tube (U) before emerging into the space above the surface of the liquid anaesthetic in the bottle. The open end of the tube (U) is covered by a metal hood (H) which can be positioned as required by moving the rod (R) attached to it up or down.

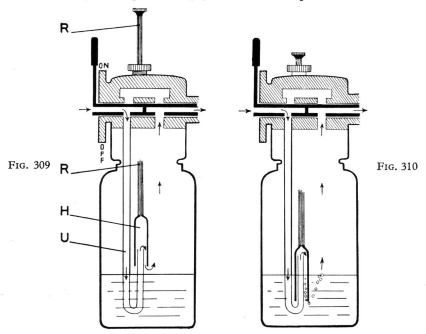

FIG. 309   FIG. 310

Fig. 310—As the hood is pushed downward, the path which the gases must take is deflected nearer and nearer to the surface of the liquid ether. Finally, when the open end of the hood is depressed below this level the gases must bubble through the liquid ether on their way to the outlet. With the tap in the ON position and the hood fully depressed, the whole gas flow bubbles through the maximum depth of ether and a maximum concentration of ether vapour is picked up.

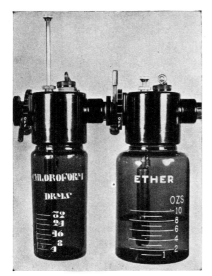

FIG. 311. Boyle's bottles.

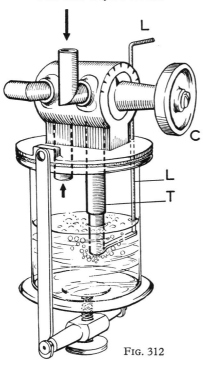

FIG. 312

Fig. 311—The working of these two bottles depends on the same principle, but they differ in the following details: (1) the chloroform bottle is smaller than the ether bottle; (2) the chloroform bottle is usually coloured green and the ether bottle amber; (3) the ether bottle may be surrounded by a metal container filled with tepid water to supply heat for the vaporization of the liquid ether (p. ·39).

An early Boyle-type bottle

The principle of the so-called Boyle bottle was in fact used by WALLER* in his quantitative chloroform apparatus[5] some fifteen years before the introduction of the Boyle's apparatus.[6]

Fig. 312—Shows the details of Waller's vaporizer for liquid anaesthetics.

By turning the control (C) the air from a foot pump could be diverted into the central tube (T). When the rod (L) was pulled up, the air passed over the liquid level; when it was pushed down as in the illustration, the air was forced to bubble through the liquid.

The 'modern' Boyle bottle could with advantage adopt the even regulation afforded by the control tap on Waller's vaporizer.

The bottle on the Boyle's apparatus is quite unsuitable for inclusion in a closed circuit, since the narrow bore of the gas channels would offer an

* The Waller balance, with attached chloroform bottles and controls, illustrated on p. 8 is in the possession of the Nuffield Department of Anaesthetics, to which it was presented by his daughter, Miss M. D. Waller, Ph.D., B.Sc.

intolerable resistance to respiration. In Boyle's apparatus the resistance offered by the bottle is overcome by the pressure of gases from the cylinders. After leaving the bottles the gases accumulate in the reservoir bag. The rubber tubing connecting this bag with the mask is of wide bore; thus minimal resistance to inspiration is presented to the patient.

Ether vaporizers in breathing circuits

The surface area of liquid ether exposed to the gases passing through an anaesthetic bottle can be considerably increased by the use of wicks.

Fig. 313—Wick vaporizer of the McKesson type with the indicator (arrow head) in the OFF position. The respired gases do not enter the bottle at all, but pass through the wide bore tube direct to the patient.

Fig. 314—The half-way position. Part of the gases pass direct to the patient; the remainder are directed into the bottle and through the gauze soaked in ether.

Fig. 315—When the control is turned to ON all the gases pass through the vaporizer.

Two or three thicknesses of cotton gauze held between two layers of

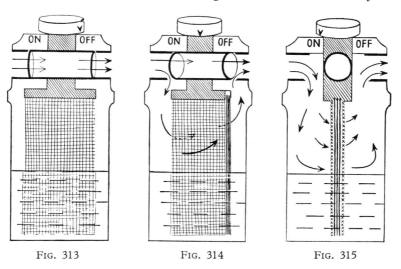

| FIG. 313 | FIG. 314 | FIG. 315 |

copper gauze dip well below the surface of the liquid in the bottle. The liquid ether rises by capillary attraction, and a large surface of ether is brought into intimate contact with gases passing through the bottle. The wide bore gas channel offers but negligible resistance to respiration, so that this type of vaporizer is suitable for all types of anaesthetic machines—closed circuit, intermittent or continuous flow. The wick should not present a complete barrier to the passage of gases. A damp wick can offer considerable resistance.

The ether vaporizer on the Coxeter-Mushin[7] absorber overcomes

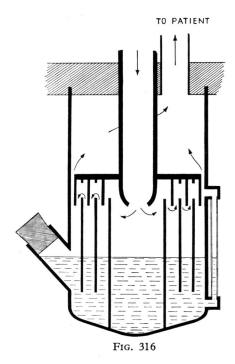

TO PATIENT

FIG. 316

two of the disadvantages sometimes found in vaporizers on other closed circuit machines, namely, the resistance to breathing caused by wicks or gauze, and the gradual falling-off of the ether vaporization, when water condenses on the cold wicks and impedes the rise of liquid ether into the meshes of the gauze. These disadvantages are overcome by dispensing with the wicks altogether. Despite this, good contact is ensured by deflecting the gases, by means of baffles, several times on to the surface of the liquid ether. The ether container is made of copper, which effectively conducts a good supply of heat from the rest of the apparatus.

The method of adding ether from a drop bottle to an anaesthetic system dates back to the beginning of anaesthetics.

Fig. 317—In 1847 MORTON patented an inhaler incorporating the dripper principle,[8] so that "the quantity of liquid required to keep up the necessary supply . . . during inhalation may be regulated by raising the valve to such height above the seat as circumstances may require".

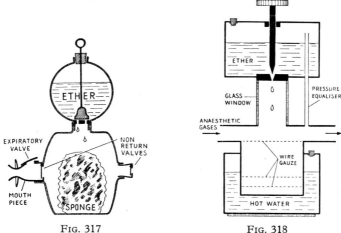

FIG. 317   FIG. 318

Ether drippers of one sort or another have been attached to anaesthetic apparatus from Morton's day to the present time. The general principle is illustrated in fig. 318.

This method of adding a liquid anaesthetic to a closed circuit is not as foolproof as might at first appear. Unlike the other vaporizers described, ether can be added to the circuit whether the patient is breathing or not. If the patient holds his breath for any reason, and ether continues to drip, the subsequent inhalation of the strong vapour which accumulates may cause violent coughing or laryngeal spasm. The rate at which the drops of ether are added to the circuit must be carefully controlled to ensure smooth induction.

REFERENCES

[1] DUNCUM, B. M. (1947). *The development of inhalation anaesthesia*, p. 275, fig. 68. Oxf.
[2] GUILFORD, S. H. (1887). *Nitrous oxide*, p. 40. Philad.
[3] MOLYNEUX, L., and PASK, E. A. (1951). *Brit. J. Anaesth.*, **23**, 81–91.
[4] MAPLESON, W. W. (1954). *Brit. J. Anaesth.*, **26**, 323–32.
[5] WALLER, A. D. (1911). *B.M.A. report of the special chloroform commission*, p. 45. Lond.
[6] BOYLE, H. E. G. (1919). *Lancet*, i, 226.
[7] MUSHIN, W. W. (1943). *Brit. J. Anaesth.*, **18**, 96–111.
[8] GOULD, A. A., and MORTON, W. T. G. (1847). U.S. Pat. 5365.

Chapter XX

EXPLOSIONS *Part* 1:

OXIDATION, COMBUSTION AND FLAMES

Combustible Anaesthetics

CERTAIN volatile anaesthetics and numerous other, closely related, compounds, commonly used in chemical laboratories and in industry, are members of a large group of combustible substances whose vapours form '*flammable*' mixtures with air or oxygen. Some of these begin to burn when heated above a certain high temperature, while others may gradually alter their character when stored at room temperature and suddenly explode violently at the slightest provocation.

The risks associated with the flammability of such substances are familiar to workers in industry, to miners and to scientists. Much information concerning explosions in these circumstances and on the precautions against ignition of flammable mixtures has been accumulated.

Scientists concerned in industrial safety measures and anaesthetists interested in avoiding explosions, are often struck by the complacency and the lack of knowledge shown by those working in operating theatres about the explosive properties of anaesthetics. This is in striking contrast to workers in factories where the risk of explosions is present; even the least trained are usually well aware of the rules drawn up to avoid ignition of flammable mixtures. The widespread ignorance of operating theatre personnel not only on combustible anaesthetics but on other flammable substances, seems regrettable in view of the profuse if sometimes inaccurate literature on this subject. In the following chapters we mainly discuss certain fundamental facts on explosions in an attempt to facilitate the study of more specialized publications[1,2] on this subject.

The Chemical Bond

In many reactions between gases the initial mixture (reactants) and the final mixture (products) consist of normal molecules. A molecule (p. 1) is composed of atoms held together by strong mutual attractions. Before atoms form a molecule, they are strongly reactive and attract one another when approaching. However, one atom can attract (bind) only a limited number of other atoms and form with these a limited number of bonds.[3]

Thus carbon (C) can attract only 4 hydrogen atoms (H) to form the molecule methane (CH_4). In chemical language: carbon is 4-valent and forms four single bonds with the 1-valent hydrogen atoms. Such bonds can be crudely visualized by endowing an atom with a number of hands equal to its valency. In one C-H bond the hand of H grasps one of the hands of C. In the methane molecule each of the four hands of C firmly grasps the one hand of each H:

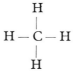

The most important feature of this type of chemical bond is that after its formation the atoms participating in the bond no longer attract any other atoms or molecules, but rather repel them. After one C and four H have firmly grasped hands, any strangers are elbowed away.

In the water molecule (H_2O or H-O-H), the 2-valent oxygen atom (-O-) has joined hands with two 1-valent hydrogen atoms (-H). Although the attraction between the O and H atoms in the water molecule is very strong, a second water molecule approaching the first one would be strongly repelled by it when the distance between the two molecules falls below a certain minimum value known as collision diameter.

Chemical Reactions

The expression:

$$WX + YZ \rightarrow WY + XZ$$

describes a particular chemical reaction in which the reactants (molecules WX and YZ) are transformed into the products (molecules WY and XZ). The letters W, X, Y, Z represent the atoms* from which the reactant and product molecules are formed.

This scheme shows that a *chemical reaction* can be also considered as a *rearrangement of bonds between atoms*. In the reactants, the bonds W-X and Y-Z hold the respective atom pairs closely together. When molecule WX approaches molecule YZ, a mutual repulsion occurs at a distance between the centres of the molecules which is often several times as large as the distance W-X (or Y-Z) between the atoms *inside* the respective molecules. In the product molecules (WY and XZ), the atoms have found new partners; the distance between W and Y is now quite small and both remain tightly bonded together in molecule WY.

* Or group of atoms which remain together during the reaction.

Atom X is now part of molecule XZ, and in a collision with molecule WY the atom X can no longer approach closely to W; in other words, molecules WY and XZ repel one another in a collision.

Heat of Reaction and Bond Energy

When atoms attract one another and form a bond, energy is released. Conversely, the splitting of a bond requires energy which has to be supplied from outside.

Example

In the hydrogen molecule (H-H) the energy of the single bond between the two hydrogen atoms is high: 103·2 kcal have to be supplied to one mole of hydrogen gas to 'dissociate' every molecule into its two H-atoms. The magnitude of this dissociation energy may be better appreciated by the following comparison. The dissociation of 2 grams of hydrogen molecules into hydrogen atoms requires as much energy as the heat which raises the temperature of 1000 g water from 0 °C to boiling point.

We considered previously a chemical reaction as a rearrangement of bonds between individual atoms making up the molecules of reactants and products. From this it will be understandable without strict proof that the difference between bond energies of products and reactants determines whether heat is liberated or taken up during the reaction. If the bond energies of the products are greater than those of the reactants, the difference will be liberated as heat: the reaction is **exothermic.**

Example—Reaction of hydrogen with chlorine gas

This reaction is represented in the general scheme (p. 285) by choosing H atoms for W and X, Cl atoms for Y and Z. One then obtains:

$$H_2 + Cl_2 \rightarrow 2 \cdot HCl + 2 \times 22 \text{ kcal}$$

If one mole of hydrogen and one mole of chlorine molecules combine to yield two moles of hydrochloric acid gas, a quantity of heat equal to 2×22 kcal is liberated. Dividing both sides of this chemical equation by 2, one obtains on the right one mole of HCl, and the respective *heat of reaction* becomes 22 kcal.

It was shown above that the bond energy of H-H is 103·2 kcal/mole. The Cl atoms in the chlorine molecule are less strongly bound and the respective bond energy is 57. In the product molecule (HCl), the H and the Cl atoms are strongly attracted and the bond energy is similar to that in H_2, i.e. 103 kcal/mole. For the formation of one mole HCl from half a mole H_2 and half a mole Cl_2 we have the following rise in bond energies:

$$103 - \tfrac{1}{2} \times 103\cdot2 - \tfrac{1}{2} \times 57 = 22\cdot9$$

This theoretical value agrees closely with the measured heat of reaction of the process given on p. 286. The positive result ($+ 22$ kcal/mole) indicates that heat is liberated in this (exothermic) reaction.

Reactions with Oxygen (Oxidation)[4]

The commonest chemical reaction in nature is that between oxygen and other molecules, known as *oxidation*. Most oxidations are accompanied by liberation* of energy in the form of heat and are therefore exothermic reactions.

The energies needed both to support life and to propel a steam locomotive are derived from oxidation processes. As in the examples of general chemical reactions, we can consider the reaction of oxygen with other molecules as a regrouping of atoms leading to more stable arrangements (product molecules) with liberation of heat. In the oxidation of hydrogen, water molecules (H_2O) are formed in which two hydrogen atoms are linked by single bonds to one O atom (H-O-H). The chemical equation:

$$2\cdot H_2 + O_2 \rightarrow 2\cdot H_2O$$

can be interpreted as a breaking of the bonds between the H atoms in the H_2 molecules, between the O atoms in the O_2 molecule, and the formation of new bonds between one O and two H in each of the two water molecules:

the sum of the two O-H bonds in one H_2O is   : 218   kcal/mole;
the bond energy of a single H_2 is again : 103·2 kcal/mole
and the bond energy of one O_2 is   : 117   kcal/mole.

The difference of bond energies between products and reactants becomes:

$$2 \times 218 - 2 \times 103\cdot2 - 117 = 114 \ (\text{or } 2 \times 57)$$

From this it follows that 57 kcal should be liberated for every single mole of water vapour formed by the oxidation of hydrogen.

Combustion

We shall shortly see that the oxidation of hydrogen is usually a fast process during which the mixture heats up to high temperatures. The heat of reaction of such oxidation processes is more generally known

---

* There are, however, several oxidation processes during which heat is absorbed instead of liberated. One of these *endothermic* reactions is the formation of nitrous oxide from nitrogen and oxygen molecules; over 19 kcal has to be supplied to the reactants from outside when 1 mole of N_2O is formed.

as HEAT OF COMBUSTION.* The experimental value for the heat of combustion liberated during the formation of 1 mole H_2O is nearly 56 kcal. The appropriate chemical reaction equation is:

$$H_2 + \tfrac{1}{2}O_2 \rightarrow H_2O \text{ (g)} + 58 \text{ kcal}$$

In this as in all other chemical combustions it is important to indicate the state of the various molecules. The reactants (H_2, O_2) are obviously gases. The product (H_2O) is here assumed to be in the form of vapour, as indicated by the letter g ($=$ gas).

This distinction is of some importance as heats of combustion are frequently given for *liquid* water as the end product. The value for the heat of combustion is then greater because the latent heat of vaporization of water is liberated during its condensation: 10·5 kcal per mole of water condensed.

The heat of combustion of 1 mole of hydrogen to liquid water becomes therefore:

$$58 + 10\cdot5 = 68\cdot5 \text{ kcal/mole.}$$

In this process 2 g hydrogen have been oxidized by $\tfrac{1}{2} \times 32 = 16$ g oxygen to 18 g liquid water. Therefore, in the production of 1 gram of liquid water $68\cdot5/18 = 3\cdot8$ kcal or 3800 cal are liberated. Compare this large amount of heat with the heat required to raise the temperature of this 1 gm H_2O from ice point to boiling point!

It can easily be shown that most of the water formed by the combustion will condense to liquid if the products are cooled to room temperature:

Example

Assume that the initial mixture of 1 mole H_2 and $\tfrac{1}{2}$ mole O_2 exerted a total pressure of 1 atm. At room temperature one mole of an ideal gas exerts a pressure of 1 atm when contained in a volume of 24 litres. The $\dfrac{3}{2}$ moles of reactants were therefore in a vessel of $\dfrac{3}{2} \times 24$ litres capacity. The one mole of (fictitious) water vapour formed by the combustion and cooled to room temperature, would exert a pressure of 1 atm in a volume of 24 litres; in the vessel of $\dfrac{3}{2} \times 24$ litres it would exert a pressure of

$$\dfrac{24}{\dfrac{3}{2} \times 24} = \dfrac{2}{3} \text{ atm}$$

---

* Furthermore, *combustion* can be defined as that reaction between oxygen and fuel molecules which yields H_2O and CO_2 as products. On the other hand, *oxidation* may lead to a variety of complicated products (e.g. ether to aldehydes) which themselves could be further oxidized under different conditions. From this point of view, a combustion can be considered as the complete oxidation of a molecule.

However, at room temperature the saturation pressure of water vapour is only about $\frac{1}{30}$ atm, and most of the water vapour will condense to liquid, ($\frac{2}{3} - \frac{1}{30} = \frac{19}{30}$ out of the initial $\frac{2}{3}$) or 95% of the total vapour.

Mechanism of Oxidations

At room temperature the reaction between oxygen and other combustible molecules fortunately does not take place merely on contact. A piece of sugar exposed to the oxygen in the air does not combust spontaneously. Yet, the same lump of sugar can be readily oxidized by the tissue cells, thereby yielding a considerable amount of heat (heat of combustion of 1 gram glucose = 3·7 kcal). Similarly, coal is safely exposed to the open air at normal temperature, although in our grates it is readily oxidized to provide warmth (1 kg carbon oxidized to CO_2 yields 7800 kcal).

In spite of the strong affinity between oxygen and molecules containing carbon and hydrogen atoms—shown by the great amount of heat liberated when their combustion takes place—reaction between them with a measurable speed occurs only under certain conditions. At room temperature in, say, a mixture of ether vapour and oxygen, the molecules of ether and oxygen repel one another during collision. This zone of repulsion forms an intangible barrier round each molecule; it must be overcome and changed to strong mutual attraction before the reaction (combustion) can occur.

One way in which the repulsion barrier can be overcome and the reaction initiated is by inciting particularly violent collisions between oxygen and the combustible molecule ('fuel'). Although both slow and fast collisions occur in a gas at any temperature, the proportion of fast collisions (with high energy) rises rapidly with increasing temperature. The energy which has to be imparted to the colliding molecules to initiate reaction is known as the ACTIVATION ENERGY. In the exothermic combustions considered by us, this energy is regained later on in the course of the reaction.

Considering again the special reaction scheme:

$$WX + YZ \rightarrow WY + XZ$$

we know from previous discussion that complete dissociation of

$$WX (\rightarrow W + X) \text{ and of } YZ (\rightarrow Y + Z)$$

could immediately lead to a very rapid union of the atoms to form the product molecules: WY and XZ.

In general, however, the activation energy is well below the sum of the bond energies of the reacting molecules. Instead of complete dissociation into their atoms, the reacting molecules have only to be deformed to a certain degree before the regrouping of bonds and the formation of the product molecules take place.

Mechanical analogy of a chemical reaction

The relationship between the activation energy and the heat of combustion can be illustrated in the following manner:

Fig. 319—   *Model*

A lake (A) is situated high above a river (B). The residents in a nearby town propose to generate electricity by utilizing the potential (hydraulic) energy possessed by the water in A owing to its height above B. Before this can be done, however, the water in A must first be lifted from level (*l*) to a higher level (*h*), so that it can overcome the hill (C) which forms a ridge between A and the mountain slope.

Reaction Mechanism

The reactants: oxygen and combustible (fuel) molecules are represented by A. Under room conditions (*l*) no reaction takes place. The energy needed to lift the water from A over C represents the *activation energy* which has to be supplied to molecules in the initial mixture before reaction can take place. When the oxidation has taken place and the heat of combustion is released, the final products of combustion are at a low energy level represented by that of river (B).

The *heat of combustion* is represented by the difference in level between A (*l*) and B. The *activation energy* temporarily expended to lift the water from lake (A) over hill (C), i.e. from *l* to *h*, is regained during the descent from the top of C down the mountain slope.

The hilly ridge (C) represents the repulsion barrier between the molecules of the initial mixture. In many chemical oxidations this barrier is overcome by heating the mixture. One of the effects of heating a gas is to increase the proportion of very fast-moving molecules; these can then overcome the barrier which leads to formation of the product molecules with liberation of the heat of combustion. In the pictorial analogy, the heating of the molecules in the initial mixture is represented by raising the lake level from *l* to *h*. In the violent collision between such 'activated' molecules, they penetrate much deeper into their mutual repulsion barrier. The reacting molecules are thereby deformed, the distances between certain atoms in each of them are stretched and the bonds holding together the atoms in a given

Fig. 320

Fig. 321

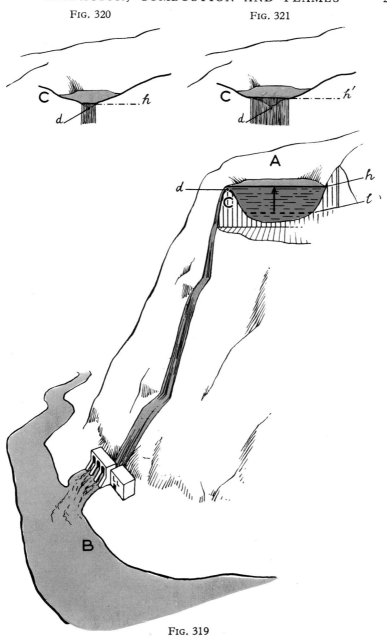

Fig. 319

molecule are weakened. The violent collision also permits closer approach between atoms of *different* molecules until they begin to attract one another, thus forming the new bonds of the product molecules.

In biological oxidation processes the barrier between oxygen and the carbohydrate or fat molecule is overcome, not by heating but by the activity of enzymes. These are in some ways comparable to the catalysts used in many industrial chemical processes. Although the mechanism of their action is very complicated, they may be said to deform the reacting molecules at normal temperatures to such a degree that the repulsion barrier disappears and reaction becomes possible owing to the great reduction in activation energy.

Effect of Temperature on Combustion

The speed with which reaction takes place is considerably influenced by the temperature of the combustible mixture. An empirical rule given by ARRHENIUS states that:

> *the speed of a reaction is doubled when the temperature of the initial mixture is raised by* 10 °C.

Figs. 320 and 321—will help to visualize this rule. The ridge (C) is assumed to dip in a certain region, forming a (saddle-) pass leading from A down the mountainside to B. When water from A is lifted just to the lowest dip (*d*) in the ridge (C), only a small trickle of water flows through the lowest part of the shallow dip (fig. 320). In other words, the reaction rate is slow.

In fig. 321 the water from A is shown to be lifted somewhat higher above the lowest point of the pass (*d*). This small increase in the height of *h* above *l* results in a much greater flow-rate of water streaming through the pass down the hill; the stream through the saddle or dip (*d*) in the ridge (C) is much wider.

Described in molecular language, the proportion of activated fuel and oxygen molecules (endowed with high energy) which are able to overcome the mutual repulsion barrier rises rapidly with temperature.

It can be easily shown that the Arrhenius rule gives indeed a very fast rise of reaction rate with temperature. As a rise in temperature of 10 °C doubles the rate, a rise by 40 °C would give already a 16-fold increase in rate ($2 \times 2 \times 2 \times 2 = 2^4 = 16$). A temperature rise of 230 °C would give a ten million times greater reaction rate.*

---

* Generally: $2^a = 10^L$ where $L = 0.301 \times a$; for $a = 23$ one obtains $L = 6.92 \simeq 7$. Thus $2^{23} \simeq 10^7 = 10 \times 10^6$, or ten million.

The reader familiar with logarithmic notation will recognize that 0.301 is log 2.

The mountain analogy of a chemical reaction also helps to understand the fact (p. 290) that the activation energy is frequently well below that of the bond energies of the reactant molecules. This statement is symbolized by the high mountain walls surrounding the lake (B) except at the pass (d). Any other passage from A to B leading high over those walls would represent a complete separation of the bonds in the reactant molecules before the new bonds in the product molecules are formed.

Activation energy and bond energies of reactants

Under certain circumstances the difference between activation energy and bond energies of the reactant molecules can be very large indeed. The following example refers to a reaction of a free atom with a molecule. Although free atoms do not occur amongst the initial reactants, they are of great practical significance because many combustion processes involve such reactive atoms (and also bits of molecules with free valencies called *radicals*) as intermediary steps in the reaction process.

$$H + Cl_2 \rightarrow HCl + Cl + 45 \text{ kcal}$$

This reaction of a hydrogen atom with a chlorine molecule liberates 45 kcal per mole (height of lake A above river B). The activation energy (A.E.) of this reaction is only about = 2 kcal; in other words, the level (l) is very near the lowest part (d) of the mountain pass. If the reaction of H with Cl-Cl would require initially a complete separation of the two Cl atoms, the activation energy would be equal to the dissociation energy of the chlorine molecule (= 57 kcal), i.e. almost 30 times as large as the actual activation energy.

Influence of activation energy on reaction rate

The critical influence of the magnitude of the activation energy on the reaction rate may be appreciated from the following example:

Assume a reaction proceeding with a certain rate (R) at a temperature of 530 °C (= 800 °K), and that the activation energy of the process is A.E. = 20 kcal.

If the activation energy were 28 instead of 20 kcal, the reaction rate can be shown to decrease from R to R/150, i.e. the reaction rate would be less than 1% of the previous rate R.

The reaction rate can be expressed as that fraction of the initial mixture (reactants) transformed into products in unit time. Theory shows that the reciprocal of the rate $\left(\dfrac{1}{R}\right)$ is proportional to $10^{(A.E./4 \cdot 6T)}$; T is the temperature in °K, and A.E. is here expressed in cal/mole.

Combustion and isothermal oxidation

Considering the great effect which temperature may exert on the rate of a reaction, it will be understandable that the heat of reaction liberated during the process may have a vital influence on the character of the reaction. If the heat liberated is removed quickly enough, the temperature of the reacting system will remain more or less constant and there will be no increase in reaction rate due to temperature increase of the reactants.

If the reaction rate is sufficiently slow, the liberated heat will obviously have time to escape from the reaction vessel. Such slow reaction of oxygen with oxidizable molecules is known as *isothermal oxidation*.

If the reaction rate is too fast for the heat of reaction to escape as soon as liberated, the mixture will heat up to high temperatures and we talk generally of a *combustion*. The definition of explosions comprising the phenomena of deflagration and detonation will be given later on.

Even without much theoretical discussion will it be understandable that a reaction of oxygen with a fuel (say methane) can proceed at practically *constant* temperature if the reaction rate is sufficiently slow. In practice the vessel would have to be small (e.g. 1 litre) to ensure that the heat of combustion does not accumulate in the vessel but can escape as fast as it is produced.

A useful indicator for the **reaction rate** is that time (t_h) which elapses until one-half of the initial mixture in a given volume has been transformed by reaction into the final products. If t_h is of the order of hours one would expect an isothermal oxidation, if t_h is of the order of seconds one would expect combustion or explosion.

Molecular Collisions in a gas mixture

If a certain reaction can only occur during the collision of *two* molecules, it is known as 'bimolecular'. One factor determining the rate of this reaction will be obviously the number of collisions in a given time. The enormous frequency of collisions in a gas at normal temperature and pressure will be apparent from the following example:

Consider a mixture of two gases, a and b, each exerting a partial pressure of $\frac{1}{2}$ atm. If every single collision between a pair of molecules (a and b) would lead to a chemical reaction, half the initial mixture would be transformed into the final products in a fantastically short time—in far less than one-millionth of a second. Under certain assumptions for size and weight of the two kinds of molecules (a, b), the half time of the reaction turns out to be: $t_h \sim 10^{-9}$ s, or one-thousandth of a millionth of a second.

The fact that at room temperature and normal pressure the rate of oxidation processes and of other reactions in gases is often nil or very slow, shows that practically all collisions between a and b are *ineffective*. In such 'elastic' collisions the molecules bounce off one another without undergoing any chemical change.

The molecular theory of gases states that the *average* energy in a head-on collision of two molecules is approximately: $2 \times T$ cal/mole, where the temperature T is expressed in °K. At room temperature this energy is 2×300 cal/mole, or 0·6 kcal/mole. As mentioned before, collisions with smaller and larger energies occur in the gas at a given temperature, but the number of molecules with much higher energies than the average is very scarce. For example, the frequency of collisions with four times the average energy is less than 2%, while only one collision in ten thousand has an energy greater than ten times the average.

These remarks will explain why bimolecular reactions may proceed quite slowly if only those pairs of molecules can react, which collide with an energy equal to or greater than the activation energies in Table 8.

Rate of bimolecular reaction

In the following we consider a fictitious reaction:

$$\text{molecule } a + \text{molecule } b \rightarrow \text{products}$$

with the partial pressures $p_a = p_b = \frac{1}{2}$ atm in the initial mixture.

TABLE 8

Activation Energy A.E. (in kcal)	Temperature of initial mixture		
	27 °C (300 °K)	180 °C (450 °K)	330 °C (600 °K)
	Half time (t_h) of reaction		
15	1 min	10 ms*	$\frac{1}{7}$ ms
20	$2\frac{1}{2}$ days	3 s	9 ms
25	28 years	12 min	$\frac{1}{2}$ s
30	—	2 days	38 s

* 1 ms = 1 millisecond = 0·001 s.

Various activation energies are given in table 8 for this type of reaction; the respective reaction rates represented by the time it takes for one-half of the initial mixture to react have been entered. The reactions in mixtures at three different temperatures are compared. The reactions are assumed to proceed isothermally, i.e. the liberated heat is conducted away to the outside of the container as quickly as it is formed. This assumption is, of course, quite inappropriate for reaction rates with a half time (t_h) of a few seconds and less.

Effect of the composition of a mixture on its combustion

The composition of a combustible mixture may vary between wide limits. The mixture corresponding exactly to the chemical equation describing the combustion process is known as the **stoichiometric** mixture. In a stoichiometric mixture the combustion can be *complete*: all fuel and oxygen molecules contained in the initial mixture are completely transformed into the product molecules.

The molecules of most organic compounds of interest to anaesthetists contain only three kinds of atoms: H, C and O; the general combustion equation in a stoichiometric mixture of these can therefore be written* as:

1 mole **fuel** + b mole **oxygen** → products (consisting of CO_2 and H_2O)

The fuel content of any mixture can be expressed as the ratio of the fuel moles to the total number of moles present in the mixture: this ratio gives also the volume of the fuel (say, under a pressure of 1 atmosphere) divided by the total volume of the mixture (p. 61). Multiplication of the fraction by 100 gives then the fuel concentration (f) in % v/v.

Stoichiometric mixtures

(i) in OXYGEN

In the special case of a stoichiometric mixture, the fuel concentration (f_{st}) is given by:

$$f_{st} = \frac{1}{1+b} \times 100 \ \%v/v \qquad . \qquad . \qquad . \qquad (1)$$

Example—*Combustion of hydrogen in oxygen.*

$$1 \cdot H_2 + \tfrac{1}{2} \cdot O_2 \rightarrow 1 \cdot H_2O$$

number of mole oxygen $b = \frac{1}{2}$; one obtains from Eq. 1 the stoichiometric fuel concentration $f_{st} = \dfrac{1}{1 + \frac{1}{2}} \times 100 = \dfrac{100}{1 \cdot 5}$

$$= 67 \ \%v/v.$$

(ii) in AIR

In fuel mixtures with **air** we have to remember that for every volume of oxygen a $\dfrac{79}{21}$-fold volume of nitrogen is also present (air con-

---

* In practice, the oxidation process even in a stoichiometric mixture may be far from complete. See also footnote on p. 299.

tains 21 %v/v of oxygen). In a stoichiometric mixture of fuel and air, the fuel concentration (f_{st}') is given by:

$$f_{st}' = \frac{1}{1 + b + \frac{79}{21}b} \times 100 = \frac{1}{1 + 4 \cdot 76 \times b} \times 100 \, \%v/v \quad (2)$$

Example: Find the stoichiometric concentration of hydrogen mixed with air.

From the preceding explanation it will be obvious that the left side of the combustion equation becomes now:

$$1 \cdot H_2 + \tfrac{1}{2} \cdot O_2 + \tfrac{1}{2} \times \frac{79}{21} \cdot N_2$$

The concentration of hydrogen (fuel) in this mixture follows therefore from (Eq. 2):

$$f_{st}' = \frac{1}{1 + 4 \cdot 76 \times \tfrac{1}{2}} \times 100 = \frac{100}{3 \cdot 38} = 29 \cdot 6 \, \%v/v.$$

These two examples show that the highest concentration of hydrogen which can be completely combusted in air is less than half the corresponding concentration in a mixture with pure oxygen. The following examples for combustion of hydrocarbons in oxygen and air will demonstrate that the ratio of f_{st}' in air to f_{st} in oxygen is generally much less favourable.

Examples of stoichiometric mixtures

For simplicity's sake we have assumed that air is composed of (1/5) oxygen and (4/5) nitrogen. Therefore 1 volume of oxygen is contained together with 4 volumes of nitrogen in 5 volumes of air. Eq. 2 is simplified to:

$$f_{st}' = \frac{1}{1 + 5b} \times 100 \, \%v/v \quad . \qquad . \qquad . \quad (2a)$$

(a) METHANE/OXYGEN: $CH_4 + 2 \cdot O_2 = CO_2 + 2 \cdot H_2O$
  i.e. 1 vol. methane + 2 vol. oxygen
  or $f_{st} = \frac{1}{1 + 2} \times 100 = 33 \, \%v/v$ methane in oxygen can be completely combusted.

(b) METHANE/AIR: $CH_4 + 2 \cdot O_2 + 8 \cdot N_2 = CO_2 + 2 \cdot H_2O + 8 \cdot N_2$
  1 vol. methane + 10 vol. air (containing 2 vol. O_2)
  or $f_{st}' = \frac{1}{1 + 5 \times 2} \times 100 = 9 \, \%v/v$ methane in air can be completely combusted.

(c) ETHER/OXYGEN: $(C_2H_5)_2O + 6 \cdot O_2 = 4 \cdot CO_2 + 5 \cdot H_2O$
i.e. 1 vol. ether vapour + 6 vol. oxygen

or $f_{st} = \dfrac{1}{1 + 6} \times 100 = 14$ %v/v ether in oxygen can be completely combusted.

(d) ETHER/AIR: $(C_2H_5)_2O + 6 \cdot O_2 + 24 \cdot N_2 = 4 \cdot CO_2 + 5 \cdot H_2O + 24 \cdot N_2$
1 vol. ether vapour + 30 vol. air (containing 6 vol. O_2)

or $f'_{st} = \dfrac{1}{1 + 5 \times 6} \times 100 = 3$ %v/v ether in air can be completely combusted.

These examples explain why a given volume of the stoichiometric fuel/**air** mixture develops *considerably less heat* than the stoichiometric fuel/**oxygen** mixture. In the case of diethyl ether the mixture in air (d) with the highest heat content can deliver only $\frac{3}{14} \simeq \frac{1}{5}$ of the heat of the mixture in oxygen (c) with the highest heat content.

'Rich' and 'lean' mixtures

If the fuel concentration (f) in a mixture with oxygen or air is greater than the stoichiometric concentration (f_{st} or f'_{st} respectively) the combustion cannot be complete. Some fuel will be left over amongst the products. These mixtures are called 'rich'.

In 'lean' mixtures, on the other hand, f is smaller than f_{st}, or f'_{st} respectively, and there is a fuel deficit. Although the combustion of the fuels in these mixtures can be complete, oxygen will be left over amongst the final products.

In all mixtures with a fuel concentration different from the stoichiometric value, the heat of combustion generated by a given quantity of the fresh mixture will be smaller than that developed by the same volume of a stoichiometric mixture.

Examples

(i) Given 1 litre of a *stoichiometric mixture of methane in oxygen* with a total pressure of 1 atm.

We know that $f_{st} = \frac{1}{3} \times 100 = 33$ %v/v (a, p. 297). The partial pressure of methane is therefore $\frac{1}{3}$ atm and that of oxygen $\frac{2}{3}$ atm.

In an ideal gas under room conditions:

1 mole is contained in 24 l at a pressure of 1 atm
$\frac{1}{3}$ mole ,,   ,,   ,, 24 l ,,   ,,   ,, $\frac{1}{3}$ atm
$\frac{1}{72}$ mole ,,   ,,   ,, 1 l ,,   ,,   ,, $\frac{1}{3}$ atm

The mixture therefore contains $(\frac{1}{3} \times \frac{1}{24}) = \frac{1}{72}$ mole of methane and $\frac{1}{36}$ mole of oxygen.

If one mole of methane combusts to water vapour and CO_2, the heat of combustion liberated in the process equals 192 kcal. The mixture in our example liberates: $\frac{1}{72} \times 192 = 2.7$ kcal.

Substituting the molecular weights of methane (16) and oxygen (32), it will be seen that the total weight of the mixture equals: $\frac{1}{72} \times 16 + \frac{1}{36} \times 32$, or slightly more than 1 gram. The large amount of heat liberated by this 1 g of combusting mixture may be appreciated by stating that a piece of brass weighing 40 g could be made red-hot by the same amount of heat.

(ii) We consider next a *rich* mixture of: 80% CH_4 + 20% O_2. As 2 vol. of O_2 are required for every vol. of CH_4, only $\frac{1}{2} \times 20\% = 10\%$ CH_4 can be completely combusted by the available oxygen. There will be $80 - 10 = 70\%$ CH_4 left over amongst the final products.

The heat liberated in one litre of this rich mixture will be only 10/33 of that liberated in the stoichiometric mixture, i.e.

$$\frac{10}{33} \times 2.7 = 0.8 \text{ kcal.}$$

(iii) In comparison, a *lean* mixture of: 10% methane + 90% oxygen would again yield only: $\frac{10}{33} \times 2.7 = 0.8$ kcal. As 20% O_2 is required to combust the 10% methane in the mixture, a surplus of: $90 - 20 = 70\%$ of oxygen will remain in the final mixture.*

Fig. 322—expresses graphically the various relations between the heat liberated and the composition of fuel mixtures with air or oxygen. Mixtures of the same volume and under the same total pressure are compared. Increasing density of shading on the drawing represents increasing fuel concentrations of the mixtures.

The heat liberated during the combustion of a fixed volume of any of the mixtures is represented by the height of the sloping lines above the horizontal base.

If the fixed volume is chosen so that the stoichiometric mixture (St. M) in oxygen contains *one mole fuel*, the height of the peak of the large triangle would represent the *heat of combustion per mole* of fuel.

The graph also demonstrates that:

(1) In lean mixtures the heat liberated is the same for fuel/oxygen

---

* In conformity with the procedure applied generally in this book, the description of reaction processes and statements on combustion products have been oversimplified. Thus, in a *rich* mixture the available oxygen will not simply transform the fraction of fuel determined by the chemical equation of the combustion process into carbon dioxide and oxygen; a much smaller portion of the fuel molecules may be combusted completely, while other fuel molecules may be transformed into various oxidation products (e.g. ethyl ether into acetaldehyde, etc.).

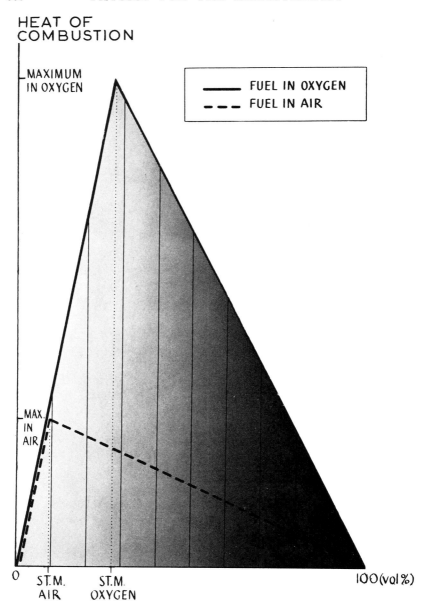

HEAT OF
COMBUSTION

MAXIMUM
IN OXYGEN

FUEL IN OXYGEN
FUEL IN AIR

MAX.
IN
AIR

0   ST.M.   ST.M.   100(vol%)
      AIR   OXYGEN

FUEL CONCENTRATION

Fig. 322

as for fuel/air, until the fuel concentration reaches the stoichiometric value in air ($f = f'_{st}$).

(2) The heat liberated in the stoichiometric fuel/oxygen mixture is much higher than that in the stoichiometric fuel/air mixture (compare the peak of the solid line triangle with the peak of the broken line triangle).

Heat liberated by combustion of various mixtures

From the preceding discussion, one can derive the following general relations between the composition of a fuel/oxygen (or fuel/air) mixture and the heat liberated by the combustion. All mixtures are now assumed to be contained in a vessel of 24 l at a pressure of 1 atm.

H = heat of combustion per one mole of fuel (see table 9, col. 4).

f_{st} = fuel content (vol %) of stoichiometric mixture.

f_l = fuel content (vol %) of any lean mixture ($f_l < f_{st}$).

f_r = fuel content (vol %) of any rich mixture ($f_r > f_{st}$).

Q_{st}, Q_l, Q_r = heat liberated in the combustion of stoichiometric, lean and rich mixtures.

With these definitions one derives:

$$Q_{st} = H \times f_{st} \qquad \cdot \qquad \cdot \qquad \cdot \qquad \cdot \qquad (3)$$

$$Q_l = Q_{st} \times \left(\frac{f_l}{f_{st}}\right) \qquad \cdot \qquad \cdot \qquad \cdot \qquad \cdot \qquad (4)$$

$$Q_r = Q_{st} \times \left(\frac{100 - f_r}{100 - f_{st}}\right) \qquad \cdot \qquad \cdot \qquad \cdot \qquad (5)$$

The fraction in the expression for Q_r (Eq. 5) is the ratio of the oxygen concentration in the rich mixture to that in the stoichiometric one. This is understandable as in rich mixtures the oxygen concentration determines the amount of fuel which can be combusted.

From the expression for Q_l it is apparent that the ratio: f_l/f_{st} determines the amount of heat which is liberated in a lean mixture compared to the maximum possible value Q_{st}. For that reason the heat liberated and other properties of combustible mixtures are frequently plotted on a graph in which the abscissa is graduated in this ratio; i.e. the division 'one' on the abscissa represents a stoichiometric, values below 'one' a lean and values above 'one' a rich mixture in this scheme.

Example

Apply the foregoing expressions to determine the heat liberated by the combustion of various mixtures of *diethyl ether* in oxygen and air. For convenience sake volumes of 24 l of the mixtures under a pressure of 1 atm are considered. Division of results by 24 would give the heat liberated in 1 litre of the mixtures. The heat of combustion for 1 mole is $H = 608$ kcal.

(i) One mole of diethyl ether requires $b = 6$ mole of oxygen for complete combustion; the stoichiometric fuel concentrations are therefore:

IN OXYGEN   IN AIR

$$f_{st} = 14\cdot3\% \qquad\qquad\qquad f'_{st} = 3\cdot4\%$$

The heat liberated during the combustion of these stoichiometric mixtures is:

$$Q_{st} = 608 \times \frac{14\cdot3}{100} = 87 \text{ kcal} \qquad Q'_{st} = 608 \times \frac{3\cdot4}{100} = 20\cdot7 \text{ kcal}$$

(ii) Considering next a *lean* mixture of $f_l = 2\%$ ether, the heat liberated will be:

$$Q_l = 81 \times \left(\frac{2}{14\cdot3}\right) = 12\cdot2 \text{ kcal} \qquad Q'_l = 20\cdot7 \times \left(\frac{2}{3\cdot4}\right) = 12\cdot2 \text{ kcal}$$

(iii) In a *rich* mixture of $f_r = 30\%$ the heat developed is:

$$Q_r = 81 \times \left(\frac{100 - 30}{100 - 14\cdot3}\right) = 71 \qquad Q'_r = 20\cdot7 \times \left(\frac{100 - 30}{100 - 3\cdot4}\right) = 15\cdot0$$

This example confirms once more the conclusions drawn from fig. 322: for fuel concentrations below the stoichiometric concentration in air, the heat developed in mixtures with oxygen and in those with air is the same. For fuel concentrations above the stoichiometric concentration in air, the heat developed in mixtures with air is small compared with that in oxygen; in the example (iii) the ratio of the amounts of heat developed is as 15/65.

In order to facilitate the assessment of heat which can be liberated by the combustion of various mixtures, Table 9 opposite lists the heat of combustion[5] per mole of fuel as well as the stoichiometric concentration of fuel mixtures with oxygen and with air. A few simple combustible compounds as well as most combustible anaesthetic agents are entered; they are all assumed to be in the gaseous state. The heat of combustion values in column (4) imply water *vapour* in the end product; if the water is assumed to be condensed, the number of moles of water formed according to the chemical equation (column 3) multiplied by $10\cdot5$ kcal/mole (see p. 288) has to be added to the values in column (4).

The table shows that the heat of combustion rises with the size of the molecule; if molecules were formed from the same material, the heat of combustion *per gram* might be expected to be constant. This assumption is, of course, much too crude, but it will be seen from column (5) that one gram of certain molecules, which are composed of hydrogen and carbon only, has a heat of combustion of approximately 11 kcal.

TABLE 9

HEAT OF COMBUSTION AND STOICHIOMETRIC CONCENTRATION OF FUELS

(1)	(2)	(3)	(4)	(5)	(6)	(7)
			HEAT OF COMBUSTION		STOICHIOMETRIC CONCENTRATION	
FUEL	Mole of Oxygen per mole fuel (b)	Mole of water formed (w)	$\dfrac{kcal}{1\ mole}$ of fuel	$\dfrac{kcal}{1\ g}$	f_{st} vol % in: Oxygen	f'_{st} Air
Hydrogen H_2	$\frac{1}{2}$	1	57·8	28·7	66·7	29·6
Carbon (graphite)	1	–	94·0	7·9	–	–
Methane CH_4	2	2	192	11·9	33·3	9·5
Ethyl alcohol C_2H_5OH	3	3	305	6·6	25	6·5
Acetylene C_2H_2	$2\frac{1}{2}$	1	300	11·5	28·6	7·7
Ethylene C_2H_4	3	2	316	11·3	25	6·5
Cyclopropane C_3H_6	$4\frac{1}{2}$	3	460	10·9	18·2	4·5
Diethyl ether $(C_2H_5)_2O$	6	5	608	8·2	14·3	3·4
Divinyl ether $(C_2H_3)_2O$	5	3	557	8·5	16·7	4·0
Ethyl chloride C_2H_5Cl	3	2	320	5·0	25	6·5

Transition from isothermal oxidation to thermal explosion

So far we have excluded the possibility that a reacting mixture is heating up itself. We assumed that the rate of heat production was sufficiently small for the heat to be conducted away to the walls of the container; the process was described as isothermal oxidation.

What happens if the heat generated at the beginning of the reaction is only partly carried away to the walls of the vessel?

Even a small amount of heat left behind in the mixture will raise its temperature and thus increase the reaction velocity; consequently the rate of heat production will also rise. Increasing temperature of the mixture will, however, also lead to increasing heat loss to the walls of the vessel which are at lower temperature.

The preponderance of one or the other of these two factors will decide if the temperature increase in the mixture comes to a halt or not. If the temperature rise persists, the reaction velocity and heat production increase very rapidly and a steady oxidation process is no longer possible: it is replaced by an EXPLOSION. The explosion process is preceded by a rapid rise of the reaction velocity, although there is a limit set by the gradual consumption of the reactants: the exploding mixture becomes increasingly diluted with the combustion products.

If a vessel containing fuel/oxygen mixture is gradually warmed, oxidation may become measurable at some elevated temperature. A slight increase in temperature will raise the oxidation rate but the oxidation may still proceed at a constant rate while the walls of the vessel are kept at a certain temperature. A further slight rise in temperature may then lead to *explosion* as will become clear from the following

Example: A stoichiometric mixture of hydrogen ($H_2 + \frac{1}{2}O_2$) under a total pressure of 1 atm is enclosed in a small vessel ($\sim \frac{1}{4}$ l). The experiment is repeated with fresh mixtures for various temperatures (t °C) at which the walls of the vessel are maintained.

The oxidation rate is expressed as '% reaction in 1 minute'. Thus a reaction rate of 0.1% in 1 minute signifies that one part in one thousand of the original mixture is combusted to water within one minute.

TABLE 10

t (°C)	510	519	527	535	543	548	553	556
Rate	0·1	0·2	0·5	1	2	4	8	EXPL.

The entry in the last column signifies that a tiny increase in temperature of the walls above that in the previous column leads to an EXPLOSION: the oxidation no longer proceeds at a constant rate. Although the reaction still begins with a moderate rate (about 16% in 1 min), the heat developed can no longer be given off to the walls quickly enough, and the *temperature in the vessel rises rapidly.* As we know from p. 292, the rate of reaction will speed up tremendously. The reaction rate increases from a few % per minute to complete combustion within a small fraction of one second. The heat of reaction has no longer time to escape and the mixture will heat up accordingly.

The example will also help to understand the meaning of SPON-TANEOUS IGNITION TEMPERATURE of an evenly heated mixture, i.e. 556 °C in this particular experiment. The fact that the ignition temperature of a given mixture is not a universal constant should also be understandable: the walls of a small spherical vessel must be raised to a higher temperature than those of a larger vessel before onset of explosion. The heat developed during the reaction in the smaller vessel is much less than in the larger vessel, and it can also escape more easily to the walls. The temperature rise in the mixture comes thereby to a halt and the oxidation can proceed still at a constant rate in the smaller vessel, while explosion would occur in the larger vessel under the same conditions.

Combustion and Flames[6]

The terminology of fast oxidation processes is not quite strict. A reasonable generalization is that under suitable conditions most oxidations in mixtures which are neither too rich nor too lean lead to a rapid production of heat, and usually to the emission of light as well. Such vigorous oxidation can be called a COMBUSTION. When the combustion is associated with the emission of an appreciable amount of light or other radiation, the oxidation process is spoken of as a FLAME.

In the case of a wax candle with a central wick, the vigorous oxidation is initiated by the heat from a lighted match which melts the wax and supplies the heat of activation to its vapour. From then on the heat developed by the reaction between the wax and the oxygen of the ambient air is sufficient to maintain the combustion process at the end of the wick. The combustion process at the tip of a candle represents the special case of a 'static flame'; although there is plenty of wax present to be burned, the flame does not spread to envelope the whole candle but is confined to a particular site.

Static flames also occur in lean mixtures of a fuel with air or oxygen if a suitable, external heat source is present. In the following illustrations (figs. 323–5) a fine wire spiral (similar to that in an electric light bulb) is located at the centre of a glass flask. On closing a switch in the leads from a battery, the wire is heated and becomes red hot. The experiments are viewed in a dark room.

Fig. 323—the glass flask is filled with a very lean mixture, containing only 1% fuel vapour and 99% air. Although the mixture is non-flammable, a small luminous zone around the wire indicates that combustion of the fuel takes place. In the neighbourhood of the hot wire the temperature and therefore the rate of reaction is high, and the heat liberated produces this 'aureole'. If the switch would be opened, the aureole and the associated combustion process would *disappear*.

Fig. 324—a less lean mixture has been introduced into the flask and the static flame is larger and brighter. This corresponds to an increased amount of heat liberated by the combustion process in the neighbourhood of the red hot wire. Opening of the switch would again extinguish the static flame because the heat developed by the weak mixture is not sufficient to ignite the next outer layer.

Fig. 325—a richer mixture has been introduced. As soon as the switch is closed and the wire heated, a much brighter flame of an altogether different character is seen spreading away from the wire. The bright luminous zone is shown approaching quickly the walls of the flask, while the inner region has again become darker. The flame would continue to travel outwards even if the switch were suddenly opened; the mixture containing 4% of the fictitious fuel is said to be **flammable**.

Self-propagating flames

This process (fig. 325) introduces us to a different class of flames of considerably greater interest to the anaesthetist.

Example:

A horizontal tube—say 100 cm long and 2 cm in bore—is filled with a mixture of 10 %v/v coal gas and 90% air. A lighted match is approached and inserted into the end of the tube.

A flame is produced which *travels rapidly throughout the length of the tube*. Even if the match is quickly removed after igniting the mixture, this type of flame will continue to travel through the fresh mixture, leaving in its wake the combustion products.

Such a combustion accompanied by a self-propagating flame is known as DEFLAGRATION; the gas mixture in which a deflagration can occur is said to be *flammable*.

Flame propagation

The flame which travels is not a material thing; it is simply the zone in which explosive oxidation takes place under liberation of heat and

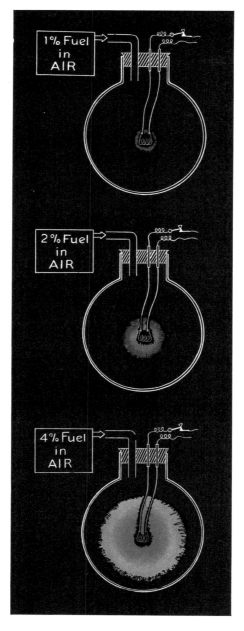

Fig. 323

Fig. 324

Fig. 325

light, advancing into the fresh mixture at a certain speed. A comparison with the spreading of other waves is helpful. In a normal sound wave travelling at a speed of 330 m/s, the air practically does not advance at all; only a disturbance of the air particles is propagated with that speed.

We shall see later that the speed of many deflagrations in gaseous mixtures is of the order of 1 m/s,—far below the speed of sound.

The spreading of a self-propagating flame can be visualized as follows: when the flame approaches a layer of fresh gas mixture, the temperature of this layer rises until the oxidation velocity in it exceeds a certain value, when the reaction will assume an explosive character. Thus this layer becomes itself the flame front; the heat of combustion liberated in it will warm the next adjacent layer of fresh mixture sufficiently to initiate a similar, fast reaction in it. The combustion is thus kept spreading and the visible effect is a self-propagating flame.

One way of describing the condition for the spreading of a self-propagating flame is that any layer of fresh mixture adjacent to the flame front must be heated above the IGNITION TEMPERATURE.

Ignition of Flammable Mixtures

The temperature to which a vessel containing the flammable mixture has to be heated before deflagration occurs is known as the *spontaneous ignition temperature* (see example on p. 305). Although oxidation does occur in the mixture at much lower temperatures, this is a slow process which produces no significant temperature rise and is therefore known as isothermal.

Of more immediate interest to the anaesthetist is the **local ignition** where only a small region of the whole flammable mixture is initially brought to ignition. Sources of such local ignition can be the following:

(*a*) extraneous flame (lighted match, etc.)
(*b*) hot wire (cautery, etc.) and arc (switches)
(*c*) electrical spark (due to frictional electricity, etc.)

Under suitable conditions any of these sources may start a self-propagating flame, travelling through a flammable gas mixture long after the source of ignition has become extinct.

Heat balance in deflagrations

When considering more closely the conditions leading to deflagration in gaseous mixtures, the fate of the heat released by the combustion must be considered. The heat of combustion produced in any given volume of a burning mixture is dissipated as follows:

(1) Heating of contiguous layers of fresh mixture.
(2) Leaking away by conduction and radiation through the walls of the container.
(3) Stored as heat content of hot, burnt gases (combustion products).
(4) Heating up of molecules in the mixture which take no part in the reaction (e.g. nitrogen in the air).

The auspices for a self-propagating flame are good if the loss of heat (2) is small, if no or few diluent gases (4) are present and if the fuel concentration is not too far away from the stoichiometric value. If conversely only little heat can be produced by the combustion of a particular mixture, or if the losses (2) are great, the combustion—even when started—may die out as soon as the source of ignition is withdrawn.

Generally speaking, the *composition* of the fresh mixture will be the major factor which determines the possibility of a deflagration spreading after ignition.

Deflagration in a gas stream

The possibility of deflagration in a given mixture is closely connected with the FLAME SPEED in it. If the flame speed approaches zero, there will obviously be no deflagration in this mixture. The fuel concentration of the fresh mixture—or rather the ratio f/f_{st}—is likely to influence decisively the flame speed.

A homely example of the influence of fuel concentration on flame speed can be derived from a study of the Bunsen burner. Although at first sight the combustion on the burner seems to resemble the static flame of a candle, it is actually a *deflagration* which is kept steady in space by maintaining a flow of fresh gases up the burner tube.

The coal gas passes from the rubber tubing through the small constriction ('jet') just visible inside the air entrainment opening at the lower end of the burner tube (fig. 326). The fast gas stream escaping from the jet entrains a quantity of 'primary' air which is controlled by rotation of the ring perforated by a hole.

Coal gas consists mainly of hydrogen and methane with a small amount of carbon monoxide; about five volumes of air are required for every volume of gas to ensure complete combustion. In many burners only up to $2\frac{1}{2}$ vol. of air per vol. of coal gas can be entrained, so that the

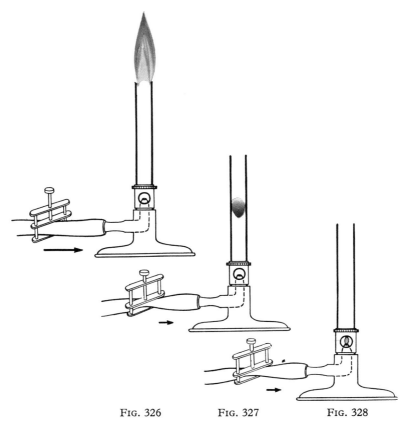

mixture travelling up the tube is quite rich ($f/f'_{st} \simeq 2$). Additional air*
is diffusing from the surroundings into the mixture at the top of the
burner tube.

In the above three illustrations the primary air opening is kept
widely open, and the composition of the mixture flowing up the tube
is assumed to remain constant.

Fig. 326—a fast stream of coal gas (long arrow) escapes from the
burner jet, entrains air and the mixture is ignited at the top. The flame
will continue to burn at the top of the burner tube.

Fig. 327—the gas supply is gradually reduced (see shorter arrow)
by tightening the screw clamp on the rubber tubing. The flame gets
gradually smaller and will finally travel down the tube *against* the flow
of the fresh mixture.

* Known as 'secondary air'.

Fig. 328—looking through the air entrainment opening, a small flame can now be seen burning at the jet. To the unwary the burner appears to be out of action, but any attempt to pick it up may result in blistered fingers.

Flash-back in gas burners

The ignition of the mixture at the top of the burner starts a deflagration; a flame begins to travel through the fresh mixture at a certain speed. However, in a burner the flammable mixture is not at rest, and the flame cannot travel down the tube as long as the flow velocity of the gas mixture exceeds the flame speed in this particular fuel/air mixture.

A crude simile would be a ship capable of a given speed trying to enter a fast-flowing river from the estuary. If the speed of the ship is smaller than the water velocity in the river, it will not be able to travel upstream. However, it could remain stationary (with engines 'full ahead') close to the mouth of the river where the water velocity has been reduced sufficiently by spreading out into the estuary.

When the gas supply is gradually reduced (fig. 327) a situation occurs in which the *linear velocity* of the flammable mixture up the tube is *smaller than the flame speed* in this mixture. The flame is now able to travel from the top of the burner down the tube against the flow, and may continue to burn at the jet.

This *'flash-back'* can be avoided by reducing the size of the air entrainment opening whenever the coal gas supply is diminished. This manoeuvre will produce a richer mixture flowing up the tube in which the flame speed is less than previously (e.g. p. 328, Table 17); the flame can no longer travel down the tube against the stream of fresh gases.

Flame propagation through Tubes

A long, horizontal tube is filled with a flammable gas mixture which has been ignited at the left end. A flame begins to travel through the tube and is observed at a certain moment some distance away from the site of ignition.

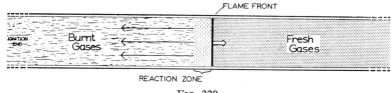

FIG. 329

Fig. 329—ahead of the FLAME FRONT is the fresh gas mixture at rest. In a layer behind the front, chemical reaction takes place which is completed at the end of a narrow zone. The heat of combustion heats the gases in the zone to a high FLAME TEMPERATURE. Further back, behind the reaction zone, are the burnt gases (combustion products), still fairly hot, but losing heat rapidly to the walls of the tube.

We visualize once more the process of flame propagation by considering the layer of fresh gas just adjacent to the flame front at a certain moment. Owing to the large temperature difference, heat will be quickly conducted from the flame zone into the adjacent layer of fresh gases; when the temperature in the layer exceeds the ignition temperature, the rate of reaction in it will accelerate rapidly. The heat of combustion raises the temperature of the layer to the flame temperature. This layer becomes then itself the flame front, which has thus advanced.

Conditions in a self-propagating flame

Some numerical values may help to visualize the events in a flame front. Certain flame zones have an estimated width[7] of about 0.01 cm. Even if the deflagration travels at the moderate speed of 50 cm/s, it sweeps across this layer within $\dfrac{0.01}{50} = \dfrac{1}{5000}$ s. At the same time the reactants contained in this layer are converted into the final products, i.e. the whole explosive combustion is completed within 0.2 millisec. Also during this short period the temperature of the layer will rise from room temperature to 1500 °C and above.

Owing to the high temperature in the reaction zone, both pressure and volume of the gases in it will tend to increase because the product of pressure and volume is proportional to the absolute temperature.* In the arrangement of fig. 329 the tube is assumed open at the site of ignition; the pressure, therefore, can equalize with the atmosphere to a large extent and will be only slightly above atmospheric. The volume alone will increase in proportion to the high temperature. Consequently the burnt gases expand and stream away (see single line arrows) in a direction opposite to the flame propagation (white arrow).

If T_F = flame temperature   and
T_O = temperature of reactants well ahead of the flame,
the following approximate relation can be derived:

$$\frac{\text{flame speed}}{\text{burnt gas velocity}} = \frac{\text{specific vol. of reactants}}{\text{specific vol. of burnt gas}}$$

* (a) from p. 98 : $p_0 \times v_0 = (22\cdot41/M)$ at $T = 273°K$
(b) from p. 114: $v = v_0 \times (T/273)$ [Charles]
(c) from p. 115: $p = p_0 \times (T/273)$ [Gay Lussac]
combining (b) with (c): $p \times v = p_0 \times v_0 \times (T/273)$
and substituting (a): $p \times v = (T/273) \times (22\cdot41/M)$.
Therefore: $p \times v \propto T$.

The specific volume of an ideal gas at constant pressure is proportional to the absolute temperature, and the relation becomes:

$$\frac{\text{flame speed}}{\text{burnt gas velocity}} = \frac{T_O}{T_F}$$

or   burnt gas velocity $=$ flame speed $\times \dfrac{T_F}{T_O}$

Example: Assume temperature of reactants $T_O = 300\ °K\ (27\ °C)$
       ,,   flame temperature $T_F = 2100\ °K$
       ,,   flame speed: $0\cdot5\ \text{m/s}$
Then the burnt gas velocity will equal

flame speed $\times \dfrac{T_F}{T_O} = 0\cdot5 \times \dfrac{2100}{300} = 0\cdot5 \times 7 = 3\cdot5\ \text{m/s}$

Ignition at the closed end of a tube

The high flow velocity of the burnt gases compared with the flame speed in a deflagration is of practical importance when ignition takes place at the *closed* end of a tube. In such an arrangement the burnt gases can no longer freely expand and stream backwards; instead, they will push the fresh mixture forward in the direction of flame propagation.

The flame will now travel through a gas which itself is streaming in the direction of flame propagation. As seen by a stationary observer from the outside, the flame travels along the tube at a speed which is the *sum* of the normal flame speed through a mixture at rest plus the flow velocity of the streaming gas. In other words: the explosion of a flammable mixture in a tube ignited at a closed end proceeds much faster than in the case of ignition at an open end.

It will be apparent that flame speed is not a simple property of a given flammable mixture, but depends on many extraneous factors. In fact, 'steady' flames spreading at a constant speed of the order of 1 metre/sec throughout a flammable mixture are the exception rather than the rule in other than laboratory conditions.

If the tube is too *narrow*, heat losses from the combustion zone to the walls will be excessive, and a self-propagating flame may be unable to travel through the flammable mixture (see fig. 374, p. 410).

On the other hand, the tube must not be too *wide* either, if the flame is not to accelerate to excessive speeds or to show other non-steady features. Deflagrations with flame speeds up to one or a few m/s are characteristic for many fuel mixtures with low oxygen content, e.g. for those with air.

The erratic behaviour of deflagration flames may explain the considerable variation in the relatively mild 'explosions' which have occurred after accidental ignition of anaesthetic vapours mixed with *air*.

Limits of Flammability[8]

We saw in the discussion of oxidations in general (p. 298) that these do not only occur in stoichiometric mixtures. Similarly, deflagrations in flammable mixtures occur not only at the stoichiometric concentration, but also in lean and in rich mixtures.

Lower Limit (L.L.)

If flame propagation is studied in various mixtures in which the fuel concentration is gradually reduced from f_{st}, while the total pressure is kept constant (e.g. 1 atm), a *lowest* fuel concentration is reached below which no flame will travel through the mixture. In still weaker mixtures combustion (or oxidation) still occurs in proximity to a suitable ignition source, but ceases as soon as the source is extinguished. A flame cannot travel through these weak mixtures because too few molecular reactions are taking place in each unit volume, and the heat production is too small to heat adjacent, fresh gas layers above the ignition temperature. The weakest fuel mixture through which a flame will propagate, represents the LOWER LIMIT OF FLAMMABILITY.

TABLE 11

Type of fuel mixed with oxygen	Lower Limit	Stoichiometric concentration
	fuel %v/v	fuel %v/v
Methane	6·5	33·3
Ethyl ether	2·1	13·3

The values in Table 11 show clearly that deflagration can still take place in very lean mixtures ($f \simeq \frac{1}{6} \times f_{st}$). The exact numerical values of these lower limits may vary considerably with the size and shape of container, with the nature of the ignition source and with other extraneous factors (see pp. 313 and 328).

Upper Limit (U.L.)

If, on the other hand, various mixtures with increasing fuel concentration are tested with suitable ignition sources, self-propagating flames can be produced until the fuel concentration has reached a certain upper value. Beyond this UPPER LIMIT OF FLAMMABILITY no deflagration occurs; such very rich mixtures are non-flammable. Oxidation can still take place in them, but the lack of oxygen keeps the rate of heat production at too low a level for a flame to travel away from the ignition source.

TABLE 12

Type of fuel mixed with oxygen	Upper Limit	Stoichiometric concentration
	fuel %v/v	fuel %v/v
Cyclopropane	60	18
Divinyl ether	85	16·7

According to Table 12 a deflagration is still possible in these mixtures with fuel concentrations from three to five times higher than the stoichiometric value. The same reservations regarding the validity of the numerical data hold as were already mentioned in connection with Table 11.

Simple hypothesis for the chemical heat content of L.L. and U.L. mixtures

Instead of taking the fact of two limits of flammability for granted, we shall try to get a better insight into the nature of such mixtures. The way has already been prepared by our study of the heat which may be liberated in the combustion of lean and rich mixtures (p. 302).

Each of the boxes (i) on the left in figs. 330–3 represents a small unit volume of different mixtures of a fictitious fuel with oxygen. *White* spheres represent oxygen molecules, *black* spheres the molecules of a combustible substance, or fuel (F). The boxes (ii) on the right represent the end products of the combustion processes.

In order to simplify the picture, the product is assumed to be formed by the union of one fuel molecule with one oxygen molecule according to the reaction equation:

$$1 \text{ vol. F} + 1 \text{ vol. O}_2 = 1 \text{ vol. (F·O}_2)$$

The stoichiometric fuel concentration for this fictitious combustion process is

$$f_{st} = \frac{1}{1 + 1} \times 100 = 50\% \text{ v/v}$$

and the limits are assumed to be: L.L. $= 10\%$; U.L. $= 90\%$.

The pressure in the boxes (i) on the left is assumed constant; it is proportional to the total number of spheres per unit volume which has been kept constant at 20.

Fig. 330—in this stoichiometric mixture of 10 black and 10 white spheres, 10 combustion processes are possible: $f = f_{st} = (10/20) \times 100 = 50\%$. The combustion of this mixture yields a maximum of heat.

Fig. 331—the concentration of oxygen in this mixture is slightly in excess of that required for complete combustion; fuel concentration: $f = (8/20) \times 100 = 40\%$.

Nevertheless, a flame is assumed to be capable of travelling through such mixtures, since the 8 combustion processes per unit volume occurring in a certain time generate enough heat to raise the temperature of an adjacent volume above its ignition temperature. A surplus of 4 oxygen molecules is left amongst the combustion products.

Fig. 332—here the mixture is very lean, and only 2 combustion processes occur per unit volume. The heat generated is just insufficient to ignite the next volume. This and leaner mixtures are non-flammable. $f = (2/20) \times 100 = 10\%$; the lower limit of flammability of F is L.L. $= 10\%$.

Fig. 333—represents a rich mixture, and again only 2 combustion processes can take place per unit volume; this and any richer mixtures are assumed to be non-flammable. $f = (18/20) \times 100 = 90\%$; the upper limit of flammability is U.L. $= 90\%$.

The discussion of the fictitious examples of limits of flammability in figs. 332 and 333 is based on the following assumption:

in both limiting mixtures the heat which can be liberated by combustion (chemical heat content) is the same.

Whether such a hypothesis is justified to any degree will have to be decided from experimental data (p. 320); for the moment it will help to understand the effect of a third, inert component (diluent) in the mixture on the limits of flammability.

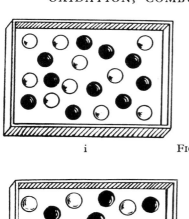
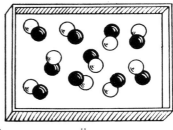

i   Fig. 330   ii

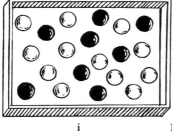
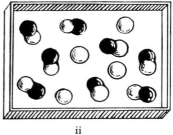

i   Fig. 331   ii

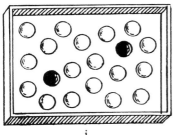
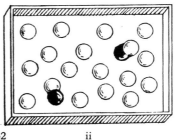

i   Fig. 332   ii

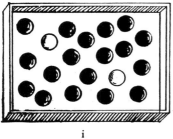
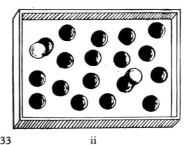

i   Fig. 333   ii

L.L. and U.L. mixtures of the fictitious fuel with Air

Diluent is the generic term for any compound which does not participate in the combustion process. The commonest diluent is introduced whenever oxygen is replaced by air in a mixture with fuel; in this case the ratio of diluent (nitrogen) to oxygen remains fixed at $(79/21) \simeq (4/1)$.

In flammable mixtures of fuel-oxygen, heat production near the L.L. is determined by the number of available fuel molecules, because there is an abundance of oxygen present. In the mixture of fig. 332, the total amount of fuel (10 %v/v) combined with 10 %v/v oxygen, leaving a large surplus of the latter amongst the final products (ii).

If the oxygen (90 %v/v) in the initial mixture (i) were replaced by 90 %v/v air, the oxygen content would be reduced to $\simeq (1/5) \times 90 = 18\%$. This amount is ample to combust the total fuel (10%) of the mixture.

Comparison of hypothetical limits in air and oxygen

For the following it is preferable to enlarge the size of the boxes of the fictitious mixture (p. 317) so that the number of the representative balls in the initial mixtures (i) is increased from 20 to 100. This merely multiplies the various combustion processes mentioned on p. 316 by a factor 5; i.e. there would be 50 processes in the stoichiometric mixture of fig. 330, 10 in the lean mixture of fig. 332 and also 10 in the rich mixture of fig. 333. In the mixture containing 90% air, the number of combustion processes would again be 10.

If the L.L. composition of fuel-oxygen and the L.L. mixture of fuel-air would have the same chemical heat content (i.e. liberate equal amounts of heat by combustion) we could conclude that:

the Lower Limit of flammability (expressed in fuel %v/v) is the same in oxygen and in air.

The U.L. of flammability cannot be found simply by replacing oxygen with air in the rich mixture. The U.L. of the fuel-oxygen mixture of the fictitious example contained 10 %v/v oxygen; replacing this by air would leave us with only $= (1/5) \times 10 = 2\%$ oxygen.

If deflagration at the U.L. in the fuel-air mixture again requires at least 10 combustion processes (same number as for oxygen), the U.L. mixture in air must contain 10% oxygen, but this amount is contained in 50% air. Therefore, the U.L. mixture of this particular fuel in air would contain 50% fuel and 50% air. In the fuel-air mixture another $4 \times 10 = 40$ additional balls (say grey) representing nitrogen would have to be added. As the total number of balls (in boxes i) has to be kept constant at 100, room is left for $100 - (10 + 40) = 50$ black balls; fuel concentration at U.L. in air $= \dfrac{50}{100}$ or 50%.

After the reaction in the U.L. mixture of fuel-oxygen, $90 - 10 = 80$ fuel molecules (black balls) are left amongst the products in the final mixture (ii). After the corresponding reaction in the U.L. mixture of fuel-air, $50 - 10 = 40$ fuel molecules and 40 nitrogen molecules are left amongst the products.

The limits of deflagration for this fictitious fuel can now be summarized in Table 13; for comparison the stoichiometric mixture concentrations have also been entered.

TABLE 13

Combustion: $1 \, F + 1 \, O_2 \rightarrow$ Products $(F \cdot O_2)$

Properties of Mixture	Mixtures of Fuel	
	with OXYGEN	*with* AIR
	fuel concentration in % v/v	
Lower Limit	10	10
Stoichiometric	50	17
Upper Limit	90	50

Simple theory of limits for the general combustion process

So far we have limited ourselves to the special case of combustion in which one fuel molecule requires one oxygen molecule ($b = 1$; p. 315). However, a discussion of the general case with different values of b would not alter the trend of our conclusions reached so far. Nevertheless, there are some significant differences when studying the combustions with other values of b, e.g. cyclopropane where $b = 2 \cdot 5$.

The concentration at the U.L. of fuel-oxygen *no longer* equals $(100 - \text{L.L.})$, but is considerably less. From a closer study of the general case, the following conclusions can be drawn when comparing this crude theory with experimental data:

Mixture composition at the Lower Limit of flammability

    Theoretical: The L.L. for mixtures of a fuel with OXYGEN and with AIR are the same.

    Experimental: Numerical values of L.L. for mixtures of a given flammable gas with oxygen and with air lie, in fact, closely together (see Table 14).

The L.L. of the fictitious example was taken rather high in order to simplify the drawing (10%; fig. 332). Many anaesthetic and other common, flammable mixtures have values of L.L. ranging from 2% upwards. In other words, only two combustion processes need to occur amongst 100 molecules of the initial mixture in order to propagate a flame at the L.L.

Mixture composition at the Upper Limit of flammability

Theoretical: The U.L. of deflagration for mixtures of a fuel with OXYGEN is considerably higher than that for fuel-AIR mixtures. In the fictitious example (Table 13) the value is 90% compared to 50%. If b of the combustion process is greater than 1, both the U.L. in oxygen and in air would have been less than the above values.

The range of deflagrations in mixtures with oxygen is much wider than the range in mixtures with air.

Experimental: The U.L. for fuel-oxygen mixtures is indeed much higher than for fuel-air mixtures.

There exists, however, the following discrepancy. The U.L. concentration of fuel both in air and oxygen is lower than predicted from the simple assumption of an equal number of combustion processes required for L.L. and U.L. mixtures of a given fuel. (Because the experimental U.L. is lower than the theoretical U.L., more oxygen will be present in the U.L. mixture and therefore more combustion processes can occur.)

Furthermore, the U.L. in oxygen usually corresponds to many more combustion processes than the U.L. in air for a given fuel; this is equivalent to saying that the chemical heat content of the U.L. fuel-oxygen mixture is considerably higher than that of the U.L. mixture of fuel-air. Furthermore, the U.L. mixture has a higher chemical heat content than the L.L. mixture; this holds both for fuel-oxygen and for fuel-air mixtures.

The number of combustion processes at the L.L. and U.L. in oxygen and air.

These findings will become clearer from the following

Example: Flammable mixtures of cyclopropane with oxygen and air. The number of possible combustion processes in mixtures containing a total of 100 molecules are given in Table 14. These numerical values are also proportional to the heat liberated in the combustion of the various mixtures. The U.L. and L.L. values are based on experimental data.

The increased number of combustion processes required to ensure self-propagating flames at the U.L. compared with the L.L., and the

TABLE 14

Mixtures	At Limits of Flammability Lower	Upper	In Stoichiometric Mixture
Cyclopropane	Number of combustion processes		
with OXYGEN	2·5	9	19·2
with AIR	2·4	4	4·7

larger number necessary in the fuel-oxygen mixtures compared with fuel-air, may become comprehensible by considering the components which are warmed by the heat of combustion, thereby reducing the final flame temperature.

At the U.L. of fuel-oxygen many more fuel molecules are left over in the final mixture than in the combustion at the U.L. of fuel-air which mixture contains many nitrogen molecules (see p. 319). The specific heat of fuels is usually much higher than that of nitrogen* so that a given number of combustion processes (i.e. amount of heat) raises the mixture containing much surplus fuel to a less high temperature. If, therefore, the temperature which can be produced by the combustion of mixtures at the L.L. and U.L. is decisive for the possibility of flame propagation, the elementary assumption that in all limiting mixtures of a certain fuel the same number of combustion processes is required, will have to be modified.

By a similar argument the slightly increased number of combustion processes required at the U.L. compared with those at the L.L. in fuel-air mixtures can be made understandable. There will be again a surplus of fuel in the final mixture at the U.L. (although much less than at the U.L. of fuel-oxygen). The greater heat capacity of this surplus of fuel, compared with that of nitrogen and oxygen at the L.L. necessitates a few more combustion processes at the U.L. compared with the number of processes at the L.L.

Simple rule for L.L. mixtures of flammable anaesthetics[9]

So far we have limited the comparison of the number of combustion processes at the L.L. and U.L. in mixtures with air and oxygen to a *given* fuel. Yet it is permissible to inquire if there are any relations between the L.L. and U.L. of *different* fuels. An obvious hypothesis

* e.g. specific heat per 1 mole of substance at 1000 °C:
ethylene ~ 25 cal; nitrogen ~ 8 cal

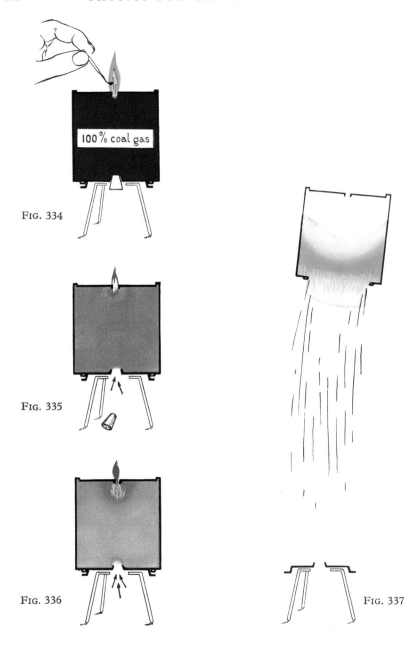

FIG. 334

FIG. 335

FIG. 336

FIG. 337

100% coal gas

would be that the heat liberated in the combustion of any fuel-oxygen (or -air) mixture at the L.L. should be adequate to heat the mixture to some *minimum* FLAME TEMPERATURE.

The problem is greatly simplified by the crude assumption that the specific heat of the final mixture formed by combustion at the L.L. is the same for all fuels under consideration. This assumption is not too far fetched as most of the molecules in the final mixtures will be oxygen (or nitrogen and oxygen respectively) because the L.L. concentrations of most fuels are quite low. The postulate assumes then the form:

the heat liberated by the combustion of a unit volume containing the Lower Limit concentration is the same for any fuel.

This heat is easily calculated by multiplying the molar fuel concentration at the L.L. with the heat of combustion of the particular fuel.

TABLE 15

HEAT LIBERATED BY THE COMBUSTION OF EQUALS VOLUMES (24 l) OF MIXTURES CONTAINING FUEL CONCENTRATIONS AT THE LOWER LIMIT OF FLAMMABILITY

Fuel mixtures with air	*L.L. Concentrations fuel % v/v*	*Heat liberated in 24 l (kcal)*
Methane	5·0	9·6
Ethylene	2·7	8·5
Cyclopropane	2·4	11·0
Diethyl ether	1·8	11·0
Divinyl ether	1·7	9·5

It will be appreciated from Table 15 that the postulate is confirmed reasonably well by experimental data. The heat liberated by combustion of L.L. fuel mixtures is in the region of 10 kcal per 24 litres.

Transition from static flame to deflagration by dilution of a very 'rich' mixture

The combustion processes in rich fuel mixtures which are gradually diluted can be observed in the following, simple

Experiment: An empty tin with a press-in lid is provided with small holes both in lid and base. The tin has been filled with coal gas and is placed inverted on a small tripod; a cork occludes the hole in the lid.

Fig. 334—a lighted match is applied to the upper hole (i.e. in base of tin) and a *static* flame begins to burn above this hole. As the interior of the tin is filled with pure fuel (f = 100%) no flame can spread into it.

Fig. 335—the cork in the lower hole (lid of tin) is removed. Owing to the draught produced by the flame, air enters through the lower hole to replace the gas burning away at the top. The fuel in the tin is thus diluted with air (f decreases). The lowered fuel concentration is indicated by a lighter shade of colour. The fuel concentration in the tin decreases towards the upper limit of flammability. A self-propagating flame is not yet possible, but an aureole grows inside the tin below the upper hole. At or above the upper hole the gas is strongly diluted with outer air; its concentration is between the limits of flammability and it can continue to burn. It also forms the heat source for the steadily growing static flame inside the tin.

Fig. 336—air continues to enter through the lower hole. When the fuel concentration in the tin has decreased to the upper limit, the flame shrinks and the aureole inside increases in size and brightness. Finally, the flame disappears completely inside the hole at top and

Fig. 337—a moment later a loud bang occurs; the tin moves upwards by 'rocket propulsion', leaving the lid behind on the tripod.

Shortly before this event, the fuel concentration in the lower part of the tin had fallen well below the U.L. and a fast deflagration became possible. The range of flammability in coal gas* for a flame travelling downward through the mixture is from $f = 10$ to $19 \%v/v$ approximately. Part of the contents of the tin must therefore have been diluted below $f = 19$ before the deflagration could occur.

Experimental Limits of Flammability

The comprehensive Table 16 of flammability limits is inserted here, although certain conditions for the data in it will be explained in later sections. The limits are given for mixtures with air, oxygen and nitrous oxide; substances supplying oxygen for combustion are often known as *supporters* of combustion. As help in visualizing the position of the limiting mixtures relative to those with maximum chemical heat content, columns 8, 9 and 10 giving the stoichiometric fuel concentrations in the various supporters have been added.

---

* The combustible components (vol %) of coal (or town) gas are approximately: hydrogen 40 , methane 25 , carbon monoxide 15.

TABLE 16
LIMITS OF FLAMMABILITY IN AIR, OXYGEN AND NITROUS OXIDE

(1)	(2) (3) (4) Lower Limit in			(5) (6) (7) Upper Limit in			(8) (9) (10) Stoichiometric Mixture in		
	Air	O_2	N_2O	Air	O_2	N_2O	Air	O_2	N_2O
Hydrogen	4·0	4·6	5·8	74	94	86	30	67	50
Methane	5·0	5·4	4·0	15	59	40	9·5	33	20
Ethylene	2·8	2·9	1·9	28	80	40	6·5	25	14
Cyclopropane	2·4	2·4	1·6	10	63	30	4·5	18	10
Diethyl ether	1·8	2·1	1·5	[36]	82	24	3·4	13	8
Divinyl ether	1·7	1·8	1·4	[27]	85	25	4·0	17	9
Ethylchloride	4·0	4·0	2·1	15	67	33	6·5	25	14

The values in columns 2 and 3 confirm our earlier findings of nearly equal lower limits in mixtures with air and with oxygen.

REFERENCES

[1] LEWIS, B., and ELBE, VON G. (1951). *Combustion, flames and explosions of gases*, New York.
[2] JOST, W. (1946). *Explosions and combustion processes in gases*, New York.
[3] SPEAKMAN, J. C. (1955). *An introduction to the electron theory of valency*, 3rd ed., Lond.
[4] LAIDLER, K. J. (1950). *Chemical kinetics*, New York.
[5] ROSSINI, F. D. et al. (1953). *Selected values of physical and thermodynamic properties of hydrocarbons and related compounds*, Pittsburgh.
[6] GAYDON, A. G., and WOLFHARD, H. G. (1953). *Flames: their structure, radiation and temperature*, Lond.
[7] BEHRENS, H. (1950). *Z. phys. Chem.*, 195, 329–36; cf. p. 334.
[8] COWARD, H. F., and JONES, G. W. (1952). *Limits of flammability of gases and vapours*, U.S. Bur. Mines, Bull. No. 503.
[9] JONES, G. W. (1938). *Chem. Rev.*, 22, 1–26.

CHAPTER XXI

EXPLOSIONS *Part* 2:

DEFLAGRATIONS AND DETONATIONS IN FUEL MIXTURES

Speed of Deflagration

THE character of deflagrations in any fuel mixture varies within the range of flammability. Near the L.L. and U.L., the self-propagating flame tends to die out, while the most powerful deflagration tends to occur for fuel concentrations near the stoichiometric value.

This statement finds a more quantitative expression in terms of FLAME SPEED; when this has its maximum value the effects of a deflagration are most pronounced.

Fig. 338—a row of vertical tubes (100 cm long) are filled with increasingly rich fuel/air mixtures. The composition of the mixtures in the various tubes can be read underneath from the horizontal scale. At the lower ends of the tubes, wires are inserted which can be heated by an electric current.

In the first three tubes on the left containing lean mixtures, and in the two tubes on the right containing rich mixtures, the wires are kept permanently heated. As these mixtures are supposed to lie below the L.L. and above the U.L. respectively, only static flames are possible in the neighbourhood of the heated wires.*

In all the other tubes the wire was heated for a short moment only at zero time in order to ignite the flammable mixtures. The position of the self-propagating flames is shown one second later.

In this fictitious fuel the flame speed rises from about 45 cm/s at the L.L. (f = 4%) to a maximum of 85 cm/s at f = 8%, and decreases in richer mixtures to 55 cm/s at the U.L. (f = 11%).

The part of the tubes shaded with short lines indicates the burnt gases (final products) left behind in the wake of the advancing flames.

Change of flame speed with composition of mixture

A practical example of the change of flame speeds with fuel concentration is given in Table 17 for Ethylene-Air mixtures. The values refer to flames travelling upwards in vertical tubes of 2·5 cm internal diameter. In the second row of the table, the fuel concentrations are expressed

---

* In an actual experiment, the flames in mixtures near the U.L. would appear bright and 'smoky', because incomplete oxidation leads to the formation of incandescent carbon particles. In fig. 338 the flames below L.L. and above U.L. are both in mauve to symbolize their static character.

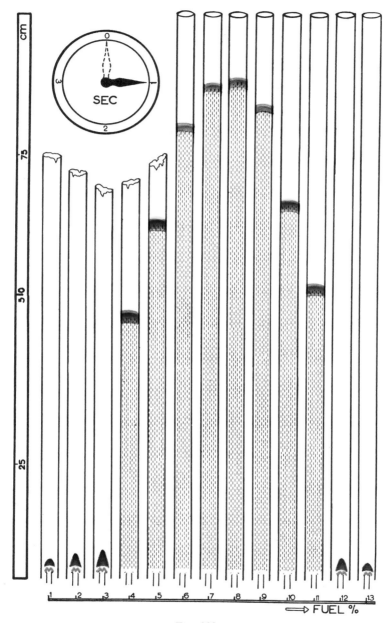

Fig. 338

relative to that of the stoichiometric mixture in air; lean mixtures are here represented by numbers below 1, rich mixtures by numbers above 1 (see also p. 301).

The flames travel fastest in mixtures with f = 7·2 %v/v, i.e. in mixtures which contain one-tenth more fuel than the stoichiometric one. The table shows that the L.L. of deflagration occurs at about one-half the stoichiometric value. The same ratio holds approximately for various other fuel/air mixtures.

At the upper limit the flame speed is only one-sixth of the maximum value, and the concentration is over three times greater than the stoichiometric concentration.

TABLE 17

SPEED OF DEFLAGRATION IN ETHYLENE-AIR MIXTURES

Ethylene $\dfrac{f\,\%v/v}{f/f_{st}}$	3·5 0·53	4·0 0·61	6·0 0·92	7·2 1·10	9·4 1·44	23 3·52
Speed (cm/s):	26	40	110	140	70	22

If the speeds of deflagration in METHANE/Air mixtures are measured under similar conditions, a maximum speed of 65 cm/s is found at f = 10·3 %v/v; here $f/f_{st}' = 10\cdot3/9\cdot5 = 1\cdot08$.

At the limits (L.L. = 5·8%; U.L. = 13%) the speeds are approximately one-third of the maximum speed.

Direction of flame propagation

The speed and character of a deflagration are decisively influenced by environmental conditions (see p. 313). The following comments refer to flammable mixtures contained in tubes.

For a tube of given size, the limits of flammability depend on the position of the tube and on the site of ignition.

Fig. 339—this vertical tube is filled with a fuel/air mixture, and at zero time the filament near the lower end has been heated by closing the switch in a battery circuit. Within a short time (say, 1 s) a flame is travelling up the tube into the fresh mixture with a speed indicated by the white arrow. The switch is now opened, and in

Fig. 340—the filament has again cooled down. Nevertheless, the flame has continued upward into the fresh mixture and has reached the upper end of the tube within another few seconds.

In the following illustrations we consider another tube filled with the same fuel/air mixture, but this time with the igniting, hot filament arranged at the upper end.

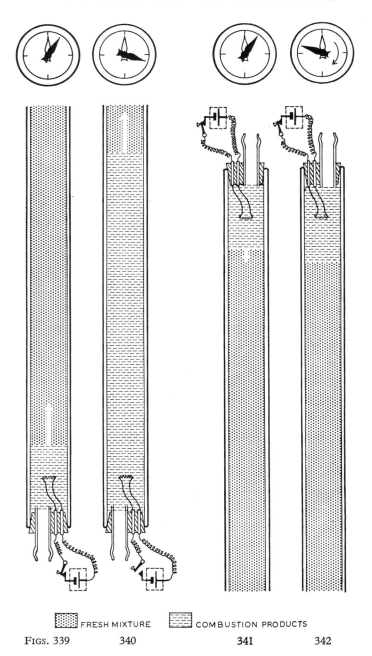

FRESH MIXTURE   COMBUSTION PRODUCTS

FIGS. 339   340   341   342

Fig. 341—at zero time the switch has been closed, the filament heated and within a second or so a flame has begun to travel downward. Within this short time the flame is seen slowing down as indicated by the shorter length of the white arrow compared to that in fig. 339.

Fig. 342—the switch is still closed and the clock shows that a much longer time has passed than in fig. 340. Nevertheless, the flame has not advanced much beyond its position in fig. 341 and is now completely extinguished.

During the upward propagation (fig. 339), the hot combustion gases tend to rise because their density is smaller than that of the cool, fresh mixture above the flame front. The resulting convection currents mix some of the hot gases with the fresh mixture and thereby increase the flame speed. The same convection process also *extends the limits* of flammability compared with those in downward propagation or in a horizontal tube. Table 18 gives a practical example for Ethylene/Air mixtures.

TABLE 18

LIMITS OF FLAMMABILITY AND DIRECTION OF FLAME PROPAGATION IN MIXTURES OF ETHYLENE/AIR

Fuel concentration *% v/v*	*Direction of flame propagation*		
	Upward	*Downward*	*Horizontal*
at L.L.:	3·3	3·6	3·3
at U.L.:	25·6	13·7	18·2

Although the effect of the direction of propagation is small at the lower limit of flammability, it can be very significant at the upper limit. It is thus possible that a given mixture which is non-flammable when ignited in a vertical tube at the top, may support a lively deflagration when the ignition takes place at the lower end.

In the case of the fictitious fuel mixture of figs. 339 et seq. it was assumed that its composition is near the U.L. for upward propagation.

DETONATIONS

Under certain conditions explosions occur in gaseous mixtures which are extremely violent compared with the relatively mild deflagration processes discussed so far. These phenomena are known as *detonations*, and the flame speed in them is very high.

Gaseous mixtures of combustible substances with a *high oxygen content* are prone to detonate when ignited. If the fuel concentration of such oxygen-rich mixtures is not too near the lower or upper limits of flammability, the rate of combustion, and consequently the rate of heat production, can accelerate quickly to very high values. Owing to the fast liberation of heat in each successive layer and the correspondingly high temperature produced in it, insufficient time is available for the pressure to equalize.

The pressure in the flame front rises, therefore, *to considerable values*. A steep pressure wave (comparable to a breaker in sea waves on the coast) impinges on the adjoining layer of fresh mixture and, similar in action to a piston, heats this by compression. This heating by compression is extremely rapid and raises the temperature of the layer far above its ignition temperature so that the rate of reaction in it becomes extremely rapid.

From now on the initiation and propagation of the combustion is continued by the high temperature developed whenever the compression wave reaches a layer of fresh mixture.

A simile for deflagration and detonation

The difference between a deflagration and a detonation may be illustrated by the following crude analogy:

Imagine a crowded sports field. At one corner a man whispers to his neighbour some interesting fact. This first neighbour hands on the information to a second neighbour also in a whisper. The second person again hands on the message which thus travels through the crowd at a steady, slow rate until everybody in the field has heard the news. Such a method of propagation could be likened to a mild *deflagration*.

Suppose that in the same field the message whispered by the first person is overheard by two or three neighbours. Each of these in their turn hands on the message to two or three others. Here and there, however, are people who either do not hear the message or who may hear the same message from two of their neighbours; in other words, certain messages are wasted. The resultant effect is that at every step the message is spread on the average by, say, three persons at a time. The message travels at a *faster* rate than in the first example, but still at a fairly moderate and steady speed. This might be compared to a strong deflagration.

The members of another assembly are assumed to be equipped with much stronger voices. The man who first spreads the message has a loud voice and shouts the message to his fellows. The message is heard by, say, twenty people who in their turn transmit it by shouting to some four hundred other persons. Very soon the whole field would be in a state of pandemonium. The message has spread across the assembly with extreme rapidity, and this might be likened to a *detonation*.

In the first two examples where the message is whispered close to the ears of the nearest neighbours, the speed of propagation of the message depends on personal contact. In a deflagration the ignition of the fresh mixture is caused by the relatively slow process of heat conduction.

In the last example, however, personal contact was unnecessary because the message travelled across the field practically with the speed of sound.

Physical principles of a detonation

The mechanism whereby the detonation is propagated through a tube is roughly as follows:

Assume that a flame has already begun to travel through the mixture. The heat generated in the combustion zone behind the flame front is great and quickly produced, so that the adjoining layer of fresh mixture is heated up to a higher temperature than the initial temperature of the preceding layer. In accordance with Arrhenius' rule, the rate of reaction and heat production in this second layer will be considerably higher than in the preceding layer; this second layer has now become the flame front with a considerably higher temperature. The next (third) layer of adjoining, fresh gas will therefore be heated to a higher temperature than that reached by the second layer. This process continues, and it will be understandable that in a short time very high temperatures are produced in the advancing flame. At the same time, pressure disturbances begin to travel ahead of the flame.

Propagation of small pressure disturbances through a gas

Any localized, small increase of pressure in a gas is propagated through it with the velocity of normal sound; such a pressure pulse might be produced by tapping a rubber membrane stretched over the open end of a tube filled with air or any other gas. As the gas molecules are responsible for the transmission of the pressure wave, it is not surprising that the speed with which the wave is propagated is close to the value of the *average molecular velocity* at the ambient temperature.

In air at normal conditions the speed with which any small pressure disturbance is propagated, is approximately 330 m/s. This is the speed of sound.*

In a normal sound wave as produced during speech or in any noise of moderate intensity, the transmitted pressure wave is extremely small. When the pressure wave sweeps across any point in the tube, the local pressure rise above atmospheric in the gas is usually much smaller than 1 mm H_2O.

One can expect that the speed of sound will rise with increasing

* 1200 km/h or 750 m.p.h.

temperature of the gas in the same way as the molecular velocity rises. This relation can be expressed as:

$$\frac{\text{speed of sound at T}}{\text{speed of sound at T}_0} = \sqrt{\frac{T}{T_0}}; \quad T \text{ in } °K$$

If the gas is heated from room temperature to 900 °C, the speed of sound in it will be increased by approximately

$$\sqrt{\frac{1200}{300}} = \sqrt{4}, \quad \text{or 2-fold.}$$

Propagation of large pressure disturbances

The picture is very different if the pressure disturbance at the beginning of a gas column is high; this could be produced by suddenly pushing a piston into the end of the tube with a velocity approaching molecular velocity, i.e. several hundred metres/sec. The resultant pressure wave will travel through the tube at speeds far above normal speed of sound.

The strong pressure wave compresses the gas rapidly and thereby raises its temperature very considerably. This temperature rise alone would cause an increase in the speed of propagation. Furthermore, the pressure sets the gas into motion at a high velocity. Any subsequent pressure waves will therefore travel not only in a much hotter gas but also in a gas which is streaming with high velocity in the same direction. Finally a narrow zone of high pressure travels at supersonic speed: this is known as a SHOCK WAVE.

The speed of propagation of the pressure wave as seen by an observer watching from outside the tube is the sum of the sound velocity in the heated gas plus the stream velocity of the gas itself. This is an example of the law of super-position of velocities.

Another example of this super-position law is the following: An observer standing next to a railway track is watching a train travelling with a velocity (v_t). A passenger is running with a velocity (v_p) forwards along the corridor of his coach. The outside observer will note that the traveller is moving with a velocity: $(v_t + v_p)$ relative to the landscape. If the passenger is running at 10 miles/hour along the corridor in a train travelling at $v_t = 20$ miles/hour, the passenger is moving at $10 + 20 = 30$ miles per hour relative to the landscape.

Shock waves[1]

In real life, shock waves in air are easily produced by letting off a high explosive bomb, or by an aeroplane exceeding the local speed of sound.

Example: It is assumed that the air is initially at rest under a pressure of 1 atm and at a temperature of 0 °C. A shock wave is assumed to be travelling through the air and is raising the pressure momentarily to 10 atm at any point across which it is sweeping.

This shock wave compressing the resting air ahead of it travels at a

SHOCK SPEED $= 980$ m/s   (1550 miles/hour)

The air is put into motion with a

STREAM VELOCITY $= 720$ m/s   (1140 miles/hour)

While the air ahead of the shock front is at 0 °C, it is raised just behind the front to a

SHOCK TEMPERATURE $= 430$ °C

According to assumption, the pressure in this shock wave is 10 atm (147 lb/in²). The air reached by the front of the shock wave is compressed, and its SPECIFIC VOLUME is reduced in the ratio 1 to 4 compared with that of the resting air. This compression is much less than expected from the 10-fold pressure increase, because of the high temperature rise which counteracts the compression.

The example shows that the stream velocity of the air behind the shock, and even more the speed of the shock itself, are much higher than sound velocity in the undisturbed air (330 m/s); the shock process is 'supersonic'.

The energy for compressing, heating and putting into motion the resting air will gradually weaken the shock wave, unless it is sustained by a 'vis a tergo'. The latter could be supplied by a fictitious piston being pushed from the back along the tube with a velocity equal to that of the streaming air.

Detonation: fast Combustion propagated by a Shock wave[2]

In the case of a *detonable* fuel/oxygen mixture, the heat liberated in the combustion can supply the energy necessary to maintain the shock wave. A considerable proportion of the energy expended by the shock front is used for producing a supersonic stream of gases in the direction of the wave propagation.

Values for the heat liberated in the combustion of fuel/oxygen mixtures which are not too far from stoichiometric, are in the region of 1 kcal/1 g of mixture. If all this heat could be transformed into kinetic energy of streaming, burnt gases, their velocity could approach 2500 m/s. Of course, only part of the heat is used for maintaining a fast stream of burnt gases immediately behind the shock front, but the estimate shows that the energy is adequate to produce the supersonic stream velocities observed in experiments on detonation.

One significant *difference between a normal shock wave in a non-reacting gas and a detonation* is that the steep pressure front is followed by a very narrow combustion zone in which the temperature rises to twice or more the value at the shock front.[3]

Fig. 343—is a schematic representation of the essential features of a detonation travelling through a detonable mixture, and should be

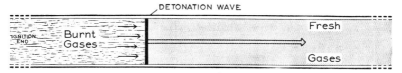

DETONATION WAVE

IGNITION END   Burnt Gases

Fresh

Gases

FIG. 343

compared with fig. 329 (p. 311) describing a deflagration.

The very high speed of the detonation wave is represented by the long, double arrow pointing into the fresh mixture. The detonation wave itself is indicated by a thick, black band which also recalls the analogy of a moving piston (p. 333). The front edge of the black band represents the *shock front* which compresses and heats the fresh gas mixture. Within the width of the black band the combustion proceeds and is completed at the left edge where the temperature is much higher than at the front edge.

The high pressure accelerates the gas towards the right: *note the contrast to the movement of the burnt gases in a deflagration.*

The stream velocity of the gases is highest at the front edge of the wave where it may reach 80% of the speed of the detonation wave itself; at the end of the combustion zone (left edge of black band) the stream velocity of the gases may have fallen to one-half of its value at the front edge.

A short distance behind the detonation wave the burnt gases move already much slower owing to frictional losses and cooling; this situation is indicated by using relatively short arrows for the streaming, burnt gases behind the detonation wave.

Pressure and Temperature in Detonations

Fully developed detonations travelling through detonable gas mixtures in tubes show the following range of characteristic values:

(a) Speed of detonation wave: 2000 to 3000 m/s
(b) Max. temp.   „   „   :   2500 to 3500 °C
(c) Max. pressure „   „   :   20 to 30 atm

The pressures in (c) represent static values which could be measured by a suitable gauge attached to the wall of the tube. If the detonation wave meets an obstacle, these pressures are augmented by the *impact* of the fast stream of the compressed gases following immediately behind the front of the wave.

The total pressure exerted on an obstacle will be therefore a multiple of the pressures listed in (c).

This aspect may be of considerable practical importance in assessing the destructive effects of a detonation in anaesthetic mixtures.

Example:

Assume a static pressure of 25 atm in a detonation front, and that the total impact pressure is three times this value.

If this detonation wave strikes an obstacle of 20 cm² area (corresponding to a circle of 5 cm diameter), the force exerted on it will be:

$$20 \text{ cm}^2 \times (3 \times 25) \frac{\text{kg}}{\text{cm}^2} \simeq 1500 \text{ kg}, \quad \text{or } 3300 \text{ lb}$$

Limits of Detonability

Just as in the case of deflagration, there are lower and upper limits of detonation in all detonable gas mixtures. For very lean and for rich fuel/oxygen mixtures the heat liberated becomes inadequate to maintain a powerful shock wave; beyond these limits we have again normal deflagration flames travelling through the mixtures. Within these limits the speed of detonation varies relatively little, compared to the changes in speed of deflagrations between the limits of flammability. The practical significance of this feature is that detonations are equally destructive throughout the range of detonability.

For the anaesthetist a comparison of detonations in *oxygen-rich* mixtures with deflagrations in mixtures of an anaesthetic vapour with *air* is of particular interest.

Fig. 344—gives a schematic comparison of the limits of detonation in Ether/Oxygen with the limits of deflagration in Ether/Air mixtures. The range and speeds of deflagration (blue line) in Ether/Air mixtures is very small compared with the range and speeds of detonation in Ether/Oxygen mixtures (red line).

In order to view the deflagration on this chart, a cylindrical magnifying glass is used which enlarges the speed scale by 170x and leaves the concentration scale unaltered. The enormous difference between the two processes will be apparent without further discussion.*

---

* The range of deflagration shown is correct for flames travelling downward through a tube. The mauve line near the 20 vol.% mark represents the range of 'cool' flames (see p. 343).

The speeds of detonation entered for ether concentrations above 40% are not based on experiments, and the continuation of the curve beyond the black line drawn from the word 'detonation' is speculative. The main purpose of this illustration is to stress the great difference between deflagration in the mixtures with air and detonation in mixtures with oxygen.

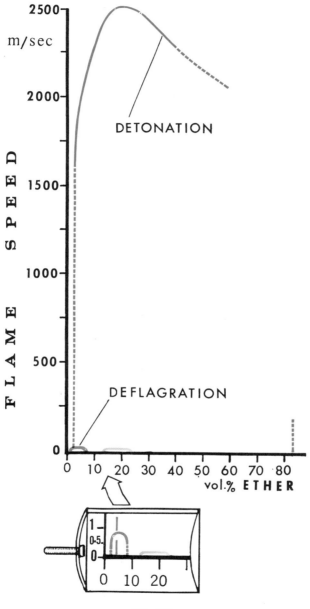

FIG. 344

When the fuel concentration beginning with a very lean mixture in oxygen is increased above the lower limit of flammability, deflagrations will occur in increasingly richer mixtures until the L.L. of detonability is reached. For a wide range of richer mixtures, detonations are possible until the U.L. of detonability is reached. Mixtures with still higher fuel concentrations further permit the passage of deflagrations until the U.L. of flammability is reached.

These various transitions are shown in Table 19 for Acetylene/ Oxygen mixtures for which consistent, experimental values are available.[4] Even though acetylene is nowadays used only for welding and other industrial purposes, it had some vogue as an anaesthetic in former days.

The stoichiometric concentration can be derived again from the combustion equation where $b = 2\frac{1}{2}$ (number of moles of oxygen required to combust one mole of fuel).

$$f_{st} = \frac{1}{1 + 2\frac{1}{2}} \times 100 = \frac{200}{7} = 29\%$$

TABLE 19

DEFLAGRATION AND DETONATION LIMITS IN FUEL/OXYGEN MIXTURES

	DEFLAGRATION				detonation		DEFLAGRATION		
	L.L.				L.L.	U.L.			U.L.
Acetylene (vol. %)	3·5	4·7	7·4	11·0	15	60	63·5	70	88
Speed (m/s)	0·4	2·2	9·7	22	~ 2500		31	4	0·2

The table has been simplified by giving an average value for the speed of detonation within the range of detonability. The change of speed of detonation with concentration is, however, fairly small:

$$f = 25\% \quad \text{speed} = 2330 \text{ m/s,}$$
$$f = 50\% \quad \text{speed} = 2920 \text{ m/s}$$

Initiation of a detonation[5]

If the ignition of a detonable mixture occurs near the closed end of a tube, the expanding combustion products set the fresh gases into motion so that the flame travels through an accelerating gas stream. The flame speed is thereby increased, and conditions for the formation of a high pressure shock wave are so favourable that a proper detonation sets in very quickly.

If the ignition of a very detonable mixture occurs near the open end of a tube, a measurable time interval will elapse during which the flame speeds up from a deflagration to a true detonation.

Fig. 345—Gradual establishment of a detonation.

1st clock: a certain time interval (say $\frac{1}{4}$ s) has elapsed after a spark jumped across the gap of the sparking plug used as ignition source, and an accelerating deflagration flame (blue) has advanced by one metre.

2nd clock: in about one-half of the first time interval the flame has travelled three times as far. This rapid acceleration has led to the formation of a fully developed detonation.

3rd clock: the detonation has travelled through the intervening 16 metres of the mixture in a very short time —say $\frac{1}{100}$ second or

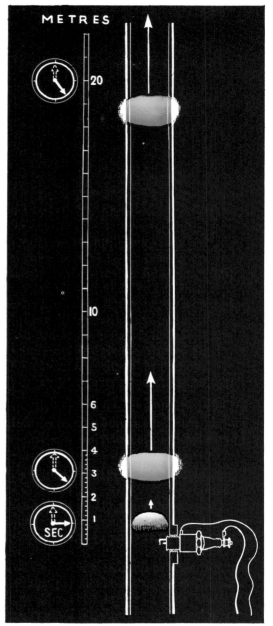

Fig. 345

less. Up to the 20 metre mark the tube is now filled with combustion products.

The detonation wave is illustrated as a bright, fairly wide zone; this is only done to indicate the high temperature and powerful associated radiation (mainly infra-red) produced. The actual width of the combustion zone behind the shock front (see fig. 343) is extremely narrow, and is of the order of the molecular mean free path—say 1000 Å, or 10^{-5} cm.

Why detonations do not occur in mixtures of anaesthetic vapours with AIR

A reader familiar with the literature on detonations may be surprised at the omission by us of any discussion on detonations in mixtures with low oxygen content—say fuel/air mixtures. The following example will show that their inclusion would only confuse the issue for the anaesthetist owing to the exceptional conditions necessary for their production.

Large *petrol storage tanks* and the associated duct systems occasionally contain vapour/air mixtures; their accidental ignition is known to have caused extremely violent explosions and structural damage. In imitation of these conditions, propane/air mixtures were filled into large pipes, about 30 cm in diameter and up to 50 metres long.[6] When the mixture is ignited near the closed end, a deflagration with a speed of a few m/s begins to travel; owing to the expansion of the burnt gases, the fresh gases begin to stream away from the closed end and the flame is accelerated. The flame speed reaches 100 m/s after travelling a few metres. By this time the combustion process has become too fast for the pressure to remain constant, and pressure waves travelling ahead will lead to a true detonation by the time the flame has travelled some 10 metres from the site of ignition. It will be obvious that in a short tube of, say, 1 metre length no detonation could have occurred.

In an extremely narrow range of ETHER/AIR mixtures contained in *wide, long* pipes, detonations can also be produced by *very powerful ignition* sources.[7] However, in the relatively narrow, short breathing tubes or ducts of anaesthetic machines detonations in ether/air mixtures do not occur.

The HISTORY of detonations is closely linked with the characteristics which we have just discussed. In most investigations of flammable gas mixtures during the century following the study of oxygen by LAVOISIER, PRIESTLEY and SCHEELE, small containers of a few cm³ capacity were used. Only after scientists began to study flammable mixtures in large vessels or in long tubes did they find the transition from deflagration into detonation. The pioneer work in this field was done by BERTHELOT and VIEILLE[8] in 1881.

EXPLOSIONS IN ANAESTHETIC MIXTURES

Ether/Air

Only mixtures in the narrow range from 1·8 to 6·5 %v/v of ether in air support normal, self-propagating flames travelling *downward* through a tube. There is a much wider range of combustion processes for other external conditions. Considering in the first instance normal deflagrations, their speed is slow near the limits, and the effects of the deflagration will be very mild. In between the limits lies a mixture yielding the highest speed; when ignited at the open end of a normal pipe (say with a diameter of 10 cm or less) the speed will be below 1 m/s—but it may be a multiple of this value if ignition is near a *closed end* of the duct. The pressures produced when the tube is open at one end are quite negligible; the main harm which can be caused by the deflagration will be due to the flame temperature. For many deflagrations in vapour/air mixtures the temperatures are in the range from 1500 to 2000 °C.

The mixture with the highest flame speed is also the easiest to *ignite*; the composition of this mixture lies on the 'rich' side of the stoichiometric mixture ($f'_{st} = 3·4\%$) at a value of about 4·5 %v/v ether, i.e. at $1·3 \times f'_{st}$. The flammable mixtures near the U.L. and L.L. are the most difficult to ignite; if the source of ignition is an electric spark, the energy required to ignite the limiting mixtures is at least five times that necessary for the most flammable mixture at 4·5%.

Cool Flames[9,10]

Even a short study of the literature on flammability limits of diethyl ether would impress the reader with the apparently considerable variations of the values quoted in it. The main reason is the existence of the somewhat mysterious '*cool flames*'. They can travel through very rich mixtures of diethyl ether, and of some other organic vapours, with air at a total pressure of 1 atm, when the fuel concentration is *above* the upper limit of normal deflagration. While the normal deflagration is a combustion process leaving in its wake mainly CO_2 and H_2O, the cool flame is a *partial oxidation process* travelling through the fresh mixture; in the case of ether some of the final products are acetic acid and acetaldehyde. The name of the process indicates that the temperature is quite low compared with that in a deflagration, and the light emission is correspondingly feeble. For this reason cool flames can be usually observed only in a darkened room.

Propagation of Cool Flames

The temperature in these cool flames may be only a few hundred degrees Celsius, and the mechanism of propagation must be very different from the thermal process used to explain deflagration. In fact, cool flames are propagated by very reactive fragments of molecules (radicals) which require only a very low activation energy to react with the fresh mixture. In order to continue the process, the reaction must also generate further radicals: this mechanism is known as a CHAIN REACTION.

Chain reactions

The pattern of a chain reaction is:

$$R + c \to P + c' \; ; \qquad c' + R \to P + c \; ; \text{etc.}$$

with R = reactant and P = product molecules. The chain carriers: c, c', etc., may be radicals or atoms. The single reaction process does not only yield the products (P) but generates another chain carrier which continues the reaction.

Some explosions, and present-day power generation by nuclear fission, are based on **branched chain reactions.** However, in nuclear fission R and P represent atomic nuclei, chain carriers (c) are neutrons, and the energies liberated are million times greater than in a chemical explosion.

The pattern of a branched chain reaction is for example:

$$R + c \to P + 2 \cdot c \; , \qquad 2 \cdot c + 2 \cdot R \to 2 \cdot P + 4 \cdot c \; , \text{etc.}$$

The single process generates *two* new carriers, each of which initiates another reaction yielding again two more carriers. It is apparent that the chains proliferate and the reaction rate accelerates rapidly.[11]

Some characteristic features of Cool Flames are:

(i) Ignition by electrically heated wires or small gas flames, but *not* by electrical sparks of moderate energy.

(ii) Propagation much influenced by shape and direction of duct or tube; do not travel downward through tubes of normal size.

(iii) The speed is less than that of normal deflagrations; in diethyl ether it may be only a few cm/s.

(iv) Occur only in fuel-rich mixtures ($f > f'_{st}$); they are easiest produced and travel best through mixtures in which the fuel and oxygen concentrations are roughly equal, e.g. 20 %v/v ether with 80% air.

From the characteristics of cool flames it will be understandable that data on their range have to be linked closely with information on size, position and other features of the tube in which they are ignited.

In a *vertical* tube with ignition at the lower end, the range of cool flames joins up without interruption on to the upper limit of deflagration and extends up to f = 40% and beyond.

In *horizontal* tubes there may be a large gap between the U.L. of deflagration and the L.L. of cool flames in which no flames can be propagated through the mixture.

As a practical example we give in Table 20 the limits of deflagration and cool flames in a glass tube of 2·5 cm internal diameter, under certain conditions of ignition.

TABLE 20

LIMITS OF DEFLAGRATION AND COOL FLAMES IN ETHER/AIR MIXTURES

DIRECTION OF PROPAGATION			
Upwards	*Horizontal*		*Downwards*
Deflagration and Cool Flames combined	*Deflagration*	*Cool Flames*	*Deflagration*
Range (vol % ether) 2·0 to 47	Limits (vol % ether) 2·0 to 6·2	Limits (vol % ether) 14 to 25	Limits (vol % ether) 2·0 to 6·2

The various luminous combustion and oxidation processes which can occur in ether/air mixtures are illustrated in figs. 346–50.

Fig. 346—a horizontal tube is filled with a lean ether/air mixture

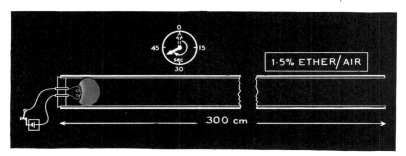

FIG. 346

below the lower limit of flammability. A wire at one end of the tube is heated electrically, and a static flame (aureole) forms around it. If the current were switched off, the static flame would disappear. Even if the wire is kept hot, the static flame may soon disappear as it can only be maintained by fresh mixture diffusing, or being carried by convection currents, into the neighbourhood of the wire. A clock indicates that the flame has not travelled away from the wire although a long time has elapsed.

Fig. 347—a similar tube has been filled with a mixture which is somewhat richer than the stoichiometric value. At zero time the switch

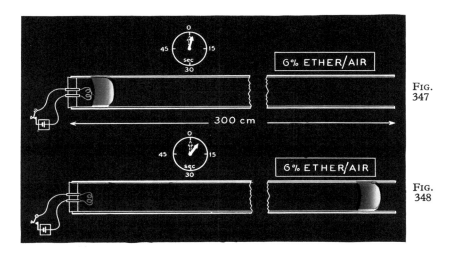

FIG. 347

FIG. 348

to the battery has been closed and within a very short time a bright flame has formed near the hot wire. The switch is now opened and

Fig. 348—illustrates the situation a few seconds later. The wire has cooled down considerably, but the bright flame has continued to travel throughout the 300 cm long tube.*

Fig. 349—a similar tube has been filled with a very rich mixture far above the U.L. of normal deflagration and the switch has been closed at zero time. Some seconds later a faint luminosity seems to 'grow away' from the heated wire; the switch is now opened and

Fig. 350—shows the situation many seconds later. The hot wire has

---

* For this arrangement of the site of ignition illustrated here, the U.L. of deflagration in a 5 cm wide tube is approximately 9 %.

by now cooled to room temperature and a ghost-like, cool flame has slowly travelled along part of the tube.

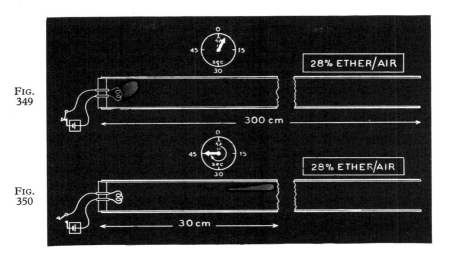

FIG.
349

FIG.
350

Ether/Oxygen

As mentioned in the general discussion on detonations, there is a wide range of mixtures of these two components in which the combustion process may be a violent detonation. The whole range of flammability is much wider than in ether/air mixtures and extends from $f = 2$ to over 80%; detonations have been experimentally observed between approximately 3 and 33%.

Detonable ether/oxygen mixtures can all be ignited by electric sparks. Mixtures near that of greatest detonability are ignited by very feeble sparks. For diethyl ether the most detonable mixture is $f_i \simeq 15\%$; the respective spark energy is less than $\frac{1}{100}$ of that required to ignite a mixture of 5% ether in oxygen. (See also p. 377.)

On the other hand, ether/air mixtures are not easily ignited by a spark; furthermore, the most easily ignited ether/air mixture requires a spark energy comparable to that of the least ignitable ether/oxygen mixture.

The contrast between the effects of igniting a mixture of ether/**air** and another with the same concentration of ether in **oxygen** is quite extraordinary, as will become apparent from a comparison of figs. 351–3 with figs. 354–5.

Fig. 351—A flammable ether/air mixture fills the long, horizontal glass tube. Ignition is by an electrically heated wire near the left end. At zero time the wire is already heated to ignition temperature. A short interval elapses before the cross section of the tube is filled with a deflagration flame. The switch is now opened.

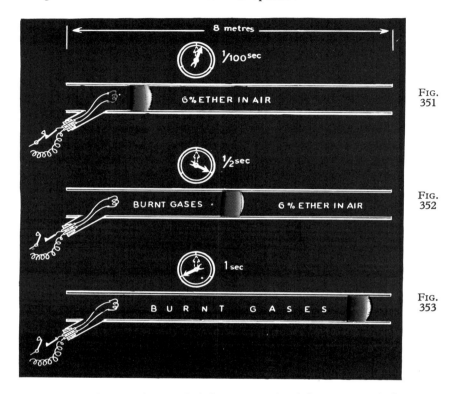

FIG.
351

FIG.
352

FIG.
353

Fig. 352—the wire has cooled down, but the deflagration is independent of the ignition source and has travelled through part of the tube.

Fig. 353—the deflagration has continued to travel at a fairly uniform rate through the fresh mixture.

It should be noted that the illustrations are quite schematic; thus the deflagration speed in an actual experiment of this kind would be far less if the tube were open near the ignition end. The speed which could be derived from these figs. might occur in a tube which is closed at the ignition end, but such a flame would not travel at uniform speed. The purpose of this representation is to stress the fact that even a rapid deflagration is a much slower affair than the detonation discussed in the following figs. 354–5.

Fig. 354—the tube is filled with a *detonable* ether/oxygen mixture. In order to correlate this experiment with fig. 351, a hot wire is again

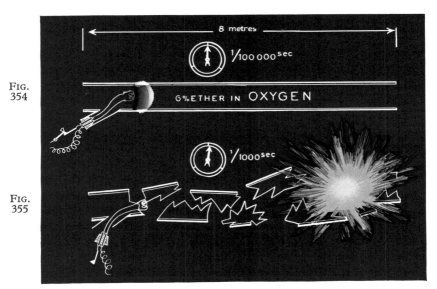

FIG. 354

FIG. 355

shown as ignition source, although in practice an electrical spark could be used. At zero time the wire temperature is assumed to exceed the ignition temperature; within a very short time interval a rapidly accelerating deflagration has formed which will shortly develop into a full detonation.

Fig. 355—within one (or a few) milliseconds the detonation has raced through the long tube which has begun to disintegrate.

Comparison of the clock dials in figs. 354–5 with those in figs. 351–3 shows that the detonation is practically over before the deflagration in the air mixture has started to move away from the vicinity of the ignition source.

Comparing the effects of a deflagration in *ether/air* mixtures with those of a detonation in *ether/oxygen* mixtures, one can predict of the former that its harmful effects to the patient would be those of burning. The main harm caused by a detonation in ether/oxygen mixtures would not only be due to the high pressure wave but also to the very elevated flame temperature.

In this connection it should be mentioned that the shock front of a detonation can continue to travel into a non-flammable or inert mixture. Although the pressure wave travelling through this will be quickly weakened (attenuated), it may still cause dangerous injuries. Thus a breathing tube with mask, containing a detonable mixture, might be placed over the mouth while the patient's respiratory tract still contains only air. If the mixture in the tube should be accidentally ignited, the detonation wave would end in the face mask, but a pressure shock wave could still travel down the respiratory tract and cause injuries of trachea or lungs by 'blast'. If the respiratory tract itself is filled with detonable mixture, the patient would also be badly burnt by the extremely high flame temperature.

Cyclopropane/Oxygen

Cyclopropane is almost invariably administered with pure oxygen. Such mixtures detonate over a wide range within the limits of flammability. The following Table 21 lists the various combustion processes possible in mixtures of cyclopropane with oxygen and with air. The wide range of flammability of mixtures with pure oxygen would be gradually reduced if the mixture were diluted with air.

TABLE 21

EXPLOSIONS IN MIXTURES OF CYCLOPROPANE

WITH OXYGEN	WITH AIR	
Deflagrations and Detonations combined	*Deflagrations only*	
Range (vol. % cyclopropane)	Limits (vol. % cyclopropane)	
	L.L.	U.L.
2·5 to 60	2·4	10·3

As in other flammable anaesthetics, mixtures of cyclopropane in air give relatively mild deflagrations compared with the destructive detonations which may result when oxygen-rich mixtures are ignited.

The apparatus used for administering cyclopropane is the closed circuit, and ideally no mixture should escape into the air. Explosions may often be due to leaky connections, even though the anaesthetist might not be aware of such faults. The explanation given for certain accidents was that sparks from an X-ray machine passed through the walls of rubber tube or breathing bag. From a technical point of view this seems not very likely. However, sparks due to the equalization of static potential differences just when the face mask is close to the patient is quite another matter and have certainly caused a number of explosions. These always took place in oxygen-rich mixtures of cyclopropane, the patients suffering from marked blast effects.

On the other hand, no explosion has ever been reported from, say, a leaking cyclopropane cylinder. Were cyclopropane administered with air, fewer explosions would have occurred and probably none with fatality. At least one author[12] has described a technique for the administration of cyclopropane with air.

Divinyl Ether mixtures with oxygen and air

This substance is said[13] to be more explosive than diethyl ether in mixtures with air; low concentrations of only 2 %v/v in air are stated to deflagrate rapidly, although this may need confirmation. Measurements giving unusually high flame speeds for 5% mixtures were made in completely closed tubes.

Explosions in closed vessels

This may be the place to point out that all flammable mixtures when ignited in closed vessels show much higher combustion rates and associated flame speeds than are found for the same mixtures in open tubes. The hot combustion gases tend to expand and thereby cause turbulent flows in the gas mixture which greatly speed up the flame. Furthermore, the pressure rise due to the high temperature of the burnt gases usually speeds up the reaction rate. The peak pressure during the combustion of a 5% divinyl ether/air mixture in a closed vessel exceeds 100 lb/in² (7 atm).

The U.L. in mixtures with air given in Table 22 deserves some comment. Although much less prone than diethyl ether to produce cool flames at atmospheric pressure, divinyl ether in a wide, vertical tube ignited from the lower end shows these in a range from f = 20 to 26%. Of further interest is the very wide range of flammability in mixtures with pure oxygen; the value for the U.L. refers to spark ignition near the closed end of the tube.

TABLE 22

EXPLOSIONS IN MIXTURES OF DIVINYL ETHER

WITH OXYGEN	WITH AIR
Deflagrations and Detonations combined	Deflagrations and Cool Flames
Range (vol. % D.V.E.) 1·8 to 85	Limits (vol. % D.V.E.) 1·7 to 27

The very high vapour pressure of this substance at room temperature (see p. 70) makes it liable to leak from the storage bottles. Particular care is therefore necessary to store it away from any source of ignition.

Ethyl Chloride

Contrary to erroneous views expressed occasionally,[14] this substance is very flammable.

Experiment

A large bowl is partly filled with water. A few cm³ of ethyl chloride are sprayed on to the water and a lighted taper is approached to the surface. The ethyl chloride vapour burns brightly in air and a pungent smell of hydrogen chloride is noticeable.

Mixtures of ethyl chloride with oxygen are explosive, although such explosions are extremely rare in general anaesthesia. This rarity is probably due to the fact that ethyl chloride is usually mixed with air

TABLE 23

EXPLOSION LIMITS IN MIXTURES OF ETHYL CHLORIDE

WITH OXYGEN		WITH AIR	
(E.C. vol.%)		(E.C. vol.%)	
L.L.	U.L.	L.L.	U.L.
4·0	67	3·8	15

instead of with oxygen, and is also used only for a few minutes during induction of anaesthesia. The vapour has already departed from the scene by the time the diathermy machine or other sources of ignition are started.

However, numerous deflagrations have been reported when ethyl chloride was sprayed on the skin in the vicinity of a source of ignition, e.g. when it was used for anaesthetizing the skin before application of cautery at that spot.

The limits in Table 23 are for upward propagation in vertical pipes of 5 cm diameter; the ignition was at the lower, open end.

Flammability of chlorinated hydrocarbons

Ethyl chloride is a chlorinated hydrocarbon; yet other compounds of this class, e.g. carbon tetrachloride, are even used as fire extinguishers. Whether a chlorinated hydrocarbon can form flammable mixtures with oxygen or not, depends on the number of chlorine atoms relative to the number of hydrogen atoms contained in the molecule, and also on the molecular structure. The structure of a few chlorinated hydrocarbons and their explosive properties are listed in Table 24.

TABLE 24

	Formula	Properties of mixtures with oxygen or air
METHANE	CH_4	flammable
METHYL CHLORIDE	$CH_3 \cdot Cl$	flammable
CHLOROFORM	$CH \cdot Cl_3$	non-flammable
CARBON TETRACHLORIDE	$C \cdot Cl_4$	non-flammable
ETHYLENE	$H_2 \cdot C = C \cdot H_2$	flammable
TRICHLOROETHYLENE	$Cl_2 \cdot C = C \cdot HCl$	practically non-flammable
ETHANE	$H_3 \cdot C - C \cdot H_3$	flammable
ETHYL CHLORIDE	$H_3 \cdot C - C \cdot H_2Cl$	flammable

Trichloroethylene

While many mixtures of ethylene are very flammable, trichloroethylene is unlikely to be ignited under *clinical conditions*. Some confusion regarding the practical significance of explosion in oxygen-rich mixtures of high vapour strength may have been caused by a publication[15] which inverted the usual emphasis on the absence of explosive risks in trichloroethylene mixtures. This article stressed that only below 28 °C could one consider trichloroethylene as non-flammable. This is chemically quite correct, but somewhat obscures the main point that such strong vapour mixtures are extremely unlikely ever to accumulate in an anaesthetic apparatus.

Example

At 20 °C: Pressure of saturated vapour $= 60 \text{ mmHg}$

Maximum concentration of vapour $= \dfrac{60}{760} \times 100 = 7 \cdot 9 \%$

At 28 °C: Pressure of saturated vapour $= 95 \text{ mmHg}$

Maximum concentration of vapour $= \dfrac{95}{760} \times 100 = 12 \cdot 5 \%$

The lower limit of flammability of trichloroethylene in pure oxygen is L.L. $= 10 \cdot 3 \% \text{v/v}$. Even in a saturated mixture of the vapour with pure oxygen at 28 °C the explosion would be very mild because the concentration is so near to the L.L.

The upper limit in mixtures with oxygen is U.L. $= 64\%$ which corresponds to a saturation temperature of 72 °C! Such combinations of high temperatures and saturated vapours are, of course, never met with in clinical practice even in the tropics.

Mixtures of trichloroethylene with AIR are always *non-flammable*. The air must be enriched with oxygen to reach an oxygen concentration of at least 33% before it becomes flammable. In this case the lower limit becomes L.L. $= 13 \cdot 3\%$ which corresponds to a saturation temperature of 32 °C. One must not overlook in this connection that even in an anaesthetic bottle the concentration of the vapour above the liquid is rarely as high as the saturation value at that particular temperature. In other words, the temperatures quoted above would have to be still higher in practical conditions before even the mixture in the anaesthetic bottle would approach the flammable range.

Ethylene

This gas is rapidly disappearing from anaesthetic practice; during its heyday it gave rise to a large number of violent detonations. Ethylene was invariably mixed with pure oxygen, and hardly ever used in a closed circuit, so that large quantities of highly flammable mixtures escaped into the room.

In Table 25 limits of flammability of ethylene in oxygen and in air are listed for upward propagation in a vertical tube (5 cm internal diameter).

The U.L. of detonations is probably higher than $f = 55\%$; the most violent detonations with speeds of 2500 m/s occur in mixtures with over 25% ethylene in oxygen. With a different experimental arrangement,[16] detonations were observed in a range of ethylene/oxygen mixtures from 3·5% to 92%.

TABLE 25

EXPLOSION LIMITS IN MIXTURES OF ETHYLENE

WITH OXYGEN			WITH AIR	
range of flammability	**Detonations**		*Deflagrations*	
L.L.	U.L.		L.L.	U.L.
3·1	80	9 to > 50	3	28

Deflagrations in mixtures with air are again relatively mild. The maximum flame speeds are less than 1 m/s for $f = 7\%$, when ignition takes place at the open end. As always, the range is very sensitive to size and position of tube; the U.L. for downward propagation through a tube of 5 cm diameter is approximately 15% ethylene in air.

Fuel—Nitrous oxide mixtures

If a mixture of ether with oxygen *and* nitrous oxide is compared with one containing oxygen only, it has been sometimes assumed that the former would be less explosive. The reason given was that nitrous oxide would act as a diluent, just as nitrogen does in an ether/air mixture.

This assumption is not only wrong but dangerously misleading. Nitrous oxide strongly supports any combustion process; it does *not* damp down an explosion but, in fact, enhances it. It is also as efficient as oxygen in producing detonable mixtures—say when mixed with ethyl ether.

Nevertheless, it is of interest that the oxygen in the nitrous oxide molecule does not enter into any biological oxidations; nitrous oxide does not support life.

Experiment

The high oxidation powers of nitrous oxide become apparent when thrusting a glowing piece of wood (e.g. a spill which has been lit and blown out) into a glass flask filled with nitrous oxide: the wood bursts into brilliant flames. Repeating the experiment with oxygen, it will be impossible to detect any difference in the lively combustion process.

Nitrous oxide should therefore never be mixed with a combustible agent with the intention of lessening the risk of explosion. In these circumstances the following statement will appear to be very reasonable: '*When mixed with hydrogen it (N_2O) exploded with violence like hydrogen and oxygen.*'

In this we have only translated into modern chemical terms a comment[17] by PRIESTLEY of 1780.

Stoichiometric mixtures in nitrous oxide

In comparing the combustion of a fuel molecule (F) in oxygen with that in nitrous oxide, the following significant differences will become apparent:

If the complete combustion in oxygen is given by

$$F + b \cdot O_2 \quad \rightarrow products \quad . \qquad . \qquad . \qquad . \quad (1)$$

the corresponding equation for combustion in nitrous oxide will be

$$F + 2b \cdot N_2O \rightarrow products + 2b \cdot N_2 \qquad . \qquad . \quad (2)$$

The stoichiometric concentrations† in these two cases are

$$f_{st} = \frac{100}{1 + b} \quad \% \, v/v$$

$$f_{st}^* = \frac{100}{1 + 2b} \quad \% \, v/v$$

Example

Considering the combustion of diethyl ether, one obtains with $b = 6$

$$f_{st} = \frac{100}{7} = 14 \cdot 3 \, \% v/v; \qquad f_{st}^* = \frac{100}{13} = 7 \cdot 7 \, \% v/v$$

The first impression might be that a given volume of stoichiometric mixture with nitrous oxide could produce only about one-half the amount of heat as the stoichiometric mixture with oxygen. However, the implied assumption that the heats of combustion in oxygen and in nitrous oxide are more or less equal is quite unfounded.

Heat of combustion of fuel in nitrous oxide

We recall that a combustion process can be considered as a rearrangement of bonds between atoms; also that the heat of combustion can be derived by subtracting the bond strengths between the atoms of the reactant molecules from those of the product molecules.

(i) Considering the combustion of hydrogen in oxygen:

$$O_2 + 2 \cdot H_2 \rightarrow 2 \cdot H_2O \, (g)$$

we have to subtract the sum of bond strengths of one (O-O) molecule

† The stoichiometric concentration of a fuel in nitrous oxide is indicated by f_{st}^*.

and two (H-H) molecules from that of two (H-O-H) molecules. It happens that the bond strengths of H and O atoms in the two water molecules are 2×58 kcal/mole *greater* than in the reactant molecules (O_2 and $2 \cdot H_2$). The heat of combustion of hydrogen with oxygen to 1 mole water vapour is 58 kcal/mole.

(ii) For the combustion in nitrous oxide we consider the equation

$$2 \cdot N_2O + 2 \cdot H_2 \rightarrow 2 \cdot H_2O(g) + 2 \cdot N_2$$

choosing this form in order to simplify the comparison with (i).

If the $2 \cdot N_2O$ had been formed initially from: $2 \cdot N_2 + O_2$, one would have found that the total bond strength between the N and O atoms of the resultant ($2 \cdot N_2O$) is *smaller* than that between the initial molecules ($2 \cdot N_2$ and O_2). This means that in the formation of N_2O from nitrogen and oxygen heat is *not* released but has to be supplied from the outside; the formation of N_2O is an endothermic process.

The combustion in N_2O (ii) utilizes, therefore, a supporter* which has a *higher energy* than the supporter (O_2) used in (i). This additional energy will be liberated in the reaction, and leads to an *increased heat of combustion of a fuel in nitrous oxide* compared to the heat of combustion in oxygen.

For every N_2O molecule required in the stoichiometric equation, the *additional* heat liberated is approximately 19 kcal/mole.

The general expression for the *increment* in heat of combustion compared with that in oxygen can be written as:

$$2b \times 19 \text{ kcal/mole}$$

Examples

(a) For the combustion of hydrogen, with $b = \frac{1}{2}$, the number of N_2O molecules is $2b = 1$.

The increment in heat of combustion is therefore 19 kcal/mole.

(b) For the combustion of ethyl ether with $b = 6$, the increment is $(2 \times 6) \times 19 = 230$ kcal. The heat of combustion in O_2 was found to be 608 kcal/mole (see Table 9, p. 303), and that in N_2O is therefore $608 + 230 = 838$.

The ratio of the chemical heat content in a given volume of the stoichiometric mixture of ether in N_2O to that in O_2 equals**:

$$\frac{7 \cdot 7}{14 \cdot 3} \times \frac{(230 + 608)}{608} \simeq \frac{3}{4}$$

* See p. 324.

** The first factor is the ratio of the stoichrometric concentrations (p. 354); the second, the ratio of heats of combustion in N_2O and O_2 respectively.

The values of heat liberated in stoichiometric mixtures with O_2 or N_2O are not as different as appeared at first. Another fallacious argument relating to the combustion of fuels in nitrous oxide is that N_2O could be considered as a simple mixture of two parts N_2 and one part O_2. This can be easily disproved[18]:

If the 92·3% N_2O contained in the stoichiometric mixture with $f^*_{st} = 7·7\%$ ethyl ether, were replaced by the fictitious 2:1 mixture of N_2 and O_2, it would contain $\frac{1}{3} \times 92·3 = 30·8\%$ oxygen. This quantity of oxygen could only combust $\frac{1}{6} \times 30·8 = 5·1\%$ ether instead of 7·7%.

The heat liberated by a given volume of the fictitious mixture is therefore reduced in the ratio of 0·47 to 1 compared with the actual stoichiometric mixture in N_2O. This follows from multiplying the ratio of concentrations (5·1/7·7) by the ratio of heats of combustion (608/838). The heat released in the combustion with pure nitrous oxide is therefore much higher than in the fictitious 2:1 mixture of N_2 and O_2.

Flammability of fuel—nitrous oxide mixtures

The values in Table 26 are given mainly to convey the wide range of flammability for fuel/nitrous oxide mixtures; the data are neither very

TABLE 26

LIMITS OF FLAMMABILITY IN FUEL-NITROUS OXIDE MIXTURES

	Deflagrations and Detonations combined fuel conc. % v/v		Stoichiometric Mixture	
	L.L.	U.L.	2·b	% v/v
Hydrogen	6	86	1	50
Methane	4	40	4	20
Ethylene	2	40	6	14
Cyclopropane	1·6	30	9	10
Ethyl ether	1·5	24	12	7·7
Divinyl ether	1·4	25	11	8·3
Ethyl chloride	2	33	6	14

accurate nor are they obtained under identical experimental conditions. One reason for the considerable oxidation powers of nitrous oxide is that in (O-N-N) the oxygen atom is held in place with less than half the energy compared with the (O-O) bond in the oxygen molecule. The oxygen atom becomes therefore more readily available for oxidation processes.

The ranges of flammability in Table 26 include also **detonations**. For instance, ignition of mixtures containing from 50 to 80% H_2 in N_2O leads to violent detonations, with flame speeds of about 2500 m/s. Various ethyl ether-nitrous oxide mixtures also detonate quite easily, particularly in the region of $f^* = 10\%$; if nitrous oxide is mixed with oxygen, the range is extended to higher ether concentrations.

The experiment on p. 353 showed that solids can combust in nitrous oxide as briskly as in oxygen. Fires have occurred in pressure-reducing valves in which the seating or the diaphragm consisted of combustible substances.

On the other hand, oxygen and nitrous oxide do not react with one another. This has to be kept in mind when coming across references to explosions during bronchoscopy when only these two were stated to be present. In all these cases a combustible substance must have been the real culprit. Frequently a bottle on the anaesthetic machine may have contained ether, and although the control tap was in the 'off' position, vapour could have freely escaped through the leaky tap into the ducts of the apparatus (see p. 390).

REFERENCES

[1] PENNEY, W. G., and PIKE, H. H. M. (1950). *Rep. Progr. Phys.*, 13, 46–82; cf. p. 55.

[2] BECKER, R. (1936). *Z. Elektrochem.*, 42, 457–61.

[3] EYRING, H., et al. (1949). *Chem. Rev.*, 45, 69–181; cf. p. 80.

[4] LAFITTE, P. (1938). *Chal. et Industr.*, 19, 33–7.

[5] EVERETT, A. J., and MINKOFF, G. J. (1954). *Fuel, Lond.*, 33, 184–91.

[6] STEINICKE, H. (1948). *Z. Ver. Dtsch. Ing.*, 90, 350.

[7] DICENT, V., and SHCHELKIN, K. (1944). *Acta phys.-chim. U.R.S.S.*, 19, 302–12.

[8] BERTHELOT, M., and VIEILLE, P. (1881). *C. R. Acad. Sci., Paris*, 93, 18–22.

[9] BURGOYNE, J. H. (1949). *Research, Lond.*, 2, 512–18.

[10] EGERTON, SIR ALFRED (1953). In: *Fourth Symposium (International) on Combustion*, No. 1, pp. 4–13. Baltimore.

[11] DAINTON, F. S. (1956). *Chain reactions*, cf. p. xiii. Lond.

[12] HAAS, H. B., et al. (1940). *Anesthesiology*, 1, 31–9.

[13] JONES, G. W., and BEATTIE, B. B. (1934). *Industr. Engng. Chem.*, 26, 557–60.

[14] MACDONALD, A. C., et al. (1950). *Brit. med. J.*, ii, 441–2; see also correspondence, p. 625.

[15] JONES, G. W., and SCOTT, G. S. (1943). *Anesthesiology*, 4, 441–4.

[16] ZELDOVICH, I. B. & KOMPANEETS, A. S. (1960). *Theory of Detonation*, cf. p. 136. New York.

[17] PRIESTLEY, J. (1781). *Experiments and observations relating to various branches of natural philosophy*, cf. II, p. 209. Birmingham.

[18] JORISSEN, W. P., and VAN DER DRUSSEN, A. A. (1933). *Rec. Trav. chim. Pays-Bas*, 52, 327–38.

CHAPTER XXII

EXPLOSIONS *Part 3:*

SOURCES OF IGNITION AND EXPLOSION HAZARDS

INITIATION OF EXPLOSIONS

Chemical Causes

IN former days many explosions of ether were attributed to the presence of *peroxides* occurring as impurities in the liquid. Such compounds are related to the normal hydrogen peroxide (HO-OH) in which one or both hydrogen atoms are replaced by parts of the organic molecule—say the ethyl group (-C$_2$H$_5$). Peroxides can form at room temperature in the presence of atmospheric oxygen by the action of light: this process is also known as 'autoxidation'. The peroxides are very labile and resemble in this respect the so-called detonators used in ammunition. Often the shaking of a bottle containing peroxides has led to violent explosions in chemical laboratories. Fortunately, there are numerous substances known as anti-oxidants which prevent completely the autoxidation of ether; they are always added to anaesthetic ether, and with storage in dark bottles to exclude light, the risk of formation of peroxides has been successfully abolished.

Spontaneous Ignition

The spontaneous (or self-) ignition (p. 305) of flammable mixtures occurs when the whole container with the gas mixture is quickly heated to a certain temperature; combustion takes then place almost simultaneously throughout the whole volume, after the lapse of an interval to which we shall refer shortly. As discussed in earlier sections, flammable mixtures warmed up to a suitable temperature will begin to react quickly enough and thereby heat up further. The method of spontaneous ignition is a valuable tool for the scientist, although of relatively little interest to the anaesthetist. Nevertheless, the 'ignition temperatures' quoted for anaesthetic mixtures are often based on this rather artificial procedure.

The temperature of spontaneous ignition is not a simple property of a given gas mixture. After the mixture has suddenly been heated to a temperature at which the rate of reaction is appreciable, the heat liberated will further raise the temperature until deflagration sets in. The time delay[1] after the initial heating is appropriately known as 'induction period'; according to circumstances this may vary from a

358

few millisec. to hours, particularly if the reaction is carried on by a chain of active particles (p. 342) rather than by heat transfer from the burnt gas to the adjacent fresh layer. For practical purposes only those ignition temperatures are of interest in which the induction period is reckoned in seconds—or less.

One peculiar feature of spontaneous ignition is that the minimum ignition temperature often varies little for a wide range of fuel concentrations: in order to ignite methane/air mixtures in the range between f = 3 and 12%, the mixtures have to be heated to 700–730 °C.

The **minimum ignition temperatures** for the most ignitable mixtures of anaesthetic vapours in AIR lie between 400 and 500 °C; those for mixtures with pure OXYGEN may be 50 degC or more *below* the values for air.

It will be noticed that *the minimum temperatures for spontaneous ignition are far below the flame temperatures* in the subsequent deflagration which attain 1500 °C and more.

Rich mixtures of ETHYL ETHER/AIR (above f = 10%) have exceptionally low ignition temperatures; by heating the container to only 200 °C a 'cool flame' will be initiated. Normal deflagrations, particularly in mixtures with lower ether concentrations, can only be initiated by much higher temperatures of about 450 °C.

Sources of Local Ignition

Practically all anaesthetic explosions are caused by local sources of ignition as will become obvious from the following survey; it is very unlikely that an appreciable volume would be heated evenly to the spontaneous ignition temperature. *In local ignition, heat is supplied to a small part of the whole flammable mixture;* a limited amount of heat is usually supplied during a short period.

Open flames

These sources comprise gas burners, lighted matches, etc., and ignite flammable fuel-air mixtures as well as detonable fuel-oxygen mixtures. Similar to electrically heated wires, they can be used to ignite 'Cool Flames' which are not ignited by electric sparks.

If it should seem surprising that flames are ever present when anaesthetics are handled by properly qualified staff, the following case stories may be of some interest.

Example (a):

A gasbag with ether/oxygen/nitrous oxide mixture was hanging on the trolley of an anaesthetic machine. A small spirit lamp (see fig. 95,

p. 96) warmed the fine adjustment valve on a nitrous oxide cylinder about 1 foot away from the bag. "A pinhole in the bag allowed a stream of mixture to impinge on the flame, and the bag exploded with a deafening report. My head was 2 feet away and I learnt a lesson which I will never forget."[2]

Example (b):

An Oxford Vaporiser needed refilling with ether. The ether was poured in error into the hot water compartment. A fountain of ether and water shot out of the filler opening and reached a lighted gas burner standing 2 feet away on a bench. The flame ran back to the vaporiser and set fire to the only combustible component, the rubber bellows. The occurrence was characterized by the complete absence of drama, which would undoubtedly have been present if oxygen instead of air had been mixed with ether. The ether in the vapour compartment did not catch fire because the vapour concentration in it was far above the upper limit of normal deflagration flames.

Flashpoint: This property of *liquid* fuels is of little significance to the anaesthetist, but is so frequently mentioned in publications on explosions that a short definition of the term is indicated. Flashpoint is the lowest temperature at which a liquid fuel gives off enough vapour to produce a 'flash of flame' when a small flame is passed across the surface of the liquid. It is fairly obvious that many extraneous features will influence this event; the occurrence of a flash will depend on the vapour pressure of the liquid necessary to produce a flammable vapour/air mixture above the liquid. The uncertainty of a flashpoint determination can be appreciated by merely quoting two published values for ethyl ether which are: -40 and $-29\,°C$. The corresponding vapour pressures are 19 and 38 mmHg; if the mixture above the surface were fully saturated, the respective concentrations would be $f = 2.5$ and 5% respectively.

The flashpoints for divinyl ether and ethyl chloride are also far below the icepoint, while that of ethyl alcohol is near room temperature (ca 15 °C). There is no simple relation between flashpoint and spontaneous ignition temperature of a given fuel.

Hot and incandescent surfaces

One common ignition source of this kind which has caused many industrial accidents is the glowing cigarette. An unusual incident with this has been reported in the anaesthetic literature[3] in recent years:

Fig. 356—Soda-lime had been tipped into a bucket from the canister previously used in a closed circuit for ether anaesthesia. Some time later glowing cigarette ashes were flung on it, whereupon a bright flame shot from the bucket. Ether vapour collected in the small cavities of soda-lime granules must have gradually escaped and mixed with the air

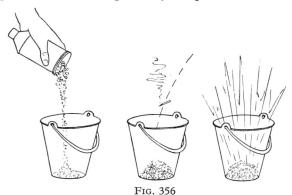

FIG. 356

in the bucket to form a flammable mixture. The incident is of interest in so far as the flame might have acted as an unsuspected source of ignition for other combustible materials in the surroundings of the bucket.

Light emission from hot surfaces

In assessing the danger of ignition by hot surfaces it is important to correlate the temperature of a solid object with the associated emission of visible radiation.

Fig. 357—A metal rod is heated at its left end by the hot flame of a blowpipe. Heat travels by conduction toward the right end, but there will be a marked temperature drop as heat is continuously lost by conduction to the outside air and by radiation. Thermometers are embedded in the rod at equal intervals in order to correlate light emission with temperature. The indications of the thermometers also show that the temperature gradient is greatest in the hottest region of the rod and tends to level out toward the right end. An iron rod heated in this fashion would emit bright yellow-white light at about 1500 °C; at 900 °C the light is bright red and at 700 °C dark red. The part of the rod with temperatures below 500 °C emits practically no visible radiation, although a hand held near this region would quickly sense the powerful infra-red radiation escaping from the hot surface.

This relation between visible light emission and temperature is quite correct for several solids—particularly carbon—but is inapplicable to hot gases. A gas burner with adequate air supply may have an almost invisible flame, although its temperature will be over 1800 °C. However, if the mixture is very rich and combustion incomplete, decomposition of the fuel may form solid carbon particles which are 'incandescent' and make the flame 'bright', e.g. candle flame.

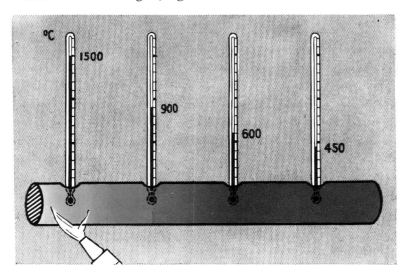

FIG. 357

It will now be obvious that the walls of many containers mentioned in the discussion of 'spontaneous ignition' would not be visibly hot for any experiment below 500 °C.

Endoscope bulbs

Such small, electric bulbs might be a potential local ignition source of the type considered in this section. However, one must not over-look that most of the low ignition temperatures quoted in literature for ethyl and divinyl ether refer to spontaneous ignition where the whole mixture was evenly heated. There is some evidence that the surface temperature of an endoscope bulb would have to be considerably higher in order to act as a local ignition source; in some of these with a supply of 3–4 volt and about 0·2 ampere, the surface temperature of the glass may be anywhere up to 250 °C. Experiments quoted in the literature[4] some twenty years ago, showed that no ignition of 'highly explodable mixtures' could be caused by these bulbs. It may be that the relative immunity from explosions during the use of bronchoscopes, laryngoscopes, etc., is partly due to this.

The situation might be quite different if the glass envelope breaks and the hot filament comes in direct contact with the flammable mixture. Even before such an accident happens, the glass envelope may get much hotter than normally if its wall is unusually thin or if the filament is very close to it. Furthermore, the bulb may be overheated without immediate fusing of the filament. It is only too easy for a nurse to turn the rheostat knob of the electrical supply to increase the voltage at the command of the surgeon who wants more light.

Cool Flame

Although this flame causes no harm by direct action, its insidious character is due to its ability to ignite detonable mixtures. We have seen that such cool flames can occur in ethyl ether/air mixtures in a range of $f = 20$ to 35% approximately. A cool flame can easily ignite detonable mixtures, and the following accident is not beyond possibility.

Fig. 358—an ether bottle has fallen off the trolley on the left and an appreciable amount of liquid ether has been spilt over the floor. The liquid evaporates and owing to its high density mixes mainly with air in the vicinity of the floor. A rich mixture spreads as indicated by the shading and reaches distant parts of the operating theatre. A faulty electric plug or the flex entering it from the portable lamp standard is 'arcing' and thus provides a hot, local ignition source. The rich mixture is accidentally ignited and a cool flame travels through it unobserved;

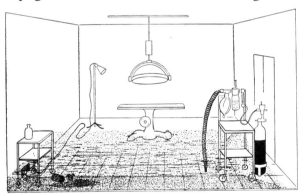

FIG. 358

it may reach the floor around the trolley on the right. Here a trickle of highly detonable ether-oxygen mixture is escaping through the breathing tube which dangles to the floor. Even though the control on the vaporizer bottle is 'off', and the needle valve at the lower end of the flowmeter is apparently closed, such unnoticed escape is not unheard of. When the cool flame reaches the lower end of the breathing tube, a violent detonation would take place.

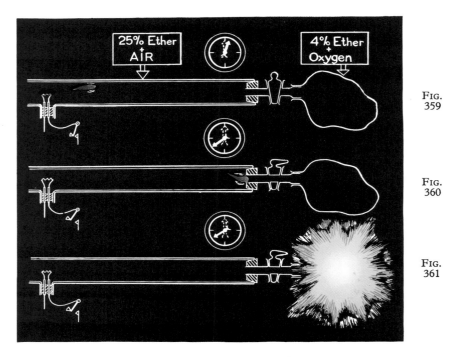

FIG. 359

FIG. 360

FIG. 361

The sequence of this kind of accident can be imitated by the following laboratory experiment:

Fig. 359—the horizontal glass tube is filled with a rich ether/air mixture of 25% (remember that $f'_{st} \simeq 3\%$ only). The right end of the tube is connected to a bag containing the detonable mixture of 4% ether in oxygen. The connecting stopcock is still shut. The filament near the left end was heated electrically at zero time, and a ghost-like, cool flame has since begun to creep along the tube.

Fig. 360—the electric switch has been opened and the wire has cooled to room temperature. The cool flame has nevertheless continued to travel slowly through the tube. In the meantime the stopcock has been opened and after a considerable time (note clock) the flame will reach the entrance to it.

Fig. 361—a moment later a violent explosion occurs: the detonable mixture of the bag has been ignited by the cool flame.

| This experiment should not be tackled by the beginner because a number of precautions must be taken. |

Ignition by hot filaments

One well-known source of this kind is the cautery. Apart from igniting anaesthetic mixtures, cautery[5] is known to have started fires when the skin was prepared with alcohol and other volatile, combustible substances. To this group of ignition sources belong also exposed filaments of broken endoscope bulbs and, furthermore, the 'arcs' which may occur whenever a switch or a flex on an electric apparatus are faulty.

The detailed mechanism of ignition by hot wires is very involved, but the following general rule can be applied to them as well as to electric sparks:

The faster the energy is supplied by an ignition source and the smaller the volume to which it is applied, the lower will be the minimum energy required to ignite a certain flammable mixture.

Two extreme situations will help to understand this rule:

(i) If a limited amount of heat is supplied very slowly, i.e. the rate of energy supply (also known as 'POWER') is very small, the heat would be conducted away without ever raising the gas temperature in the neighbourhood of the source anywhere approaching the required ignition temperature.*

(ii) If, on the other hand, a given quantity of energy is supplied instantaneously but spread out over too large a volume of mixture, the maximum temperature reached may again be rather low because a limited amount of energy is spread over a larger volume. Ignition would then only be possible if the energy is further increased.

The size, shape and material of the source, all influence the energy or temperature necessary to ignite a flammable mixture. It may happen that a fine wire heated to a certain temperature does not ignite a

---

* For ignition by a small local source of short duration—say a cautery switched on for a moment—a certain small volume of the mixture has to be raised to a high temperature before an explosion travelling through the whole mixture becomes possible. In contrast to the temperatures required for spontaneous ignition (see p. 359) these temperatures are much higher, and in the region of the flame temperature itself, i.e. instead of, say, 600 °C they might be nearer 1800 °C. Furthermore, if the source is a fine wire, the peak temperature of the wire itself may still be considerably higher.

particular mixture, while a large bar heated to the same surface temperature easily ignites it.

Electric Energy

In order to appreciate some data on explosions initiated by fine, hot wires, arcs or electric sparks, it is necessary to digress shortly, and to compare electric energy with the thermal unit of energy, the cal or the kcal.

If an electric supply source with a potential difference* of E volts is connected to a wire of resistance R ohms, an electric current of I amperes will flow through and heat the wire.**

The relation between E, I and R is given by **Ohm's law**:

$$I = \frac{E}{R} \qquad . \qquad . \qquad . \quad (1)$$

or in other forms:

$$E = R \times I ; \qquad R = \frac{E}{I} \qquad . \quad (2) \text{ and } (3)$$

Examples:

(*a*) If the potential difference across a wire is 1 volt and the current passing through it 1 ampere, then the resistance follows from Eq. 3

$$\text{with } E = 1 \text{ V}, \quad I = 1 \text{ A}, \quad R = \frac{1 \text{ V}}{1 \text{ A}} = 1 \, \Omega$$

This is actually the definition of unit resistance (1 ohm).

(*b*) If the mains voltage of $E = 240$ V is applied to a resistance of $R = 60 \, \Omega$, then the current passing through the resistance is given by Eq. 1

$$I = \frac{240 \text{ V}}{60 \, \Omega} = 4 \text{ A}$$

If an electrical supply source with a potential difference of E volts passes a current of I amperes through a wire (say in an electric fire) during a period of t seconds, the *electric energy* dissipated in the wire and appearing as heat is given by:

$$H = E \times I \times t . \qquad . \qquad . \quad (4)$$

---

* E is often called the 'voltage' of the mains; the correct scientific term is electromotive force (e.m.f.), but the expression used here helps to relate this electrical quantity to the hydraulic analogy, where E would be the pressure pushing liquid through a pipe which opposes a certain resistance to the flow.

** The unit of current is   : ampere (A)
  ,, ,, ,, potential difference is : volt (v)
  ,, ,, ,, resistance is   : ohm (Ω)

For symbols and abbreviations see: *British Standard* (1954) No. 1991: Part 1.

The unit in which the energy H is expressed is given by:

$$1 \text{ volt} \times 1 \text{ ampere} \times 1 \text{ second}$$

and is known as: 1 joule (J).

In other words, the electric energy dissipated if a potential difference of 1 V applied to a resistance sends through it a current of 1 A which is kept flowing for 1 sec, is known as 1 joule.

'Joule' is a fairly small energy unit; its relation to the familiar calorie is given by:

$$1 \text{ joule (J)} \ldots 0 \cdot 24 \text{ cal}; \qquad 1 \text{ cal} \ldots 4 \cdot 2 \text{ J} \qquad . \quad (5)$$

Example:

An electric fire (single bar type) draws a current of $I = 4$ A, when connected to the electric mains having a voltage $E = 240$ V. How much heat is generated during 5 minutes?

The energy dissipated in the wire during 5 minutes (300 s) follows from Eq. 4 and 5:

$$H = 240 \text{ V} \times 4 \text{ A} \times 300 \text{ s} = 288\,000 \text{ J} \qquad \text{or}$$
$$288\,000 \times 0 \cdot 24 = 69\,000 \text{ cal} \simeq 70 \text{ kcal.}$$

This amount of heat is about the same as that developed by the combustion of 9 g carbon.

Electric Power

It is often more important to know at what *rate* electrical energy is dissipated or at what rate heat is produced. This rate is the total amount of energy divided by the time during which it has been produced, and is generally known as '*power*' (P). It follows from Eq. 4 that:

$$P = \frac{H}{t} = E \times I \frac{\text{joule}}{\text{s}} \qquad . \qquad . \qquad . \quad (6)$$

The unit of electrical power: 1 joule/s is known as WATT (W).

Example:

An electrical light bulb for a 240 V mains supply is rated as '60 watt'. What is (*a*) the current passing through the filament and (*b*) how much energy is dissipated if the bulb is alight for three hours?

$$(a) \ I = \frac{P}{E} = \frac{60 \text{ W}}{240 \text{ V}} = 0 \cdot 25 \text{ A}$$

$$(b) \ H = P \times t = 60 \text{ W} \times (3 \times 60 \times 60) \text{ s} = 648\,000 \text{ J}$$

Only a small fraction of the electrical energy dissipated in the filament of a light bulb appears as visible light; neglecting this, one obtains for the heat production of this particular bulb:

$$0 \cdot 24 \times 648\,000 \text{ cal} \simeq 155 \text{ kcal.}$$

Example:

It may be of some interest to compare the power requirements of domestic electric appliances with the metabolic requirements of the human adult:

with a body weight of 70 kg, the requirements are approximately 70 kcal in 1 hour. If all this energy would be dissipated as heat, the corresponding 'power' would be

$$\frac{70 \times 10^3 \text{ cal}}{3 \cdot 6 \times 10^3 \text{ s}} \simeq 20 \frac{\text{cal}}{\text{s}}$$

Using Eq. 5, this power corresponds to:

$$20 \times 4 \cdot 2 \text{ J/s} \simeq 80 \text{ W}$$

Other energy and power units

The unit of electric energy consumption for which the electricity company charges the customer is not the joule but the much larger kilowatt $\times$ hour. As shown by its name, this energy unit is equivalent to an electrical power of 1000 watt supplied throughout one hour (or to 500 watt supplied throughout 2 hours, etc.). It equals, therefore, $1000 \text{ W} \times (60 \times 60) \text{ s} = 3 \cdot 6 \times 10^6 \text{ J}$, or 860 kcal.

Power rating is, of course, applied to all motor-car engines and other machinery. Instead of stating that the engine can do a specified amount of work in an unspecified time (even the weakest motor can do a lot of work when running continuously for years!), the *rate* of doing work is given. In mechanical engineering the unit is the horse power (h.p.); its relation to electric power is given by: 1 h.p. $= 746 \text{ W}$. Furthermore: 1 h.p. $= 0 \cdot 24 \times 746 \dfrac{\text{cal}}{\text{s}} = 180 \dfrac{\text{cal}}{\text{s}} \simeq 11 \text{ kcal/min}$.

Minimum energies for ignition by hot filaments

We saw earlier (p. 365) that the energy necessary for ignition is minimal if it is supplied very rapidly and not spread over more than a certain small volume. Furthermore, if wires of different diameters and lengths are used as source of ignition, the larger ones will need a greater energy input because they absorb a greater amount of *energy* in the process of being heated up:

$$= \text{mass of wire} \times \text{specific heat} \times \text{temperature rise}$$

In order to visualize the energies involved, we quote from an experiment[6] in which very short (1·5 mm) and fine wires are heated during various short periods by electric currents. The current is gradually increased until ignition occurs in the surrounding, flammable mixture of 20% hydrogen in air. If a wire of 0·02 mm diameter is electrically heated during 3 ms, the minimum energy which must be supplied to cause ignition is 7 milli-joule (mJ), or 1·8 mcal.

If the heating period is prolonged 10-fold to 30 ms, the *rate* with which electric energy is supplied to the wire cannot be simply reduced by a factor ten in order to release again the same total energy as before. In fact no ignition would occur. Instead of the 7 mJ previously needed, approximately double the energy (16 mJ) is now required to ensure ignition of the mixture.

These values are only quoted to enable a comparison to be made with the minimum energies in electric spark ignition. The minimum energy for ignition by such small wires is usually so high that the wire reaches a temperature in the region of 2000 °C, and fuses.

Some idea of the uncertainty regarding ignition by hot wires may be gathered by enumerating various possible events:

(*a*) the wire becomes oxidized when its temperature is raised by the electric current; the metal itself begins to burn and generates a much higher temperature than that due to the electric energy dissipation. The surrounding, flammable mixture is then easily ignited.

(*b*) The wire surface acts as catalyst, i.e. the reaction of fuel vapour with oxygen in contact with the wire takes place at lower temperatures than in the presence of a non-catalytic wire; wires made from platinum may have this property. It can then happen that the surroundings of the wire are filled with combustion products keeping away the fresh mixture, and the wire temperature can be raised further without starting an explosion.

SPARKS and ARCS

The mechanism of ignition by an electric discharge through the flammable mixture is scarcely less intricate than ignition by hot wires and small surfaces; only a few aspects of the problem can be considered here in any detail.

Some consolation can be gained from the fact that the multitude of contradictory statements on explosions caused by 'static electricity' or other spark sources are partly due to the hazy ideas some medical authors have on the matter, and partly to the experimental difficulties which beset this subject. For example: recent investigators of spark ignition found much of the older work valueless because too little attention had been paid to the distance and shape of the electrodes across which sparking took place, and also to the source supplying the spark.

In order to grasp some of the factors involved in the formation of static sparks and the ignition caused by them, a few principles relating to the passage of electricity through gases will be mentioned: as in previous chapters, over-simplification has been introduced for the sake of clarity.

Electric properties of molecules

Every atom consists of one positively charged nucleus and of a number of negative electrons such that the total charge is zero; similarly, molecules formed from atoms have no charge (are 'neutral'). The charge possessed by an electron is called 'elementary charge' and is the smallest quantity of (negative) electricity occurring in nature.

The hydrogen atom has a nucleus with one positive elementary charge and has one electron, while the nucleus of an oxygen atom has 8 positive charges and is surrounded by 8 electrons.

Strong forces attract the negative electrons to the positive nucleus. Only by the action of very high temperatures, fast radioactive particles, ultra-violet light, etc., can atoms (or molecules) be made to lose one or a few of their electrons. The remaining, positively charged atom (or molecule) is called a positive '*Ion*'.

The mass of one electron is only $1/1800$ that of the hydrogen atom, so that practically all the mass of atoms and molecules is concentrated in their nuclei. Owing to their extremely small mass the electrons are very mobile, compared with the heavy ions, under the influence of an external electric field.

Air and other gases are non-conductors of electricity (INSULATORS) in contrast to metals in which electrons can freely move under the influence of an externally applied, electric potential difference.

If two metal rods (electrodes) are placed in close opposition to one another in normal air, and a potential difference (p.d.) from a battery is applied to them, no electric current will flow from one to the other electrode through the air as long as the p.d. does not exceed a few hundred volts. When the p.d. is increased—possibly to several thousand volts (kilovolts or kV)—an appreciable electric current may jump as a *spark discharge*[7] across the gap between the electrodes.

Mechanical analogy of electric discharge in gases

The passage of a spark through normal air becomes possible at all, because there are always a very few (say 1000) charged particles amongst the enormous number ($\sim 10^{19}$ in 1 cm^3) of neutral gas molecules present. If the p.d. becomes sufficiently high, the charged particles begin to move more quickly—the electrons rapidly to the positive electrode, the positive ions more slowly towards the negative electrode.

The electric potential difference can be compared to the height of a mountain, and the gap between the two electrodes to the horizontal distance between mountain top and valley. A boulder rolling from the top will gather speed much quicker if the flank is steep; in other words, the *gradient* decides how quickly the boulder acquires high kinetic energy. Similarly, a charged particle is accelerated more quickly the higher the p.d. and the smaller the gap between the electrodes.

The ratio of $\dfrac{\text{potential difference}}{\text{gap distance}}$ corresponds to the gradient of the mountain, and is known as ELECTRIC FIELD STRENGTH; its unit is: $\dfrac{\text{volt}}{\text{cm}}$, or any equivalent expression.

If the field strength exceeds a value depending on the size and shape of the two electrodes, the nature of the gas and other factors, the few charged particles are speeded up to such a degree that they begin to knock electrons out of some of the neutral gas molecules which themselves become thereby positively charged ions. The electric field can now 'get a grip' on these newly formed charged particles, accelerate them (mainly the mobile electrons) until they can demolish further neutral molecules: an avalanche of electrons and ions is formed, and for a short time the gap between the electrodes becomes a good conductor of electric current.

If the source for the high p.d. has a very limited energy store, as is the case with hospital equipment charged by frictional electricity, the spark discharge across the gap will be over within an extremely short period—say one-millionth of a second (1 μs).

If the metal electrodes are not too close together, most of the spark energy will be dissipated as heat into the gas; if they are too close together, the heat would drain back into the electrodes. This aspect is of considerable importance for ignition of flammable gas mixtures; if the faces of the electrode rods, or any metal parts between which a spark passes, are large and very close together, an appreciable portion of the heat developed by the spark and by the incipient combustion may quickly drain back into the electrodes so that ignition does not take place. This process is known as **'quenching'**.

Just as the actual slope of a mountain is usually not straight and not equal to height divided by horizontal distance between top and base of mountain, so the *field strength* is not generally obtainable by dividing the total potential difference by the gap width. The field strength is fairly constant if the electrodes consist of large spheres at close distance from one another, or of two parallel metal plates (the flank of the mountain is straight).

Between small metal balls or fine, oppositely placed rods, the field strength is greatest near the electrodes: the flank of the equivalent mountain is curved; it is very precipitous near the top and less steep lower down the slope.

Minimum potential difference required for spark discharge

Table 27 gives the minimum sparking, or 'breakdown', potential difference in atmospheric air for various gap distances (g). The second column headed 'uniform field' refers to electrode rods with rounded ends and to metal spheres with diameters from about d = 2 cm upwards; it also holds for parallel plates between which the field is quite uniform (straight slope).

TABLE 27

MINIMUM SPARKING POTENTIAL DIFFERENCE IN AIR (1 atm)

Gap (g)	Electrodes	
	Uniform field	Needle points
cm	potential differ. (kV)	
0·01	0·8	
0·05	2·5	
0·1	4·5	
0·5	18	8
1·0	31	12
1·5	40	18

The smallest gap included in the table is 0·1 mm. If the gap is decreased further, the required minimum sparking p.d. does not diminish indefinitely, but reaches a smallest value of about 300 volt. However, owing to the close approach of the electrodes and the allied quenching effect, such low sparking p.d. are of little significance for the ignition of flammable anaesthetics.

Even if the field strength is constant throughout the gap (rectilinear mountain flank), its value for breakdown has to be increased when the gap is reduced; this follows from dividing the second by the first column of Table 27. For g = 0·5 the field strength is $18/0·5 = 36$ kV/cm; for g = 0·05 the field strength necessary for a spark is $2·5/0·05 = 50$ kV/cm.

Expressed in the mountain analogy: if the peak is low (p.d. = 2·5 kV), its flank must be steeper compared to that of the higher peak (p.d. = 18 kV) for a boulder to induce a sufficiently great avalanche before reaching the foot of the mountain.

Of practical importance is the much smaller breakdown p.d. between needle points (and sharp edges) compared to the p.d. required for a spark to jump between round or flat objects.

In conditions favourable for the generation of frictional electricity on hospital equipment, the potential differences rarely exceed 10 to 15 kV. The strut of a metal trolley charged to a p.d. of 12 kV might be within $\frac{1}{2}$ cm from a water pipe without a spark jumping the gap, while a small screw or wire projecting from both objects would facilitate a spark discharge.

The spark: a most economical ignition source

A spark passing between two fairly close, metallic objects, or more specifically between fine rods as in a sparking plug, represents an ideal, economical ignition source of the type discussed on p. 365. Assuming that the total available energy is limited, as is the case in any hospital equipment charged by frictional electricity, all available energy will be instantaneously dissipated* by the spark in a very small volume of the surrounding gas.

The importance of quick release of energy for ignition of a flammable mixture is illustrated in the following

Example[8]

The electrical energy dissipated by a spark is assumed to generate 1 mcal (= 0·001 cal).

If this heat is transferred to 1 mm³ (= 0·001 cm³) of air within 1 ms (= 0·001 s), it can be shown that the temperature of this small volume would rise to 1000° C.

If the same amount of heat were released slower within 10 ms, the same gas volume would be heated to only 700 °C.

This comparison shows clearly that the temperature rise in a gas near the heat source is extremely sensitive to the rate with which the heat is released.

Characteristics of spark ignition

From the anaesthetist's point of view the following features[9] of spark ignition are of main importance:

(a) The ease with which mixtures of a given fuel with oxygen or air can be ignited varies very considerably with the composition. One of the mixtures in the range of flammability requires the least ignition energy. The fuel concentration (f_i) of this **most ignitable**

---

* This statement refers to charged conductors; for the discharge of insulators see p.413.

mixture is often in the rich range for mixtures with air, i.e. f'_i/f'_{st} is greater than 1. (for ether $f'_i/f'_{st} = 1\cdot3$, see p. 341).

(b) The smallest energy required to ignite a mixture is known as 'MINIMUM IGNITION ENERGY'. Its value rises rapidly if the concentration differs from that of the most ignitable mixture (f_i). The energies may be very high when the concentrations approach the limits of flammability. This fact gives a further explanation for the relative innocuousness of mixtures near the limits.

(c) The most ignitable mixtures of fuels with OXYGEN have much *lower* minimum ignition energies than the most ignitable mixtures with air. Frequently the energy for such a mixture with oxygen is only $\frac{1}{100}$ of that with air.*

Minimum Ignition Energies

In order to appreciate the minute ignition energies required for certain flammable mixtures, we recall (p. 367) the relation between units of electric energy and of heat:

$$1 \text{ joule (J)} \ldots 0\cdot24 \text{ cal}$$

As the ignition energies of very explosive mixtures are often far below 1 J, the 1/1000th part of this unit is used instead:

$$1 \text{ milli joule (mJ)} \ldots 0\cdot24 \text{ milli calories (mcal)}$$

In order to stress the very low value of these ignition energies we consider an everyday

Example

The bulb of a small pocket torch has a filament which passes a current of $0\cdot2$ A when a battery p.d. of $2\cdot5$ V is applied to it. If the current is switched on for only 1 s, what is the dissipated energy?

From Eq. 4 on p. 366 one obtains for the electrical energy dissipated in the filament:

$$H = 2\cdot5 \text{ V} \times 0\cdot2 \text{ A} \times 1 \text{ s} = 0\cdot5 \text{ J}$$

This is the same as

$$500 \text{ mJ} \quad \text{or} \quad 120 \text{ mcal}$$

In comparison, the most detonable mixture of ether in oxygen can be ignited by a spark energy of only $0\cdot0012$ mJ, i.e. an energy which is only $\dfrac{1}{400\,000}$ of that produced by the short flash of a tiny pocket torch bulb.

* This comparison between the most ignitable mixture in oxygen and in air should not be confused with a comparison of mixtures having the same fuel concentration. Thus the ignition energies of 4% v/v ethyl ether in oxygen and in air are almost the same—yet note not only the difference between the concentrations but also the enormous difference between the energies of the most ignitable mixtures in Table 28.

The volume of mixture which can be raised by the minimum spark to a local ignition temperature of say 1000 °C is extremely small.

Example

Assume a specific heat for the most ignitable ether/oxygen mixture of about 0·5 mcal/(cm³×degC). The minimum ignition energy is 0·0012 mJ or 0·0003 mcal.

From the relation:

spark energy = specific heat × volume × temperature rise

we can calculate for an assumed temperature rise of 1000 °C the volume heated up to this value:

$$\text{Volume} = \frac{\text{Spark energy}}{\text{specif. heat} \times \text{temp. rise}} =$$

$$\frac{0\cdot0003}{0\cdot5 \times 1000} = \frac{3 \times 10^{-4}}{5 \times 10^{2}} = \frac{3}{5} \times 10^{-6} \text{ cm}^3$$

The volume is thus smaller than 1/1000 of a cubic millimetre.

The mixtures of fuel in oxygen of Table 28 are near the stoichiometric value, while those with air are richer.

TABLE 28

MOST IGNITABLE MIXTURES AND MINIMUM ENERGIES IN OXYGEN AND AIR

Fuel	Most ignitable Mixture in		Corresponding minimum Ignition Energies in	
	Oxygen (f_i)	Air (f_i')	Oxygen	Air
	% v/v		milli joules (mJ)	
Ethylene	23	7	0·009	0·085
Ethyl ether	14	5	0·001	0·200
Cyclopropane	16	7	0·001	0·180

The use of the milli joule (mJ) instead of heat units (cal or mcal) for electrical ignition is a useful convention. If the ignition is due to a wire heated for a short period, the calculation of the dissipated energy is straightforward (p. 367). For the calculation of energy dissipated in sparks jumping between frictionally charged objects which represent a limited energy source, some knowledge of electrostatics would be necessary.

Electrostatics: p.d., charge and capacitance

In this text we have limited ourselves to the kinetic and energetic aspects of explosions, and refer the reader to monographs on static electricity and electrostatics.[10, 11] In these it is shown that the CAPACI-TANCE between a charged object and earth (or between two differently charged objects) is a measure of the quantity of electricity which can be accumulated on the object by any particular potential difference. The greater the capacitance, the larger the charge which is given by the p.d. to the object in question.

Just as the ampere is the unit of flow rate of electricity (current), so the (ampere × s) serves as the unit of quantity of electricity (electric charge).*

The name for the unit of electric charge is COULOMB

$$1 \text{ A} \times 1 \text{ s} = 1 \text{ coulomb}$$

$$\text{Capacitance } (C) = \frac{\text{Electricity Charge } (Q)}{\text{Potential Difference } (E)}$$

The capacitance (C) may be that of a person standing with insulating shoe soles on a conducting floor, and E would be the potential difference between the person and the floor.

The standard unit of capacitance is the *Farad* (F); an object has this capacitance value if a charge of 1 coulomb transferred to it raises its electric potential by 1 volt. This unit is extremely large, and a much handier unit of capacitance is the so-called pico-Farad (pF); 1 pF $=10^{-12}$ F.

Many objects in an operating theatre have a capacitance of a few hundred of these smaller units. The following relations may be found useful; in these the (ampere × s) has been used again instead of the coulomb as the unit of electric charge.

$$\text{Capacitance (pF)} = 10^9 \times \frac{Q \ (\text{A} \times \text{s})}{E \ (\text{kV})}$$

$$Q \ (\text{A} \times \text{s}) = 10^{-9} \times E \ (\text{kV}) \times \text{capacitance (pF)}$$

Example: A patient lying on an insulating mattress covering the operating table may have a capacitance of 300 pF. What is the quantity of frictional electricity which must accumulate on the patient to produce a potential difference of $E = 4$ kV between him and the table?

$$Q \ (\text{A} \times \text{s}) = 10^{-9} \times 4 \times 300 = 1 \cdot 2 \times 10^{-6}$$

The charge causing a potential difference of 4000 volt is thus quite

* The hydraulic equivalents are the volume flow rate of fluid passing a section of a pipe per second, and the total quantity of fluid obtained in multiplying the flow rate by the time elapsed.

small. A current of 1 A flowing only during one-millionth of a second (or 1 mA during 1 ms) would deliver this quantity of electricity.

Energy of statically charged objects

The relation between the quantity of electricity on a charged object, its potential difference and the electrical energy stored are given by:

ENERGY $\propto$ QUANTITY OF ELECTRICITY $\times$ POTENTIAL DIFFERENCE

In appropriate units one obtains:

Energy: H (mJ) $= \frac{1}{2} \times 10^6 \times Q$ (A$\times$s) $\times E$ (kV)

Example: In the previous example the potential difference was $E = 4$ kV and the quantity of electricity $Q = 1 \cdot 2 \times 10^{-6}$ (A$\times$s). Therefore

$$H = \tfrac{1}{2} \times 10^6 \times (1 \cdot 2 \times 10^{-6}) \times 4 \simeq 2 \cdot 5 \text{ mJ}$$

This energy would be more than ample to ignite flammable mixtures listed[12] in Table 28; in order for a spark to jump between the patient and the table (or any other object connected to earth), the gap would have to be slightly less than 1 mm (see Table 27, p. 372).

TABLE 29

CHANGE OF IGNITION ENERGY AND QUENCHING DISTANCE
WITH COMPOSITION OF MIXTURE

Methane in Oxygen		Minimum Ignition Energies	Quenching Distance	Temperature of Combustion Products
f (%v/v)	f/f$_{st}$	mcal	mm	°C
10	0·3	0·010	0·7	1900
15	0·45	0·003	0·5	2350
25	0·75	0·001	0·3	2700
40	1·2	0·005	0·6	2700
50	1·5	0·110	1·6	2350
55	1·6	0·430	3·8	2200

So long as the composition of the mixture is close to the most ignitable value (f_i), the required ignition energy differs little from that of f_i. However in other mixtures (see Table 29), small changes in composition lead to very large increases in the ignition energy. The stoichiometric concentration for methane/oxygen is $f_{st} = 33\%$, and the most ignitable mixture is seen to lie on the lean side. Energies are here expressed in mcal, and the most ignitable mixture requires only one-millionth of a calorie.

Quenching of an incipient explosion

Also included is a column of '*Quenching Distances*' (see p. 371). If the distance between electrodes is decreased below these quenching distances, higher spark energies are required to ignite a given mixture. The theory of spark ignition teaches that the energy released in an extremely small volume (see p. 375) ignites the gas, but the explosion has first to grow unimpeded to a certain minimum size before a self-propagating flame can continue to travel. If the two electrodes, or any other solid objects which withdraw heat from the flame, are too close (below quenching distance) the flame cannot propagate unless a much higher, initial spark energy has been imparted to it. The more reactive a mixture, the smaller can be the quenching distance, and the flame can continue to travel even if heat-absorbing objects are close to it.

The minimum ignition energy of a given mixture changes little when the gap between the electrodes is altered,—although the required p.d. is higher for wider gaps (Table 27). However, when the gap is reduced below the 'quenching distance', much higher energies are necessary to cause ignition. For the most ignitable ether/oxygen mixture, the gap can be reduced to $\frac{1}{4}$ mm (Table 28) before the required ignition energy rises steeply; the breakdown p.d. for this gap is 1·3 kV .

The quenching effect, particularly of massive electrodes, may explain some of the erratic behaviour of ignition by frictional electricity. If the flammable mixture is not very ignitable and the capacitance of the charged object small (i.e. small amount of energy stored for the given p.d.), quenching might in certain circumstances prevent ignition of the mixture even if a spark jumps from the charged object to one at earth potential.

Electric Arcs

More powerful than sparks caused by frictional electricity are those due to certain electro-medical equipment. Before discussing these we must briefly mention another type of electrical discharge through gases which is known as an **arc**. Although there is a fairly clear distinction between 'sparks and arcs', both terms are frequently used indiscriminately.

Arcs are well known from their technical use in the arclight as well as in electric welding. The explanation of the process for an arclight holds as well for any normal domestic or hospital switch of the common variety, in which two metal contacts are separated when the switch is turned off.

Before 'striking the arc' the two carbon rods are in contact, a p.d. from an electric supply source is applied to them and a current flows across the points of contact. When the contact pressure between the rods is decreased in the process of pulling them apart, the contact area is much reduced in size; the whole current has now to flow across a few remaining 'high spots' still bridging the gap. The situation resembles one in which a large current has suddenly to flow through a few very fine wires, which it heats instantaneously to a very high temperature.

Mechanism of arc formation

The points of the electrodes (either carbon rods or the metal contacts of a switch) are heated to a very high temperature which facilitates the emission of large quantities of electrons, similar to that from the heated cathode of a radio valve. Although the gap between the electrodes may still be very small, and the applied p.d. relatively low (say 50 volt), the electrons are very rapidly accelerated owing to the high electric field strength,—given by the ratio of p.d. to gap width (see p. 371). These electrons strongly ionize the gas, the small gap becomes highly conducting and relatively large currents are passed for small values of p.d. which are often well below 100 volt. If conditions are suitable, the gap can be widened considerably without extinguishing the arc; the high temperatures of the ionized gas cause the brilliant arc light.

Comparison between arc and spark

In contrast to the arc, the electrodes in a *spark* discharge are kept apart from the beginning and remain cool; formation of ions in the gap proceeds differently and requires a much higher p.d.

The energy dissipated in an arc can be very high.[13] Although the currents may often not be above 1 A and the rate of energy dissipation consequently low, the total energy is high if the duration of the arc produced by opening a switch is of the order of 1 s. On the other hand, the instantaneous current in a spark may be very much higher but the duration is of the order of micro-seconds.

It is thus not surprising that arcs in electrical switches, motors and other electrical appliances have ignited detonable mixtures with oxygen as well as less ignitable mixtures with air.

EXPLOSION HAZARDS

Diathermy

Throughout the past eighty years, cautery[14] followed later by surgical diathermy* have been one of the chief culprits of ignition by arcs and sparks. Trouble may arise from the following causes:

* Surgical diathermy is more correctly described as: electro-surgical apparatus for electrosection and coagulation.

(a) At the active electrode, where the cutting action is produced by a high-frequency current of considerable strength, a flammable mixture can be readily ignited.

(b) In the apparatus itself. The electrical mechanism of older machines actually utilizes rows of spark-gaps which can usually be seen through ventilation holes in the cover. This feature is not present in modern high-frequency diathermy machines, but faulty insulation may still produce sparks inside them.

(c) Defective foot switches and any other switches on the apparatus may 'arc' and thus ignite flammable atmospheres, unless they are enclosed in gas-proof casing. Most gas-proof foot switches are heavy and find little favour with surgeons (see p. 395).

(d) Even when all the preceding risks are eliminated, there remains one peculiar to certain types of diathermy apparatus. In these the currents of very high frequency flowing through the patient between the electrodes may induce considerable alternating potential differences between the patient and objects in his vicinity, e.g. the operating table or the anaesthetist's hands. This is a property of currents with frequencies of many millions of cycles per second (Mc/s), far above that of the ordinary electric power supply (50 c/s). The patient may become, in a way, the transmitting aerial of a miniature wireless station which induces strong electrical potential differences in nearby objects; these p.d. may give rise to a spark at a distance from the electrodes, and such sparks possess ample energy to ignite flammable mixtures.

We have on many occasions seen and felt sparks pass between our fingers and the patient's head when surgical diathermy of that kind was applied to the lower extremities, although the manufacturer's instructions for the use of the apparatus were strictly followed. It will be obvious that safety does not lie with the distance between the active electrode and the anaesthetic apparatus near the head of the patient.

Sparks due to static electricity

Neither the principles of electrostatics nor the mechanism by which frictional electricity ('static') is generated are discussed here, since numerous elementary and advanced accounts of these phenomena have appeared in anaesthetic as well as medical and physical journals during recent years.[11,15]

Generation of static charges

The reader should, however, be made aware that 'frictional' has nothing to do with the 'generation' of electrical charges, in a mistaken analogy to the generation of heat by friction. Rubbing a plastic fountain pen with a duster, or pulling a blanket across a mattress covered with normal rubber sheet, leaves the two parts oppositely charged after separation. The main function of 'friction' is to establish a close contact between microscopically small, prominent points on the two objects. If a material A has a smaller affinity for electrons than another B, electrons cross from object A (e.g. glass rod) to object B (e.g. silk cloth). They charge B negatively and leave A with an equal but positive charge behind.

Such simple experiment is only possible because objects A and B are good INSULATORS; if they had some conductivity, the charges would be neutralized through the hands and body of the experimenter as quickly as they are produced by rubbing. The fountain pen mentioned above can be quickly given some surface conductivity by breathing on to it and will no longer remain charged. Most precautions against generation of high static potential differences on objects in an operating theatre try to ensure adequate conductive pathways between the various objects so that frictional effects never have a chance to build up appreciable potential differences.

Incidence of explosions due to static

Ignition of flammable anaesthetic vapours by static electricity has received a good deal of publicity, partly due to the somewhat mysterious origin and erratic behaviour of frictional charges, and possibly because this problematic source has been occasionally a convenient way of explaining explosions due to more obvious and avoidable sources.

Until about twenty years ago there was a striking difference in the number of reported explosions due to static in the U.S.A. and in Great Britain. A very dry atmosphere secures favourable conditions for the charging of objects by static electricity because any conducting film of moisture on objects will be absent; also elaborate air conditioning systems can rapidly produce a dry desert climate owing to some unnoticed fault occurring in the humidifying part of the plant.

Whether the majority of anaesthetic explosions are nowadays due to static electricity depends, as so often, on the manipulation of statistics. In one publication[16] the frequency of different causes of 230 anaesthetic explosions is given as follows:

Static electricity	27%
Other causes	73%

Another way of grouping explosions is in terms of the *deaths* caused by them. Rearrangement of the preceding data gives for the deaths during anaesthetic explosions the following values:

Static electricity   40%

Other causes   60%

Difference between electric sparks from various sources

The practical difference between sparks caused by, say, a faulty X-ray machine and those due to an instrument trolley charged with static electricity is the very limited energy store of the latter. This is due to the moderate electric capacitance (p. 376) of those objects which may be charged by 'static' in normal circumstances. While the faulty machine can produce numerous, powerful sparks in quick succession, the statically-charged object is likely to cause only a single spark before it has lost its high p.d. relative to earth or to differently charged objects.

In this connection it should be kept in mind that the *minimum spark energies* quoted—particularly for less flammable mixtures—represent results of tests in which a *spark was made to jump many times* across a gap before the flammable mixture was ignited. The energies of sparks which ignite flammable mixtures at the first attempt may be considerably higher.

Electric motors and switches

Motors are frequently found in operating theatres for driving suction pumps, for driving air through plenum ether vaporizers, for actuating surgical saws and for many other purposes. In former days, and occasionally even now, they were known to produce arcs at the commutator brushes or slip rings; in many ways they represent ignition sources similar to normal, unprotected switches. Motors have probably been a major source of anaesthetic explosions[17], although one rarely finds them mentioned in statistical discussions on this subject. One reason may be the relatively mild character of a deflagration in the ether/air mixtures usually involved. The damage is small and the patient rarely injured. However, the operating theatre personnel have not escaped unscathed in these explosions, although fortunately their injuries have been little more than burns and cuts from broken glassware. Motors used on saws or drills are often in unpleasantly close proximity to the patient, and any arcs produced by these can become a source of danger.

Uncommon Types of Ignition and Explosion

Ignition by compression

Explosions, or rather violent combustions, have been described as starting in reducing valves[18] attached to oxygen cylinders when the main cylinder valve was suddenly opened. The inrush of the high pressure gas into the ducts filled with gas at atmospheric pressure, can heat the latter as if it were compressed by a solid piston. The process resembles

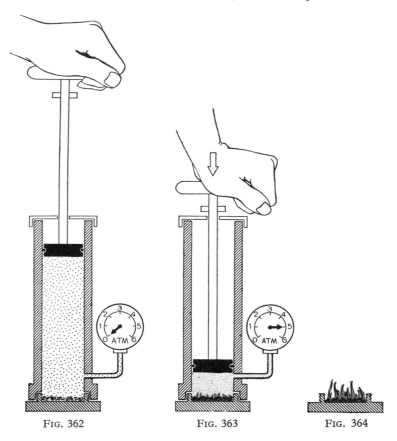

FIG. 362   FIG. 363   FIG. 364

the mechanism of the pneumatic firelighter which was in use before the introduction of safety matches.

Fig. 362—a cylinder filled with atmospheric air (gauge pressure = 0) is closed at its upper end by a piston. The detachable bottom of the cylinder contains easily ignitable, solid material such as tinder.*

Fig. 363—the piston is suddenly pushed down compressing the air, and the gauge pressure has risen to about 5 atm. The mechanical work

* A dried fungus powder mixed with saltpetre.

done in compressing the air is transformed into heat which raises the air temperature. The latter is assumed to be sufficiently high to initiate combustion of tinder in the oxygen of the compressed air. The tinder begins to glow and

Fig. 364—the small receptacle can be removed to serve as ignition source for other materials.

These illustrations must not be taken as a quantitative description of ignition by compression, as will become apparent from the following.

In an earlier application of the gas laws (a, p. 98) it was assumed implicitly that the heat generated by the work of compression was immediately conducted to the outside of the vessel. The process can easily be made isothermal by very slow compression. On the other hand, the pneumatic fire-lighter, as well as the accidental ignition caused by high pressure gas entering a reducing valve, function only if the compression takes place very rapidly.

Owing to the temperature increase, the ratio of initial to final volumes will not equal the ratio of final to initial pressures, as was the case for an isothermal volume change (p. 98). The ratio of absolute pressures (fig. 362 and 363) is $\frac{5+1}{1} = 6$; on the other hand, the *theory* of this compression process (**adiabatic,** i.e. without heat loss to the outside) shows that the volume ratio is only $\frac{3\cdot6}{1}$. The ratio of final to initial absolute temperatures is $\frac{1\cdot7}{1}$; this ratio of the temperatures can also be directly calculated with the help of the ratios for pressures and volumes from the gas laws. From $p \times v \propto T$ (footnote, p. 312) one obtains:

$$\frac{T_2}{T_1} = \frac{p_2}{p_1} \times \frac{v_2}{v_1} = 6 \times \frac{1}{3\cdot6} = 1\cdot7$$

Starting at room temperature ($T_1 = 300 °K$), we derive a final temperature of $T_2 = 500 °K$, or approximately 200 °C.

Even if the compression had been increased so that the final gauge pressure reached 10 atm, the final temperature would have only increased to 300 °C. As these temperatures are too low for ignition of most materials, the process has to be repeated a number of times by letting the piston jump back between repeated compressions. Each time the initial temperature will be higher and the final temperature higher still.

Fires in Reducing Valves

High pressure gas from a storage tank is suddenly released into the valve. The inrush of this gas compresses the low pressure gas in the ducts to 100 atm; the respective temperature rise by adiabatic compression would be about 800 °C ($T_2/T_1 = 3\cdot8$). If traces of grease, combustible dust particles and the like are present, ignition might occur and the subsequent temperature rise might also lead to the combustion of other valve components.

Investigators of such fires have not overlooked the possibility that sudden escape of high pressure gas could send powerful shock waves into the passages of the reducing valve filled at that moment with low pressure gas. It is well known that any shock wave producing a certain pressure rise where it meets the resting gas, is associated with a much higher temperature than would be produced if the gas were compressed adiabatically. The latter term implies that the piston compressing the gas does not move at high, supersonic speeds but with a speed which is much smaller than the sound velocity in the gas.

TABLE 30

COMPARISON OF TEMPERATURES PRODUCED BY SHOCK AND
BY ADIABATIC COMPRESSION

Compression ratio	Shock wave pressure	Temperatures	
		Shock	Adiabatic
(v_1/v_2)	p_2 (atm)	°C	°C
2·8	2	200	150
3·9	10	430	240
6·0	50	2000	520

The data in Table 30 are based on a shock wave travelling through air with an initial temperature of 0 °C and a pressure $p_1 = 1$ atm. For instance, if the pressure in the *shock* front is 50 atm, the specific volume of the air will be reduced in the ratio 6 to 1 and its temperature is raised to about 2000 °C. If the shock wave had been produced by a rapidly moving piston, the piston velocity would have to be over five times the speed of sound under the initial conditions of the air. If the same air had been compressed to the same extent ($v_1/v_2 = 6/1$)

by a relatively slow moving piston, under *adiabatic* conditions* in which no heat is lost to the outside, its temperature would have risen only to 520 °C and its pressure to $p_2 = 12$ atm.

In an attempt to prevent combustion in reducing valves, many designs keep the volumes of the ducts, on the high and also on the low pressure side, as small as possible. Even if the gases are raised by sudden compression to a high temperature, the heat content is then so small that the heat is quickly dissipated to the surrounding metal walls. Furthermore, in some technical valves narrow, slit-like ducts with a sudden change of direction, have been incorporated in an attempt to avoid the formation and spreading of shock waves. By eliminating organic materials from the construction of diaphragm, valve seating, etc., the risk of combustion can also be diminished.

It is well to keep in mind that probably most accidents with reducing valves have been due simply to the presence of dirt, grease and various combustible substances which should not have been there. Ignition of these may even take place directly on contact with high pressure oxygen without any appreciable additional heating.

Explosions in the absence of any external combustible agents

The human body itself cannot be neglected as the source of flammable materials. Some of these (*a*) are the naturally generated bowel gases consisting of methane, hydrogen, etc. Other combustible materials (*b*) are produced when cautery, surgical diathermy, etc., are in action; decomposition of tissues may yield ethylene, hydrogen, etc., while decomposition of water forms 'electrolytic' gas ($2H_2O \rightarrow 2H_2 + O_2$). A recent, searching survey[19] makes it quite clear that both processes (*a*, *b*) represent a real risk which has to be reckoned with.

In order to form flammable mixtures of (*a*), more oxygen than normally must be present; it has been assumed that this is introduced by swallowing, endoscopy and by breathing of high oxygen concentrations, with resulting increase of oxygen tension in the lumen of the viscus. Yet, if electro-cutting or a similar procedure is applied, the decomposition of water and the associated liberation of oxygen cannot be overlooked.

Needless to say, all well-documented accidents of this kind took place in the absence of any flammable anaesthetic: rupture of the bladder following an explosion during transurethral resection under sacral

---

* If, on the other hand, the compression had been carried out while the air retains its initial temperature (isothermal), the final pressure would have been only 6 atm,— always assuming that the air follows the ideal gas laws.

anaesthesia is only one example.[20] In this type of explosion the patient alone is always the sufferer although there have been some near misses; for instance, when a two-foot flame shot out of a sigmoidoscope!

Explosions in large confined spaces

We have stressed repeatedly the innocuous character of deflagrations in fuel/air mixtures compared with the dangerous blast effects following detonations of fuel/oxygen mixtures. This is quite correct as long as the limited volumes present in anaesthetic machines and in the respiratory tract of the patient are involved.

However, if large containers or rooms are filled with flammable fuel/air mixtures as was the case in many industrial disasters, other aspects of deflagration come into the foreground.

If *ignition* takes place *in a closed vessel*, the pressure of the combustion products will reach a considerable value owing to the high flame temperature. Pressures of 5 atm and above (70 lb/in²) may be developed and structural damage can be considerable. Even if the space is not firmly enclosed, the deflagration may be quite violent if ignition takes place near the centre of a room filled with flammable mixture. The hot gases behind the spherically expanding flame front push the surrounding, fresh mixture ahead. The flame will thus travel in a streaming gas and its speed rises far above that in a gas at rest.

In the days of open coal fires, inadequate ventilation and unawareness of explosion hazards, the risk of large-scale deflagrations was only too real. The abstract from an inquest held in 1899 needs no elaboration:

'. . . surgery is a small room (with) . . . high cupboard containing bottles of ether. . . . One nurse sat . . . (near) the fire, and the other was counting (the bottles) on one of the shelves, when an ether bottle . . . fell against another . . . and . . . broke. There was an immediate explosion, blowing out some of the window glass and setting fire to the furniture and woodwork. . . . Both nurses subsequently died of the injuries received.'[21]

Such accidents were not confined to nurses:

'Ether was upset near the fireplace by Dr. Averill whilst pouring ether from a five-pint bottle into a phial. The ether ignited and an explosion followed shaking the house, breaking the windows and the bottles in the surgery, and setting the clothes of Dr. Averill on fire.'[22]

Dangerous disposal of flammable liquids

The accumulation of flammable mixtures in a large space is not always accidental. The pernicious habit of pouring liquid ether and

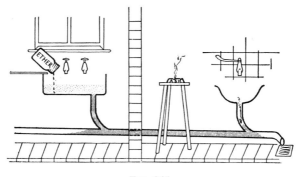

FIG. 365

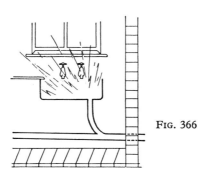

FIG. 366

other flammable liquids into sinks may lead to the following sequence of events:

Fig. 365—in the room on the left the contents of an ether vaporizing bottle are poured down a sink. Subsequently, in the room on the right a glowing cigarette end is thrown down a hand basin.

Fig. 366—shortly afterwards a brisk explosion occurs, which may be particularly noticeable in the room on the left. Under suitable conditions, the ether/air mixture in the pipes is very rich (dark shading) and a cool flame started by the glowing cigarette travels along the drainpipe to the room on the left. Here the mixture in the sink has been diluted by air currents to a normal flammable concentration (light shading), and the cool flame ignites a deflagration. Owing to the large volume the effects may be quite powerful.

This sequence is not a mere invention although references are scarce for obvious reasons: no apparent ignition source was present in the room on the left when the explosion occurred. However, this accident is known to have occurred in chemical laboratories, and even the following mystery story from an American hospital is possibly based on a similar sequence.

'. . . a technician in the Anesthesia Department . . . poured . . . ether into a worksink. A few minutes later a nurse anesthetist walked into the workroom and . . . a flame burst out of the sink and . . . reached a distance of . . . three to four feet. She was within 7 to 8 feet from the sink when the flame appeared.'[23] There were no obvious sources of ignition in this room.

All ether/air mixtures are heavier than pure air and will therefore end to spread near floor level before being stirred by air currents. This tendency may bring a flammable mixture to a source of ignition far away from the site where ether was spilt. A case is quoted[24] of an anaesthetist who usually kept an ether bottle in his coat pocket, where it spilled over one day. The ether vapour flowed on to the floor and was there ignited by a faulty X-ray machine nearby. A flame ran up his trousers, but the *patient* was none the worse for the burns suffered by the *anaesthetist*.

Explosions in the absence of flammable mixtures?

Explosions have been reported during the use of *nitrous oxide/oxygen* alone—at least, it is alleged that no other agents were used. In many of these cases, however, a vaporizer bottle containing some ether was on the anaesthetic machine, although the control tap was in the 'off' position. The following illustrations show how the escape of vapour into the ducts of the machine may accidentally become quite appreciable.

Fig. 367—just prior to turning the control to the 'off' position, a strong anaesthetic mixture had been administered to the patient; the liquid ether is therefore at a temperature well below that of the room

(R.T.). Furthermore, the vapour pressure in the bottle is accordingly low.

Fig. 368—the bottle has gradually warmed up as shown on the thermometer in the liquid ether. The saturation pressure is correspon-

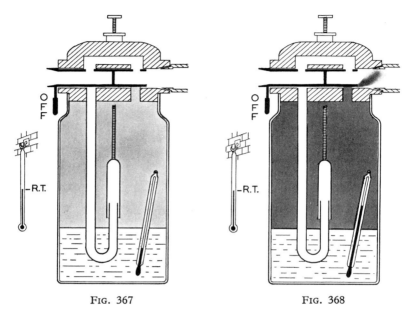

FIG. 367   FIG. 368

dingly higher; this is indicated by the denser shading above the liquid. Ether evaporates so that the total pressure in the bottle rises above atmospheric.

Although the rotor of the control occludes both inlet and outlet of the bottle, it is shown to have only a short 'land' in the barrel near the outlet. This type of tap is rarely gas-tight, and owing to the positive pressure in the bottle, ether vapour escapes into the stream of anaesthetic gases. (See also p. 392.)

REFERENCES

[1] NEWITT, D. M., and TOWNEND, D. T. A. (1938). Combustion phenomena of hydrocarbons in: *The Science of Petroleum*, IV, cf. 2862.
[2] FEATHERSTONE, H. W. (1931–2). *Proc. R. Soc. Med.*, 25, 119–22.
[3] MANNHEIMER, W. H. (1953). *Anesthesiology*, 14, 99.
[4] RUSS, S. (1938). *J. Instn. electr. Engrs.*, 83, 164–5.
[5] GREENE, B. A. (1942). *Surg., Gynec. Obstet.*, 74, 259–65.
[6] STOUT, H. P., and JONES, E. (1949). In: *Third Symposium on Combustion*, No. 35, pp. 329–36. Baltimore.
[7] MEEK, J. M., and CRAAGS, J. D. (1953). *Electrical breakdown of gases*, cf. Chapter VII, Oxford.
[8] JONES, E. T. (1928). *Phil. Mag.*, 6, 1090–1103.
[9] ELBE, G. v. (1953). In: *Fourth Symposium (International) on Combustion*, No. 2, pp. 13–20. Baltimore.
[10] SILSBEE, F. B. (1942). *Static electricity*, National Bureau of Standards, Circular C. 438.
[11] GUEST, P. G. (1938). *Static electricity in nature and industry*, U.S. Bureau of Mines, Bulletin 368.
[12] BLANC, M. V., et al. (1949). In: *Third Symposium on Combustion*, No. 40, pp. 363–7. Baltimore.
[13] FINCH, G. I. (1934–5). *Proc. R. Soc. Med.*, 28, 1130–3.
[14] CAZENEUVE, P., and PONCET, A. (1879). *Mém. Soc. Sci. méd. Lyon*, 19, 195–200.
[15] BRACKEN, A. (1952). *Med. ill.*, 6, 643–50.
[16] GREENE, B. A. (1941). *Anesthesiology*, 2, 144–60.
[17] GREENE, B. A. (1942). *Surg. Gynec. Obstet.*, 75, 73–5.
[18] RIMARSKI, W., and NOACK, J. (1940). *Autogene Metallbearb.*, 33, 69–76.
[19] GALLEY, A. H. (1955). *Proc. R. Soc. Med.* 48, 502–4.
[20] KRETSCHMER, H. L. (1934). *J. Amer. med. Ass.*, 103, 1144.
[21] ANNOTATION (1899). *Lancet*, i, 867.
[22] MEDICAL NEWS (1892). *Brit. med. J.*, ii, 1457.
[23] THOMAS, G. J. (1956). *Amer. Soc. Anesth.*, Newsletter, 20 (12), 32.
[24] GREENE, B. A. (1941). *Amer. J. Roentgenol.*, 45, 737–43.

CHAPTER XXIII

EXPLOSIONS *Part* 4:

PRECAUTIONS.
HISTORICAL NOTES.

Prevention of Explosions in general

THE only method of avoiding anaesthetic explosions with complete certainty consists in using non-flammable agents. If an inhalation anaesthetic is used, the choice is mainly limited to:

Nitrous oxide, Chloroform, Trichloroethylene and Halothane.*

It will be understandable from the hazards of escaping vapour discussed in connection with Fig. 368 that all anaesthetic vaporizing bottles containing flammable anaesthetics must be removed from the apparatus if contamination of the nitrous oxide/oxygen stream is to be avoided. A glance at the vapour pressure curve for ethyl ether (p. 69) and the temperatures in Boyle's bottles for ether (p. 35) shows that the positive pressure in the bottle may well build up to several hundred mmHg above atmospheric.

It is always necessary to consider whether the hazard of explosion in the presence of a flammable anaesthetic of choice is greater or less than the hazard of a less suitable but non-flammable anaesthetic.

This situation occurs during the administration of anaesthetics in dark X-ray rooms. Nitrous oxide with insufficient oxygen given to an adult, or chloroform administered to a child by the unexperienced may well represent a greater hazard than the risk of a mild deflagration in a slightly flammable ether/air mixture.

It frequently happens that the surgeon decides to use diathermy, cautery or to take an X-ray during the course of an operation without being able to warn the anaesthetist beforehand. It is therefore necessary to consider measures which reduce the risk of explosions to a minimum.

(*a*) The simplest measure is to stop administering the flammable and to continue with a non-flammable anaesthetic.

When the patient has been deeply anaesthetized with ether for some considerable time, the ether tension of his venous blood would be in equilibrium with a gas mixture containing between 4 and 6 %v/v ether. If the administration ceases, the alveolar ether concentration will quickly

---

* or 'Fluothane', the trade mark of Messrs. Imperial Chemical Industries (Pharmaceuticals) Ltd. for: Trifluoro-chloro-bromo ethane.

fall to this level. The rate of decrease of ether concentration in the upper respiratory tract will depend on the type of respiration; large tidal volumes will ensure rapid mixing of the alveolar gases with fresh air. However, the last portion of each breath (end-expiratory sample) will contain a higher concentration of ether than the earlier parts of the expiration.

Different observers have come to various conclusions as to when the anaesthetic concentration in the expired air has fallen below the lower limit of flammability.

One of them states[1] that expirations three minutes after the cessation of ether administration are non-flammable. An interval from 6 to 8 minutes after cessation of administration of cyclopropane is said[2] to give safety. Another observer[3] advises a simple test: a small gas sample is sucked from the pharynx into a rubber bulb syringe and then blown into a spirit flame. A 'pop' indicates an explosive mixture, while a change in colour of the flame is supposed to indicate that it is still not safe to use diathermy on the patient.

(b) Another simple safeguard against possible detonation and loss of life is the *substitution of AIR FOR OXYGEN* in the anaesthetic mixture. Ether/air explosions are characterized by the absence of detonation with its fatal blast effects. The injuries due to the relatively mild deflagrations have usually been small and consisted of burns.

'The only combustible anaesthetic mixture which is safe for the patient to receive in an operating room . . . is ether/air.'[4]

These comments do not apply to ignition of large volumes of ether/air mixtures which might form if the vapour from a broken ether bottle is quickly mixed with a large volume of room air, and is not removed by an adequate ventilating system.

(c) Preventing the accumulation of explosive vapour in a room.

Ventilation: This must be so designed that the vapour is not drawn from the head end of the patient towards the feet but in the opposite direction. Extraction ducts of ventilating systems should be sited near the floor level. In these ways explosive vapours are kept away from any electrical apparatus used by the surgeon. A general churning up of the room air should be avoided as this might bring flammable mixture into contact with sources of ignition some distance away.

In years gone by, proper ventilation was the main safeguard against explosion outside the anaesthetic apparatus; since then, the arrival of the closed circuit system and of other means for preventing escape of anaesthetic into the room have offered increased safety.

Closed circuit: Both the 'to and fro' and the circle absorbers are equally efficient in preventing escape of appreciable quantities of explosive vapours into the room. However, they offer no absolute safety and the possibility of leaks between mask and face, and of leaks in the apparatus itself is always present. The closed circuit should **never** be relied upon to prevent an explosion when a possible source of ignition is near the head.

Numerous explosions have occurred through neglecting this aspect, but views vary widely on the range at which mixtures escaping from a leak are still ignitable. Escaping ether or cyclopropane mixtures are said to have been ignited up to 1 foot (30 cm) from the leak, while one author[5] claims that ignition at only 2 inches (5 cm) is no longer possible. Such statements without careful scientific control deserve little credence[6] and, indeed, may be dangerously misleading.

Deliberate removal of expirations: By providing a metal connection to slip over the expiratory valve, a short tubing can be attached to lead the expirations through an adsorber filled with active carbon.[7] All ether vapour will be retained in the carbon which is similar to that in war-time gas masks, and an appropriate design ensures low breathing resistance. An alternative procedure utilizes an exhaust pipe leading the expirations outside the operating theatre.[8]

Prevention of Arcs and Sparks

Every electrical apparatus connected to the mains supply must be earthed. This implies that the metal casing of the motor or apparatus is connected to the earth wire of its 3-core cable. A faulty wire can not then apply dangerous mains voltage to the casing, but will simply cause a fuse to blow.

Switches: The simplest remedy would be to place all switches which are prone to produce arcs between their contacts, outside the operating theatre. As this method has numerous drawbacks, they are frequently replaced by 'Safety' switches. The tilting mercury switch (fig. 369) is one of these; any arcs occur inside a closed glass envelope and cannot come in contact with flammable mixtures on its outside.

Fig. 369—the rotation of the switch, here shown in the 'OFF' position, is limited by stops. Two sturdy metal pins are sealed from above through the glass envelope which is partly filled with mercury. In the 'off' position, only the left metal pin dips into the mercury and no current can flow between the two external wires.

Fig. 370—the switch has been turned to the 'ON' position, the glass tube is horizontal and the mercury bridges the two metal pins so that current from the external supply source can flow through the switch.

When turning the switch again to 'OFF', an arc will form when the mercury leaves the right metal pin. As the space is evacuated, the arc will be relatively feeble and is further suppressed by the rapid separation assisted by the spring on the left.

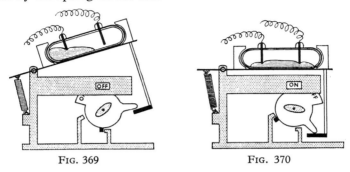

FIG. 369   FIG. 370

Another variety is known as a 'flameproof switch', and is widely used in industry together with other flameproof electrical gear. These switches suffer from the drawback of being usually very bulky. In principle they rely on a completely enclosing case as well as on packing glands for rotating spindles; the gaps between any joints and parts are made sufficiently narrow to 'quench' any flames. If flammable gases should leak inside the switch and get ignited by an arc, the flame would not pass through the narrow gaps between flanges to the outside and ignite gases in the surroundings. Industrial vapours usually contain air, and gaps of about $\frac{1}{4}$ mm are considered adequately small.[9] However, no reliance can be placed that they would stop a detonation with certainty.

As a general precaution, switches are best located high above floor level to bring them out of reach of any heavy vapours. The same holds for wall sockets; the interlocking types of these ensure that the connecting plug cannot be pulled out until the switch on the socket is in the 'OFF' position. An arc cannot occur across the contacts when this plug is inserted or pulled out.

Prevention of Static Electrification[10]

The two main factors in the generation of static electricity in operating theatres are garments made from various insulating materials and rubberware in the form of tyres, mattresses and pillows.

Formerly the main fabrics producing high static potential differences by friction (or rather by separation from one another) were wool and silk. Nowadays their number has been multiplied by numerous artificial materials such as nylon, terylene and others. Wherever conditions favour static electrification, these materials should be avoided and cotton used in their stead. Woollen blankets should at least be removed before the patient is brought near any flammable anaesthetics.

Generally speaking, static electrification is the result of a competition between the accumulation of opposite charges on two insulated objects during their separation, and the disappearance of these charges by electrical conduction to earth. Although named 'insulators', materials such as rubber, glass and many fabrics have a finite if high resistance. The slower the separation of the two insulated objects (e.g. blanket pulled off rubber mattress), giving a low rate of charge accumulation, the less will be the risk of high potential differences developing before the charges 'leak' away. On the other hand, the lower the resistance to earth, or between the objects, the smaller will be the potential difference which develops during friction of the two objects.

If a garment made of wool or cotton is taken warm from a drying cabinet, its resistance will be found to be quite high: it is a very good insulator. After exposure during an hour to normal moist room air, the electrical resistance of the fabrics (particularly cotton) will be found to have decreased owing to adsorption of moisture.[11] The great advantage of cotton over a material such as silk is that exposure to the same moist atmosphere lowers its resistance to one-thousandth of that of silk. Immediately after autoclaving or drying, cotton, and more so wool, are very good insulators and prone to generate frictional charges.

Humidification of the atmosphere

Although much discredited in many publications, this is still an important method of reducing electrification if no other measures are available.

The effect of keeping the room air humid does not consist in an increase of the electrical conductivity of the air—a statement which has sometimes been made in papers on this subject. For our purpose air is a near perfect insulator, whether dry or moist.

High humidity in the air leads to the formation of more or less continuous films of moisture on many solid objects. The moisture of the air can also react chemically with all hygroscopic substances*—the cement used for certain terrazzo floors is one of them.

Although pure water is a good insulator, traces of impurities give it an adequate degree of conductivity so that any static charges on objects

---

* Impure table salt exposed to moist air becomes 'lumpy' because small quantities of magnesium chloride contained in it are very hygroscopic.

covered with a water film are quickly conducted away to earth. For similar reasons it has been frequently advocated that anaesthetic apparatus and breathing tubes should be rinsed before use with water, or preferably with saline which is a better conductor because of its electrolyte content. The film of moisture acts then as an electrical conductor, and all parts of the apparatus are kept at the same potential. Not much reliance can be placed on continuing the electric pathway to the floor by means of a trailing chain; this has to be kept very clean to provide adequate conduction. The anaesthetist who is holding the face mask, provides an additional and better path through his body, particularly if he has leather soles on his shoes. The path to earth must be completed through the floor; many terrazzo floors have an adequately low electrical resistance; normal linoleum floors are usually excellent insulators and correspondingly dangerous.

Greater safety is offered by wearing soles of anti-static rubber, making all tyres of this material and installing a terrazzo floor resting on a well-conducting screed.

Whatever the arrangement made to dissipate frictional charges, the electric resistance to earth must not be too low; otherwise accidental contact by an individual with the electrical mains (240 volt) might cause excessive currents to flow through him, with the possibility of electrocution. If the total resistance between the electric supply and earth is approximately $0\cdot1$ megohm ($0\cdot1$ million $= 10^5$ ohms), the current passing through the body would be:

$$\frac{240\,\text{V}}{100\,000\,\Omega} = 0\cdot0024 \text{ A or approximately } 2\cdot5 \text{ milliampere (mA).}$$

This would cause only a mild shock, while halving this resistance and thereby doubling the current might lead to most unpleasant sensations. For that reason the overall resistance of all theatre equipment to earth is usually kept *above* $0\cdot1$ megohm.

PROBLEMS OF HUMIDIFICATION

The ease with which a water film forms on any object exposed to moist air, as well as the decrease in resistance of any fabric such as cotton or silk, depends on the *relative* humidity (p. 74) of the ambient air.

The **absolute humidity,** however, is of importance for the estimation of the quantity of water which has to be evaporated to raise the humidity of a room to a certain value. It is defined as:

Absolute humidity = weight of water vapour (w) in unit volume of air at given barometric pressure and temperature.

By combining Boyle's law (p. 98 and footnote on p. 312)

$$p \cdot v_o = \frac{22 \cdot 41}{M} \quad \text{for } T_o = 273 \,°K \,, \qquad p \text{ in atm, } v_o \text{ in } l/g \quad (1)$$

with Charles' law (p. 114–15)

$$\frac{v_o}{v} = \frac{T_o}{T} \qquad\qquad v_o = v \times \frac{T_o}{T} \qquad . \qquad . \quad (2)$$

one obtains

$$p \times v \times \frac{T_o}{T} = \frac{22 \cdot 41}{M} \,; \qquad p \times v = \frac{22 \cdot 41}{M \times T_o} \times T \quad . \quad (3)$$

Applying Eq. 3 to unsaturated water vapour at $T_o = 273 \,°K$, we substitute the weight of 1 mole of water: $M = 18$

$$p \times v = \frac{22 \cdot 41}{18 \times 273} \times T \quad . \qquad . \qquad . \qquad . \quad (4)$$

As we are mainly interested in temperatures of operating theatres and other warm rooms, an average value of $T = 300 \,°K$ (or $27 \,°C$) may be substituted for convenience:

$$p \,(\text{atm}) \times v \left(\frac{l}{g}\right) = \frac{22 \cdot 41 \times 300}{18 \times 273} = 1 \cdot 37 \quad . \qquad . \quad (5)$$

The absolute humidity follows then:

$$w \,(g/l) = \frac{1}{v} = \frac{p \,(\text{atm})}{1 \cdot 37} \qquad . \qquad . \qquad . \qquad . \quad (6)$$

As the partial pressures of water will be only a few mmHg, it is preferable to use this unit instead of atm; also as we are dealing with large volumes, the absolute humidity is preferably referred to cubic metres ($1 \, m^3 = 1000 \, l$ approximately). With these new units the right side of (6) has to be divided by 760 and to be multiplied by 1000, so that

$$w \,(g/m^3) = p \,(\text{mmHg}) \times \frac{1000}{1 \cdot 37 \times 760}$$

$$= p \,(\text{mmHg}) \times \frac{1}{1 \cdot 04} \simeq p \,(\text{mmHg}) \qquad . \quad (7)$$

The advantage of this representation will now be obvious: the absolute humidity is numerically equal to the partial pressure of water vapour when choosing these particular units.

Just as there is a maximum partial pressure of water vapour at any temperature, known as saturation or vapour pressure (p_s), so there is a maximum absolute humidity (w_s). This is, of course, determined by the saturation pressure, and is obtained from Eq. 7 by appending subscript($_s$) on both sides.

Example: At t $= 20$ °C the vapour pressure of water is

$$p_s = 17{\cdot}5 \text{ mmHg} \qquad \text{(see fig. 70, p. 73)}.$$

The corresponding maximum of absolute humidity is approximately: $w_s \simeq 17$ g of water per 1 m^3 of moist air.

In this connection, another handy mnemonic rule might be mentioned: if the water vapour pressure is measured in mmHg and the temperature in °C, the numerical values of the two are almost equal in the considered temperature range.

This coincidence is quite close at: t $= 27$ °C, $p_s = 26{\cdot}7$ mmHg and again at low temperatures: t $= 9$ °C, $p_s = 8{\cdot}6$ mmHg. At body temperature the deviation is already considerable: t $= 36$ °C, $p_s = 45$ mmHg.

The *relative humidity* of a gas sample is the ratio of the absolute humidity of the sample to the highest possible humidity at the given temperature:

$$\text{Relative Humidity (R.H.)} = \frac{w}{w_s} \times 100 = \frac{p}{p_s} \times 100 \text{ \%}$$

Example: At 24 °C an air sample of 5 m^3 is found to contain 44 g of water. What is the relative humidity of the sample?

The absolute humidity of this sample is:

$$w = \frac{44}{5} = 8{\cdot}8 \ \frac{g}{m^3}$$

The correct saturation pressure is $p_s = 22$ mmHg; from the approximate relation (Eq. 7) one obtains the maximum possible, absolute humidity:

$$w_s \simeq 22 \text{ g/m}^3$$

$$\text{Relative humidity R.H.} = \frac{8{\cdot}8}{22} \times 100 = 40\%$$

When a sample of moist air is heated in a closed container, its absolute humidity obviously cannot alter.

The statement that the absolute humidity of the sample does not alter when it is warmed up, is also approximately true if the sample is not in a closed container but can expand during the heating process so that the total pressure remains constant at barometric value. The partial pressures of the (unsaturated) water vapour and of the air remain then constant because their sum equals the constant barometric pressure.

According to theory, the absolute humidity changes in inverse proportion to the temperature. However, limiting ourselves to a relatively

small temperature rise, as is the case if outside air is heated in winter
to warm a room, the reduction in absolute humidity is negligible for
our purposes. Thus if air is heated through a range of 30 °C while its
pressure remains constant, the absolute humidity would decrease only
by about ten per cent.

What really matters is the enormous *decrease* in *relative* humidity
which occurs in the same circumstances. Even if the cold outside air,
e.g. t = 0 °C, p_s = 5 mmHg, is saturated with moisture, heating up
to 30 °C would reduce the relative humidity by a factor: $\frac{5}{32} \simeq \frac{1}{6}$,
because the saturation pressure at 30 °C is 32 mmHg. In other words,
the original sample with R.H. = 100% has now only a R.H. = $\frac{100}{6}$
= 16% (neglecting the expansion of the sample during the heating
process).

This fact is of practical significance where operating theatres are
air-conditioned, but in which the humidification plant is imperfect. In
winter, cold air is drawn into the air-conditioning plant, scrubbed and
warmed up. Unless the humidifier is efficient, the relative humidity
of the clean, warm issuing air may be far below that of the cold and
moist outside air. This state of affairs can obtain although considerable
quantities of water vapour have been added to the entering air in the
plant in order to increase its absolute humidity. Large volumes of
water have to be evaporated to raise the relative humidity of an operating theatre and to maintain it at a high level. This is mainly due to
the condensation of liquid water wherever the air is in contact with cold
walls and windows. The magnitude of these quantities can be appreciated by the following

Example: How much water must be evaporated into the air of an
operating theatre (10 × 10 × 4 m³, or 33 × 33 × 13 ft³) at a
temperature of 25 °C in order to raise the relative humidity from 35%
to 60%?

At 25 °C the maximum absolute humidity is w_s = 23 g/m³, and
R.H. = 35% represents an absolute humidity of

$$w = \frac{35}{100} \times 23 \quad g/m^3$$

The required R.H. = 60% represents an absolute humidity of

$$w = \frac{60}{100} \times 23 \quad g/m^3$$

By subtracting the first value of w from the second, the required increase in absolute humidity is found:

$$\frac{60 - 35}{100} \times 23 = \frac{25}{100} \times 23 = 5{\cdot}7 \text{ g/m}^3$$

The room volume is: $10 \times 10 \times 4 = 400$ m³, and the total water to be evaporated:

$$5{\cdot}7 \frac{\text{g}}{\text{m}^3} \times 400 \text{ m}^3 = 2280 \text{ g, or } 2\tfrac{1}{4} \text{ litres.}$$

In winter there may be another difficulty in maintaining a high relative humidity. A large window, constructed as it often is in certain countries, with a single layer of glass separating the theatre air from the outside, acts as a large cooling area. The inside air coming into contact with the window is cooled below its dew point (p. 75). Part of the water vapour condenses and the moisture content of the room air is lowered.

The large quantity of water which had to be added to the room air in the preceding example in an attempt to raise its relative humidity, might be easily lost again through condensation on the window. The obvious remedy would be to fit double-glazed windows with an adequate air space between the layers, a practice much used in countries with a rational outlook on fuel economy during cold winters.

Humidity in operating theatres

It is often stated that in the absence of a proper humidifying installation, a steam sterilizer in the vicinity of the theatre provides ample humidification of the atmosphere. This may be true only if the sterilizer is of large dimensions, is in constant use and in free communication with the air of the operating theatres. Nevertheless, if the walls of the rooms are badly insulated, the windows with single glazing, and the outside temperature low, very large quantities of steam would be required to maintain a high relative humidity.

According to one survey of explosions due to static electricity, most of these occurred when the relative humidity of the theatre was 60% or below.[12] In nine-tenths of the explosions the relative humidity of the room had been below 50%.

However, static sparks can be produced[13] in a relative humidity as high as 65%. A value of R.H. = 60% is now generally regarded as the lowest safe limit to reduce appreciably the risk of static electrification.

Estimates of the R.H. which can be maintained without fogging windows severely by condensation are available.[14] If the outside temperature is near freezing point (0 °C), a R.H. = 35% is possible if the windows are single-glazed, while R.H. = 65% is possible if they are double-glazed.

Hygrometric estimations in an average operating theatre will probably show quite often that the R.H. is unexpectedly low. Wherever static electrification tends to occur, an instrument for the determination of relative humidities is a useful asset.

In very warm operating theatres, relative humidities of 65% and above may be very uncomfortable and may tax the equanimity of the operating team.

Dissipation of static charges

Ionization of the room air

Certain schemes have been suggested for increasing the conductivity of the air itself, either in the whole room or at least in the neighbourhood of objects which should not become charged. Most of these methods[15] are based on the partial ionization of the air molecules by means of radioactive substances; the air thereby becomes slightly conducting, and charges on objects of different potentials can flow from one to the other, or to earth. Although used in the printing and other industries, these methods have not found general use in operating theatres.

Provision of separate conducting paths from equipment to earth

This was formerly ensured by a metal spiral in the breathing tube connecting the patient to the metal parts of the apparatus. Any electrification of the breathing bag was suppressed by enclosing it in a wire net. Conduction to the floor was continued by chains trailing from the apparatus, and the floor itself was sub-divided by numerous, grounded metal strips.

These devices, except for the trailing chains, have gone out of fashion. A 'short circuit' between a faulty electric mains cable and any part of the bare metal wires on breathing tube or bag might lead to high currents and consequent excessive heating; an explosive mixture could thus become ignited. Furthermore, the accidental contact of the mains voltage with any part of this metallic pathway might cause severe shocks or electrocution. In addition, any unobserved break in the wires might become the site of a spark when the two parts of the separated system assume a potential difference.

An attempt to overcome these drawbacks was HORTON'S 'Intercoupler'.[16] Its main feature is the introduction of fairly high resistances (1 megohm) in leads between certain persons and objects in the theatre.

These resistances are still low enough to allow rapid disappearance of frictional charges, while preventing the passage of any but very small currents even when in accidental contact with the electric power supply; overheating and powerful sparks are made impossible. The intercoupler consists of a small container with resistances from which wires lead to patient, surgeon, anaesthetist and anaesthetic trolley; from the latter a trailing chain leads to the floor which must have an adequate conductivity.

One of the disadvantages of this appliance is the wires dangling about the theatre, and this explains why it is no longer in general use in the U.S.A., where it was introduced shortly before World War II. Should a break occur in any part of the intercoupler, the risk of excessive potential differences is again present.

Use of anti-static rubber

Normal rubber is a good insulator; for instance, the normal breathing tube made from red rubber has a very high resistance. In the introduction of a slightly conducting material known as 'anti-static' rubber, the aim is again to make the electric potential of all objects the same. Since many objects in an operating theatre are earthed, all other objects must also be brought near earth potential. Persons moving about in the theatre or trolleys which are moved about, will not become charged if there are sufficiently low electric resistances between them and earth. In general the resistance of leather soles on shoes[17] is low enough for this purpose, although many authorities prefer the use of soles made from anti-static rubber with a definite and lower resistance.

The greater part of the whole pathway between patient and earth consists of rubber: face mask, breathing tube, reservoir bag, tyres of trolley wheels, etc. So-called *conductive* rubber has been in use for a long time in industry where large, undesirable frictional charges are continually produced and must be rapidly dissipated. By incorporating appreciable quantities of carbon black during the manufacture of rubber, the normally highly insulating rubber can be given a low resistance which may be many million times smaller than that of normal rubber. Tyres of large road vehicles or aeroplanes act as continuous electrification machines when running on dry road surfaces, and potential differences up to 50 kilovolt can be readily produced.[18] Conducting tyres with overall resistances well below 0·1 megohm have overcome this trouble a long time ago.

When applied to anaesthetic equipment the rubber parts must again have reasonably large resistances in order to avoid high currents when accidental contact is made with the electric power supply (see p. 397). Although non-insulating rubber had been used on anaesthetic equipment already thirty years ago,[19] such rubber parts are even now not uniformly satisfactory. The conductivity of anti-static rubber is attributed to microscopic chains of carbon particles; quite often when a breathing tube is stretched its resistance may rise considerably, and this could be explained by temporary interruption of the carbon chains.

The resistance of various anti-static rubber parts is known to increase gradually with time, so that periodical checks are necessary. These are not as easy as the measurement of, say, the resistance of an electrical fire, because there is often a large contact resistance between the rubber and any applied metal electrode.[20] The contact area between the two must be well wetted to obtain reliable readings on a resistance meter.

Safety measures must not only be applied to the anaesthetic apparatus itself. It is a reflection on the attention paid to the risk of static electrification in Great Britain that operating-theatre personnel often wear footwear with ordinary rubber soles; the resistance of the latter may be as high as 20000 megohms, while any value above 10 megohms is rather undesirable. Shuffling about on normal rubber soles can easily generate a potential difference of several kV between the person and other objects.

Maximum resistance permissible for adequate removal of charges

The overall resistance values[21] of 0·1 to 10 (sometimes 1 to 100) megohms quoted as suitable for the prevention of dangerous potential differences between various objects in a room,[22] are based on experimental observations as well as on theory. The latter is based on estimates of the maximum rate of electrification such as can be produced, e.g. by pulling a woollen blanket off a metal trolley standing on insulating tyres. It is known that the rate of electrification may correspond to a current of a few micro amperes* flowing into the insulated object and raising its potential difference relative to other neighbouring objects or to earth.

A suitable resistance must be provided between the charged object and earth, to carry away the charges as quickly as they are generated. Assuming, for example, that the p.d. of the object should not exceed 300 V if igniting sparks are to be avoided, the necessary resistance can be calculated from Ohm's law. If the rate of charging corresponds to a current of 30 micro ampere, the required resistance would be:

$$\frac{300 \text{ V}}{30 \times 10^{-6} \text{ A}} = 10^7 \text{ ohms} = 10 \text{ megohm} = 10 \text{ M}\Omega$$

* 1 micro ampere $= \frac{1}{1000\,000}$ ampere $= 10^{-6}$ A $= 1\mu$A.

In comparison to these desirable leak resistances, the resistances of a person in shoes with normal rubber soles, or of a trolley on normal rubber wheels, are much higher—possibly ten thousand times or more.

Rate of dissipation of static charges

It is sometimes useful to estimate the speed with which a high static potential of a charged object disappears if a conductive path is provided to earth. The disappearance of a p.d. from an object of given capacity proceeds exponentially.* One has therefore to choose some time during which the potential difference falls to a certain fraction of its initial value; in the following formula we have chosen the time it takes until the potential difference has fallen to 10% of its initial value.

The units of time are milli seconds, of the resistance megohms, and of the capacitance pF. In order to form some idea about the general applicability of the formula it is well to remember that most objects in an operating theatre which might become frictionally charged have a capacity of a few hundred pF. Theory shows that

$$t_{(10\%)} \text{ (ms)} = \frac{2 \cdot 3}{1000} \times \text{capacitance (pF)} \times \text{resistance (M}\Omega)$$

Example: Capacitance $C = 200$ pF; resistance $R = 100$ MΩ. This might represent the capacitance and resistance relative to earth of a person standing in shoes with leather soles on a terrazzo floor.

$$t_{(10\%)} = \frac{2 \cdot 3}{1000} \times 200 \times 100 = 46 \text{ msec, or about } \frac{1}{20} \text{ s}$$

As the absolute value of the p.d. does not enter into the formula, the same time elapses for an initial p.d. of 10000 volt to fall to 1000 volt, or for 3000 volt to fall to 300 volt.

While the foregoing example describes a situation which is unlikely to cause dangerous static sparks, the following illustrates the case of a trolley on normal rubber tyres which might easily be raised to dangerously high potentials.

Example:
Capacitance $C = 300$ pF; resistance $R = 100\,000$ MΩ

$$t_{(10\%)} = \frac{2 \cdot 3}{1000} \times 300 \times 100000 = 70000 \text{ msec, or } 70 \text{ s}$$

*The term 'exponential' is applied when the rate of change of a quantity at any moment is proportional to the magnitude of the quantity at that moment. Examples which the reader may recognize are: growth of money in the bank at compound interest, or the decay of a radio-active element. An exponential relation which does not involve time as a variable is the decrease of barometric pressure with altitude (see the curve to the right of the grey field in fig. 82, p. 86).

Thus any accidentally generated charge would persist for a long time. Continued friction, as produced by wheeling the trolley along a floor covered with normal linoleum, would raise the p.d. to very high values.

Antistatic Floors

One further link in the conductive path which must be established between anaesthetic apparatus and earth is the floor.[23, 24] Floors covered with linoleum or formed by wooden blocks may have resistances of several thousand megohms. Many 'granolithic' floors also have high resistances, but other floors formed by small stones embedded in a certain cement are very satisfactory. The anti-static properties of these 'terrazzo' floors are partly due to the hygroscopic nature of the cement. Furthermore, the sub-floor may include wire netting and carbon black. Specifications both for the laying and testing of such floors have been published.[23]

Mixtures made non-flammable by adding Diluents

This method is of very limited usefulness in clinical practice. We can roughly predict the effect of a diluent from the earlier discussion on limits of flammability; the most common diluent (nitrogen) was there added to the flammable mixture in a fixed proportion to oxygen, i.e. the limits of flammability in air were compared with those in pure oxygen. It was found that the lower limit is little affected, while the upper limit can be very greatly reduced.

The effect of such diluents is not merely due to the resultant reduction in partial pressure of oxygen in the fuel-oxygen-diluent mixture. The following experiments show this quite clearly.[25]

A small alcohol lamp is lighted and placed in a glass jar filled with air. The air is now gradually replaced by oxygen-nitrogen mixtures with decreasing oxygen content. When the oxygen concentration has decreased from 21% to slightly below 15%, the alcohol flame becomes extinguished; the limiting partial pressure of oxygen is 112 mmHg. In a second experiment the alcohol flame burns in pure oxygen at atmospheric pressure, and the pressure is gradually reduced. The flame is not extinguished until the pressure has fallen as low as 27 mmHg.

The ability of a third component (diluent) to reduce the flammability of fuel/oxygen mixtures depends both on its specific heat and its heat conductivity. In general a diluent with high values of these two properties is more efficient than others in lowering the upper limit of flammability of the fuel. The high specific heat of the diluent will swallow up part of the heat of combustion and thus reduce the flame temperature. The heat of combustion will also be better transferred to the walls of the vessel if the diluent has a good heat conductivity. The heat available to warm up layers of the fresh mixture may then become too small to ensure propagation of a flame.

Examples:
(1) The limits of flammability of cyclopropane-oxygen mixtures are: L.L. $= 2.2\%$ and U.L. $= 60\%$. A mixture of 50% cyclopropane and 50% oxygen is very detonable. If, however, 12% of oxygen in the latter mixture are replaced by helium, no flame can be propagated.[26] The mixture of

50% cyclopropane $+$ 12% helium $+$ 38% oxygen is non-flammable. Furthermore, any such mixture with an oxygen content below 38% and a correspondingly higher helium content is also non-flammable.

(2) A mixture of 20% cyclopropane plus 80% oxygen is extremely detonable. If 54% or more of the oxygen are replaced by helium, the mixtures are again non-flammable. They have an oxygen content of 26% or less.

(3) A mixture of 4% cyclopropane plus 96% oxygen is flammable. At least 84% of oxygen has to be replaced by helium to make the mixture non-flammable. Any mixture of 4% cyclopropane with helium and oxygen containing less than 12% oxygen will be non-flammable, but even if the amount of helium added were not quite high enough, the combustion process would be a very mild affair.

Certain disadvantages of the diluent method of suppressing deflagrations or explosions are obvious: low concentrations of cyclopropane could only be administered with low concentrations of oxygen, and this may be undesirable from a physiological point of view.

Another difficulty is the maintenance of the correct mixtures in anaesthetic apparatus at present in use—at least as far as the closed circuit is used. Once a machine is flushed with oxygen—say for some emergency—the accurate admixture with the diluent would have to be performed all over again.

Lately the method has found some favour in the form of miniature cylinders, containing cyclopropane and a mixture of oxygen with either helium or nitrogen as diluent, for minor surgery[27, 28].

Nitrogen is almost as efficient as helium in its suppressing action, but helium is preferred for secondary reasons. Electric sparks pass less easily through helium than through nitrogen, so that accidental ignition of a mixture with helium is less likely. Furthermore, the oxygen content of these three–component mixtures is necessarily low. Helium makes breathing easier, and partially helps to compensate for lowered oxygen concentration by facilitating increased tidal exchange.

'Quenching.'
Flame Traps

The damage caused by ignition of flammable mixtures could be greatly reduced if it were possible to prevent the spreading of the self-propagating flame from the site of ignition. One of the oldest technical applications of this principle is the safety lamp for miners; of these lamps the Davy lamp is generally known:

Fig. 371 — the naked flame of an oil lamp is enclosed by a glass cylinder surmounted by a cylinder formed from fine mesh wire gauze. The outer air has free access to the air inside the lamp through the mesh of the gauze. The lighted lamp can be used in moderately explosive atmospheres with impunity. When a flammable mixture of mine gases containing methane enters the interior, it will be ignited by the static flame of the lamp, but the self-propagating flame does not spread to the outside. Owing to the good heat conduction of the wires, the flame approaching the mesh

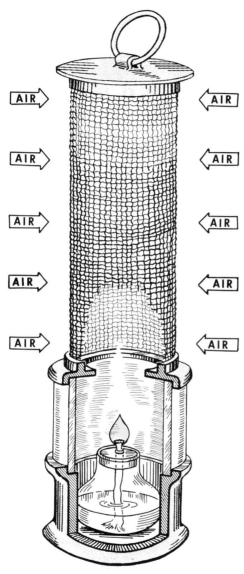

FIG. 371

from the inside is cooled to such a degree that it cannot raise the neighbouring fresh gas layer on the outside to its ignition temperature; the flame is quenched by the wire mesh.

The Davy lamp[29] serves also as a crude explosibility meter. Fig. 371 illustrates the appearance of the lamp flame when the surrounding air contains no mine gases, while

Fig. 372—shows a flame when flammable mine gases are present, although their composition is still below the lower limit of flammability. A large aureole surrounds the flame in which the flammable gases entering the lamp by diffusion and convection are combusted. This gives a visible warning to the miner that the atmosphere is unsafe, long before the methane content might exceed the L.L. value.

In highly flammable surroundings, particularly if fast air currents are travelling across the lamp, this device is unsafe and self-propagating flames may easily travel to the outside.

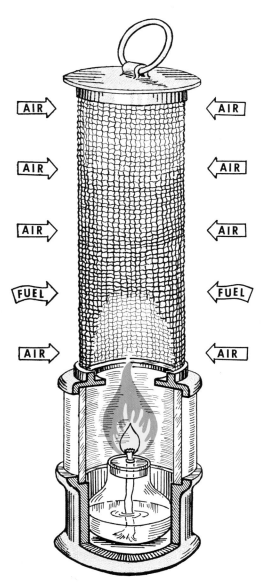

Fig. 372

We had already met the process of 'quenching' a flame at the site of ignition, while discussing spark discharge across very closely placed electrodes. A similar type of quenching at the site of ignition can be illustrated by the following example.

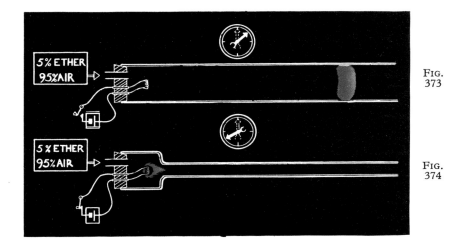

Fig. 373

Fig. 374

Fig. 373—a wide tube (say 1 cm diameter) filled with the flammable mixture carries at its left end a wire which can be heated by an electric current. At zero time the switch was closed, the wire heated to incandescence and a bright, self-propagating flame started. The switch is quickly opened, and a few seconds later the flame has travelled through the greater part of the long tube while the wire has again cooled down.

Fig. 374—the arrangement is the same as in the preceding illustration except that the wide tube has here been replaced by a much narrower tube (say 0·2 cm diameter). Although the switch has been left on and the wire kept hot for a long time, no flame has travelled along the narrow tube. Only an aureole occurs near the hot wire where fresh mixture has diffused towards it. Owing to the close proximity of the cool tube walls, heat is too quickly removed from any flame which might start to travel along it.

Many *flame traps* have been designed for industrial purposes to confine an explosion and prevent its spreading to other regions filled with flammable mixtures.

Fig. 375—a wide tube with a narrow constriction near its middle is

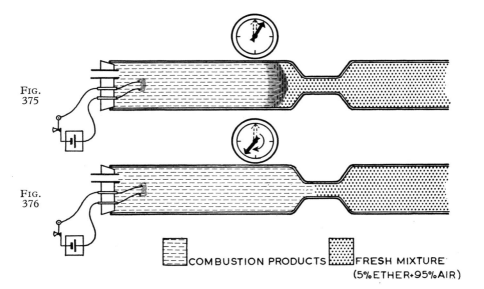

FIG.
375

FIG.
376

▒▒▒COMBUSTION PRODUCTS ░░░FRESH MIXTURE
(5% ETHER+95% AIR)

filled with a flammable gas mixture. It was ignited at zero time at the left end, and a few seconds later the flame has travelled through most of the wide tube to the left of the constriction, leaving combustion products in its wake.

Fig. 376—a long time interval has elapsed since, while the wire has been kept hot by the current from the battery. Yet the flame has disappeared, and the presence of fresh mixture indicates that the flame has not travelled through the constriction.

Flame traps have also been tried on anaesthetic apparatus,[30] either at the inlet to the breathing tube or near the face mask. However, it should be made quite clear that such traps can only stop the propagation of the slow flames occurring in deflagrations. The action of wire gauze in a flame trap is based on the high thermal conductivity of metals. On the other hand, a detonation is not propagated by simple heat conduction but by a shock wave which might pass a metal gauze without any hindrance.

It is true that technical flame traps have been made to stop even the propagation of detonations,[31] but their high flow resistance makes them unsuitable for practical use on anaesthetic machines. Such traps are sometimes made from sintered metal discs which form a kind of spongy layer, with large numbers of microscopic channels.[32]

HISTORICAL NOTES ON EXPLOSIONS

The antecedents of explosions in flammable mixtures go back a long time before the memorable year 1846. More surprising still, ignition of flammable vapours by static sparks was practised for demonstrations one hundred years earlier.

Fig. 377—On the left a hand 'rubs' a rotating insulator (sulfur ball); the frictional charges are transferred through fine wires touching the

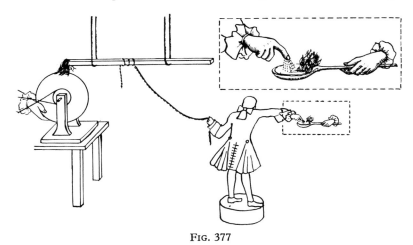

FIG. 377

ball to a metal bar suspended by insulating silk threads. A metal chain transfers them to the demonstrator standing on an insulating platform. He is charged to a high potential difference relative to an assistant standing on the floor and whose hand is shown holding a spoon filled with alcohol.

The insert shows streams of sparks jumping from the fingertip to the spoon and igniting the alcohol vapour/air mixture.

The illustration is re-drawn from one published by the Abbé NOLLET in 1745 who comments: '... the sparks ignite vapours and flammable mixtures approached to them; this is a spectacle which deserves considerable interest and one can never get tired of seeing an electrified person igniting alcohol with his fingertip.'[33] He carried out similar experiments with other flammable substances and found that it is much easier to ignite the vapours if the spoon is warmed, i.e. if the vapour pressure is raised to ensure the presence of flammable mixtures above the liquid.

It was even known that ignition is more difficult if instead of the metal spoon an insulating material (glass) is used as receptacle for the liquid:

Charged insulators give less powerful sparks than charged conductors

When a spark passes between objects at different potentials, the total charge passes from one to the other in one single spark only if both are conductors. If one of them is an insulator, the spark will neutralize only a limited area on it, because charges from further away cannot flow quickly enough to the site discharged by the spark. In other words, while the whole electric energy of charged conductors can be dissipated in one single spark, only part of the electrical energy is dissipated in one spark, if both or one of the objects are insulators.[34]

Limits of flammability

The first to elucidate the range of flammability in gas mixtures, but whose excellent work is sometimes neglected amongst the praise bestowed on J. Priestley and H. Davy, was the Honourable Henry CAVENDISH. Already in 1766 he prepared mixtures of hydrogen with air in flasks about one litre in capacity. Ignition was attempted by applying a flame to the mouth of the flask; this was done by remote control to avoid injury to the experimenter. Several of his experiments[35] are summarized in the following table 31, using modern nomenclature.

TABLE 31

Hydrogen	Air	Result of attempted ignition
1 part	9 parts	No deflagration
2	8	'Very loud noise'
3	7	'Very loud noise'
4	6	'Sound very little louder'
5	5	'Sound very little louder'
6	4	'Sound not very loud'
7	3	'Only a gentle puff'
8	2	No deflagration

Cavendish also made indirectly some observations on flame speed, by stating that mixtures between f = 20 to 40 % exploded so quickly that the light could scarcely be seen.

His work is of particular interest as until then it had not been understood that air has to be present before a flammable gas can be combusted. 'It appears from these experiments that . . . (hydrogen) . . . cannot burn without the assistance of common air.'

Ether explosions

An early link between the medical profession and ether explosions is found in the investigations by J. INGEN-HOUSZ, 'Physician to their Imperial Majesties and F.R.S.' After seeing some qualitative experiments in Holland he embarked on a close study of ignition of mixtures of ether with air and oxygen which he summarized in 1779. Following Cavendish's observations on limits of explosibility in hydrogen mixtures, he found that high concentrations of ether mixed with air cannot be exploded.

Some years previously Priestley had already noticed that oxygen-rich mixtures explode more violently than those with air. Now, Ingenhousz was pleasantly surprised to note the violent detonations in ether vapour mixed with oxygen.

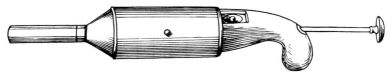

FIG. 378

The final tests were carried out with an instrument[36] re-drawn in Fig. 378—This 'air pistol' with electric ignition was constructed by

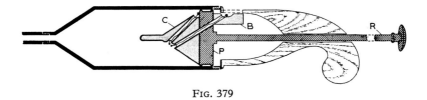

FIG. 379

the well-known instrument maker NAIRNE in London. The section Fig. 379—shows a piston rod (R) passing through the handle to the piston (P) which has a conical structure (C) attached to its inner side; the latter ensures that no dead volume remains in the pistol barrel screwed to the large cylinder, when the piston is pushed over to the left. While piston, barrel and large cylinder are of metal, the cone (C) is made of ivory to insulate the two wires leading through bores in it to the spark gap. The outer end of one wire lies in a recess of the small insulator (B) attached to the piston, the other wire is connected to the piston (P) and thereby to the cylinder. The potential from an electrification apparatus can be applied between cylinder (see small knob in fig. 378) and the other electrode, only when the piston is pulled right back, as shown in fig. 378. The end of the second wire is then exposed in the cut-out part of the handle as will be seen from fig. 379.

A small rubber bulb (elastic gum bottle) or a bladder was filled with ether/oxygen mixture and attached to the left end of the narrow barrel. The piston was pulled to the right while the bulb was gently squeezed. The large cylinder ('air box') with a length of 4 inch and a diameter of 2 inch has a volume of about 200 cm³ Finally a lead bullet wrapped in leather is rammed into the pistol barrel at the left, and a spark made to pass across the gap (ca. 2 mm).

Earlier experiments had not always gone smoothly as will become apparent from the following quotations:

'. . . the subsequent explosion tore off the various components of the pistol.'

The author was assisted by the Abbé Fontana, Director of the Cabinet of Natural History belonging to the Grand Duke of Tuscany.

'. . . Abbé Fontana wrapped a towel around the pistol for security's sake, (the ether/oxygen mixture) . . . exploded with such a strong report, that his hearing as well as mine was much hurt by it.'

REFERENCES

[1] PINSON, K. B. (1930). *Brit. med. J.*, ii, 312.
[2] GUEDEL, A. (1937). *Inhalation anesthesia*, cf. p. 151, New York.
[3] FLAGG, P. J. (1937). *Arch. Otolaryng. Chicago*, 25, 83–4.
[4] GREENE, B. A. (1941). *Anesthesiology*, 2, 144–60; cf. p. 158.
[5] HASLER, J. K. (1938). *Practitioner*, 140, 270–76.
[6] See Ref. 4, p. 148.
[7] EPSTEIN, H. G. (1944). *Lancet*, i, 114–16.
[8] BULLOUGH, J. (1954). *Lancet*, i, 798–801.
[9] BRITISH STANDARD (1946). *Flameproof enclosure of electrical apparatus* No. 229.
[10] GUEST, P. G., SIKORA, V. W., and LEWIS, B. (1952). *Static electricity in hospital operating suites: direct and related hazards and pertinent remedies*, U.S. Bureau of Mines Rep. Invest. No. 4833.
[11] BULGIN, D. (1953). *Brit. J. appl. Phys.*, 4, S. 87–91.
[12] See Ref. 4, p. 157.

[13] WOODBRIDGE, P. D., HORTON, J. W., and CONNELL, K. (1939). *J. Amer. med. Ass.*, 113, 740–44.
[14] REPORT OF COMMITTEE ON STATIC ELECTRICITY (1942). *Anesthesiology*, 3, 85–91; cf. p. 89.
[15] SLOCUM, H. C., and FINVOLD, R. (1944). *Anesthesiology*, 5, 33–9.
[16] See Ref. 13.
[17] GREENE, B. A. (1952). *Anesthesiology*, 13, 203–6.
[18] LANE, K. A., and GARDNER, E. R. (1948–9). *I.R.I. Trans.*, 24, 70–91.
[19] RITTER and RIMARSKI, W. (1928). *Muench. med. Wsch.*, 75, 314-16.
[20] BRITISH STANDARD (1953). *Laboratory tests for resistivity of conductive and anti-static rubbers* No. 2044.
[21] BRITISH STANDARD (1953). *Resistance of conductive and anti-static rubber products* No. 2050.
[22] BULGIN, D., LLEWELLYN, F. J., and THOMAS, G. (1949). *Lancet*, i, 789.
[23] REPORT OF A WORKING PARTY ON ANAESTHETIC EXPLOSIONS INCLUDING SAFETY CODE FOR EQUIPMENT AND INSTALLATIONS (1956). London.
[24] NATIONAL FIRE PROTECTION ASSOCIATION (1956). *Standard* No. 56.
[25] DOLLWIG, H. C., et al. (1917). *J. Amer. Chem. Soc.*, 39, 2224–31.
[26] REPORT OF THE COUNCIL ON PHARMACY AND CHEMISTRY OF CYCLOPROPANE (1941). *J. Amer. med. Ass.*, 116, 2502-4.
[27] HINGSON, R. A. (1954). *J. Amer. med. Ass.*, 156, 604-6.
[28] BOURNE, J. G., and MORTON, H. J. V. (1955). *Lancet*, i, 20-22.
See also:
HEWER, C. L., and LEE, J. A. (1957). *Recent advances in anaesthesia and analgesia*, cf. p. 20, London.
[29] DAVY, SIR HUMPHREY (1818). *On the safety lamp for coalminers*, Lond.
[30] CHENEY, M. B. (1929). *Curr. Res. Anesth.*, 8, 261–2.
[31] JENTZSCH, H. (1950). *Brennstoff-Chem.*, 31, 381–2.
[32] EGERTON, A. C., et al. (1953). in: *Fourth Symposium (International) on Combustion*, No. 87, 689–95. Baltimore.
[33] L'Abbé NOLLET (1745). *Hist. Acad. Roy. Sci. Paris 1749*; cf. p. 112, also Pl. I, fig. 1 and 2.
[34] BULGIN, D. (1947–8). *I.R.I. Trans.*, 23, 35–40.
[35] CAVENDISH, The Hon. HENRY (1766). *Phil. Trans.*, 56, 141–84; cf. p. 148.
[36] INGEN-HOUSZ, J. (1779). *Phil. Trans.*, 69, 376–418; cf. p. 411 and Table V on p. 418.

Chapter XXIV

PHYSICAL DATA AND CONVERSION FACTORS

L   =   Liquid.

G; V   =   Gas or Vapour.

RT   =   Room Temperature: in general 20 °C, but it may deviate by a few degrees from 20 °C if the respective property depends only a little on the temperature.

NT   =   Normal Temperature: 0 °C or 273.18 °K.

BT   =   Body Temperature; c. 37 °C.

RTP   =   Value of quantity at 20 °C and a pressure of P = 760 Torr (1 atm).

NTP   =   Quantity at 0 °C and a pressure of P = 760 Torr.

Bp   =   Boiling Point at normal atmospheric pressure (760 Torr).

[ ]   =   Any *numerical* values surrounded by such a bracket are less certain.

Row a =   The sign ' ; V' indicates that the quantity is taken at the pressure of saturated vapour.

Row b =   Theoretical specific volume under the assumption that gases and vapours at 20 °C and 1 atm obey ideal gas laws.

Row e =   The values in units (cal/ml) used in the text of the book are derived from the values given here by multiplication with the respective density.

Row k =   Coefficient of solubility = volume of gas or vapour (reduced to NTP) with a partial pressure of 760 Torr, which is being taken up by 100 ml water.

Substance:		1 Water	2 Ethyl alcohol (Ethanol)
Formula:		H_2O	$CH_3 \cdot CH_2OH$
Mol. weight:		18·02	46·07

	Property	Units		
a	Density	G; V: [g/l]	0·60 *Bp*	1·64 *Bp*
a′	Density	L: [g/ml]	1·00 *4 °C*	0·79 *RT*
b	Spec. volume	G; V: [l/g, *RTP*]	1·40	0·525
c	Boiling point	[°C; 760 Torr]	100	78·3
d	Vap. pressure abs., at 20 °C	(generally in) Torr	17·5	44
e	Heat of Vaporiz.	[cal/g]	585 *RT*	220 *RT*
f	Crit. temp.	[°C]	374	243
g	Crit. pressure	[atm]	218	63
h	Spec. heat	G; V:[cal/g, Cp]	0·46 *RT*	0·40 *25 °C*
h′	Spec. heat	L: [cal/g]	1·00 *4 °C*	0·58
i	Viscosity	G; V:[10^{-4} Poise]	1·2 *35 °C*	1·1 *100 °C*
i′	Viscosity	L: [10^{-2} Poise]	1·00 *RT*	1·20 *RT*
k	Solubility	G; V: [ml/100ml H_2O]	—	∞
k′	Solubility	L: [g/100 ml H_2O]	—	∞

3 **Diethyl** **ether**	4 **Divinyl** **ether** (Diethenyl ether)	5 **Chloroform** (Trichloro- methane)	6 **Ethyl chloride** (Chloroethane)	
$C_2H_5 \cdot O \cdot C_2H_5$	$(CH_2 : CH)_2O$	$CHCl_3$	$CH_3 \cdot CH_2Cl$	
74·12	70·1	119·4	64·5	
3·0 *Bp*	3·11 *Bp*	4·43 *Bp*	2·76 *Bp*	**a**
0·71 *RT*	0·77 *RT*	1·50 *RT*	0·90 *RT*	**a′**
0·325	0·343	0·203	0·372	**b**
34·6	28·3	61·2	12·3	**c**
442	550	160	1·32 *atm*	**d**
89 *Bp*	89 *Bp*	67 *RT*	92 *RT*	**e**
194	[190]	263	187	**f**
355	[42]	54	52	**g**
0·44 *RT*		0·14 *30 °C*	0·23 *RT*	**h**
0·53 *RT*		0·23 *RT*	0·37 *NT*	**h′**
0·72 *14 °C*		1·02 *RT*	1·05 *35 °C*	**i**
0·24 *RT*		0·58 *RT*	0·26 *RT*	**i′**
1400 *BT*	116 *BT*	405 *BT*	160 *RT*	**k**
6·9 *RT*		0·75 *RT*	0·45 *NT*	**k′**

	Substance:		7 Trichloro- ethylene (Trichloro- ethene)	8 Halothane ('Fluothane')
	Formula:		CHCl:CCl₂	CF₃·CHClBr
	Mol. weight:		131·4	197

	Property	Units		
a	Density	G; V: [g/l]	4·4 *Bp*	8·9 *Bp*
a′	Density	L: [g/ml]	1·46 *RT*	1·86 *RT*
b	Spec. volume	G; V: [l/g, *RTP*]	0·183	0·122
c	Boiling point	[°C; 760 Torr]	87	50
d	Vap. pressure abs., at 20 °C	(generally in) Torr	58	241
e	Heat of Vaporiz.	[cal/g]	58 *Bp*	35 *Bp*
f	Crit. temp.	[°C]	271	[296]
g	Crit. pressure	[atm]	49·5	[39]
h	Spec. heat	G; V:[cal/g, Cp]	0·25 *RT*	
h′	Spec. heat	L : [cal/g]	0·25 *RT*	0·19 *RT*
i	Viscosity	G; V:[10⁻⁴ Poise]	1·03 *60 °C*	
i′	Viscosity	L: [10⁻² Poise]	0·58 *RT*	0·35 *RT*
k	Solubility	G; V:[ml/100ml H₂O]	230 *RT*	
k′	Solubility	L: [g/100 ml H₂O]	0·11 *25 °C*	0·34 *RT*

	9 Cyclo- proprane	10 Nitrous oxide	11 Carbon- dioxide	12 Ethylene (Ethene)	
	$\overline{CH_2 \cdot CH_2 \cdot CH_2}$	N_2O	CO_2	$CH_2 : CH_2$	
	42·08	44·02	44·01	28·05	
	1·75 *RT*	150 *RT,V*	180 *RT,V*	108 *NT*	**a**
	0·68 *Bp*	0·79 *RT*	0·77 *RT*	0·34 *NT*	**a′**
	0·571	0·543	0·543	0·851	**b**
	—33	—88	—78 (*subl.*)	—104	**c**
	6·3 *atm*	52 *atm*	57 *atm*	—	**d**
	[48]	43 *RT*	35 *RT*	115 *Bp*	**e**
	125	36·5	31	9·6	**f**
	54	71·7	72·8	51	**g**
	0·32 27 °C	0·21 *RT*	0·20	0·36	**h**
		0·28 —123 °C	0·70	0·57 *Bp*	**h′**
	0·83 *RT*	1·46 *RT*	1·46 *RT*	1·03 *RT*	**i**
			0·071 *RT*	0·15 —100 °C	**i′**
	18·0 *BT*	39 *BT*	57 *BT*	7·8 *BT*	**k**
	—	—	—	—	**k′**

Substance:		13 Oxygen	14 Nitrogen
Formula:		O_2	N_2
Mol. weight:		32·00	28·02

	Property	Units		
a	Density	G : [g/l]	1·33 *RTP*	1·77 *RTP*
a′	Density	L : [g/ml]	1·14 *Bp*	0·81 *Bp*
b	Spec. volume	G : [l/g, *RTP*]	0·751	0·858
c	Boiling point	[°C; 760 Torr]	—183 (90·2 °K)	—196 (77·3 °K)
d	Vap. pressure abs., at 20 °C	(generally in) Torr	—	—
e	Heat of Vaporiz.	[cal/g]	51 *Bp*	48 *Bp*
f	Crit. temp.	[°C]	—119	—147
g	Crit. pressure	[atm]	50	33
h	Spec. heat	G: [cal/g, Cp]	0·22	0·25
h′	Spec. heat	L: [cal/g]	0·39 *73 °K*	0·47 *73 °K*
i	Viscosity	G: [10^{-4} Poise]	2·00 *RT*	1·74 *RT*
i′	Viscosity	L : [10^{-2} Poise]	0·19 *Bp*	
k	Solubility	G : [ml/100ml H_2O]	3·1 *RT*	1·64 *RT*

15 Air (28·96)	16 Hydrogen H_2 2·016	17 Helium He 4·003	18 Xenon Xe 131·3	
1·20 RTP	0·090 NTP	0·16 RTP	600 *10 °C, V*	**a**
0·52 Bp	0·071 Bp	0·12 Bp	1·75 *10 °C*	**a′**
0·830	11·9	6·01	0·183	**b**
—194 (78·7 °K)	—253 (20·4 °K)	—269 (4·3 °K)	—108	**c**
—	—	—	—	**d**
49	108 Bp	6 Bp	25 Bp	**e**
—141	—240 (33·2 °K)	—268 (5·3 °K)	16·7	**f**
37	12·8	2·26	58	**g**
0·24	3·40	1·25	0·04	**h**
[0·27]	2·26 *23 °K*			**h′**
1·81 RT	0·88 RT	1·96 RT	2·25 RT	**i**
0·23 *—187 °C*	0·013 *20 °K*	0·003		**i′**
1·87 RT	1·58 BT	0·88 RT	8·5 BT	**k**

Units and Conversion Factors

LENGTH

1 mile (Brit.) = 1760 yards =
    5280 ft. . . . 1·609 km
1 yard = 3 feet . . . 0·914 m
1 foot (ft) = 12 in   1 metre (m) = 100 cm
1 inch (in) . . . 2·54 cm   1 centimetre (cm) . . . 0·394 in
1 ft . . . 30·5 cm   1 m . . . 3·28 ft
1 thou (or mil) = 0·001 in   1 millimetre (mm) = 0·001 m = 0·1 cm
     1 micron (μ) = 0·001 mm
1 thou . . . 25·4 μ 1 mm . . . 39·4 thou
1 Ångstrom Unit (Å) = 10^{-10} m = 10^{-8} cm = $10^{-4}\mu$ = 0·1 mμ

AREA

1 acre = 4840 square yards
1 sq. ft (ft^2) = 144 in^2 . . . 929 cm^2 1 m^2 . . . 10·8 ft^2
1 sq. in. (in^2) . . . 6.45 sq. cm (cm^2)   1 cm^2 . . . 0·155 in^2

VOLUME

1 cu. ft (ft^3) = 1728 in^3 . . . 28·3 litres (l)
1 cu. in. (in^3) . . . 16·4 cm^3 1 cm^3 . . . 0·061 in^3

British Measures

1 gallon (Brit.) is defined as the volume occupied by 10 pounds water at 62° F.
1 gal = 8 pints = 160 fl. oz = 277 in^3 . . . 4·55 l
1 pint = 20 fl. oz . . . 568 ml
1 fluid ounce (fl. oz) = 1·73 in^3 . . . 28·4 ml
1 lit. . . . 0·22 gal = 35·2 fl. oz   1 ft^3 = 6·23 gal
480 minims = 8 fluid drachms = 1 fl. oz   1 minim . . . 0·059 ml

U.S.A. Measures

1 gallon (U.S.A.) of water at 62 °F. weighs 8·337 lb (avoirdupois).
1 gal   = 8 pints = 128 fl. oz = 231 in^3 . . . 3·78 l
1 pint = 16 fl. oz . . . 473 ml
1 fl. oz = 1·80 in^3 . . . 29·6 ml
1 gal (U.S.A.) = 0·83 gal (Brit.)   1 gal (Brit.) = 1·20 gal (U.S.A.)

Metric System

1 litre (l) is the volume of water at 4 °C which weighs 1 kilogram

1 l. = 1000·028 cm³   1 ml = 1·00003 cm³

1 cm³ = 0·999972 ml

VOLUME FLOW RATES

m^3/h	l/min	cm^3/s	gal/min	ft^3/h
0·60	10	167	2·20	21·2
1·70	28·3	472	6·23	60
1	16·7	278	3·67	35·3

LINEAR VELOCITIES

m/s	m/min	$km/hour$	ft/s	$miles/hour$
1	60	3·60	3·28	2·24
26·8	1610	96	88	60
0.305	18·3	1·097	1	0·68
0·447	26·8	1·609	1·47	1

WEIGHT

1 kilogram (kg) = 10^3 g ... 2·20 lb = 35·3 oz

1 pound avoirdupois (lb) = 16 ounces (oz) = 7000 gr

1 lb. ... 453·6 g

1 oz = 16 drachms = 437 grains (gr) ... 28·3 g

1 gram (g) = 1000 milligram (mg)

1 g ... 15·4 gr = 0·0353 oz   1 gr ... 65 mg

grams (g)	ounces (oz)	grains (gr)
1	0·0353	15·4
28·3	1	437
6·48	0·228	100

SPECIFIC WEIGHT

1 g/cm³ ... 62·4 lb/ft³

1 lb/ft³ ... 0·016 g/cm³

PRESSURE

kg/cm^2	lb/in^2	in Hg	mm Hg (Torr)	cm H_2O	millibar (mb)
0·0703	1	2·036	51·71	70·3	68·95
1	14·22	28·96	735·6	1000	980·7
0·0345	0·491	1	25·4	34·51	33·86
0·136	1·934	3·937	100	135·9	133·3
1·0197	14·50	29·53	750·1	1019·7	1000

1 ATMOSPHERE . . .
(standard)

$\left\{\begin{array}{l}\end{array}\right.$

760 mmHg (or Torr*) at 0 °C

10·30 m H_2O

1·033 kg/cm²

1013 mb

14·70 lb/in²

33·9 ft H_2O

29·92 in Hg

2116 lb/ft²

atm	lb/in^2	kg/cm^2
1	14·7	1·03
25	368	25·8
50	735	51·7
75	1100	77·5
100	1470	103·3
125	1840	129·2
150	2210	155·0
175	2580	180·8
200	2950	206·6

* In memory of the Italian scientist E. Torricelli (1608–47) who invented the mercury manometer, the pressure unit '1 mmHg' is being replaced by the expression: 1 Torr.

TEMPERATURE
Fahrenheit to Celsius (formerly: Centigrade)*

1 degree Fahrenheit = $\frac{5}{9}$ degree Celsius

$$t\,(°F) = \frac{5}{9}\,[t - 32]\,(°C)$$

For example: 60 °F $= \frac{5}{9}\,[60 - 32] = 15\cdot5\,°C$

Celsius to Fahrenheit

1 degree Celsius = $\frac{9}{5}$ degree Fahrenheit

$$s\,(°C) = [\tfrac{9}{5}\,s + 32]\,(°F)$$

For example: 20 °C = $[\tfrac{9}{5} \times 20 + 32]\,(°F) = 68\,°F$

°C	0	10	20	30	40	50	60	70	80	90	100
°F	32	50	68	86	104	122	140	158	176	194	212

Celsius to Kelvin

$$t\,(°C) = [t + 273\cdot2]\,(°K)$$

Example: 20 (°C) = $[20 + 273\cdot2]\,(°K) = 293\cdot2\,°K$

Réaumur to Celsius

$$r\,(°R) = \tfrac{5}{4}\,r\,(°C)$$

Temperature intervals

The preceding paragraphs relate to temperature *values*. When comparing temperature *intervals* the prefix '**deg**' is used, closely followed by the symbol of the temperature scale:

degC   degF   degK

For example: 20 degC = 36 degF

WIRE GAUGE AND INJECTION NEEDLE SIZES
The diameters of wires are commonly expressed in Standard Wire Gauge (abbreviations: s.w.g. or G) which is an arbitrary scale. The external diameters of injection needles, made from stainless steel, are

---

* The use of the expression 'Centigrade' in this connection is obsolete; it was abandoned by the *Conférence Genéralé des Poids et Mesures* in 1948.

nowadays related to the corresponding 'G' numbers. The other, independent characteristic of an injection needle is its length. The wall thickness and thereby the internal diameter, are determined by the external diameter for reasons of strength.

The 'designated size' in the top row of the following tables indicates the external diameters, expressed in 'G' numbers, and the length of needle in inches. All other needle measurements in these tables are given in 'mm'. In conformity with other data in this book, the values have been simplified and rounded off; accurate values and ranges will be found in 'British Standard 3387:1962'.

Hypodermic Surgical Needles

Designated Size	$18G\times2$	$19G\times2$	$21G\times2$	$21G\times1\frac{1}{2}$	$23G\times2$
Ext. Diam. (mm)	1·2	1·1	0·8	0·8	0·6
Int. Diam. (mm)	0·8	0·6	0·5	0·5	0·3
Length (mm)	50	50	50	40	50
Old Description	Serum 1	Serum 2	Serum 4	Hypo 1	Serum 6

Designated Size	$23G\times1\frac{1}{4}$	$23G\times1$	$26G\times1$	$26G\times\frac{3}{4}$	$26G\times\frac{1}{2}$
Ext. Diam. (mm)	0·6	0·6	0·46	0·46	0·46
Int. Diam. (mm)	0·3	0·3	0·24	0·24	0·24
Length (mm)	32	25	25	20	12
Old Description	Hypo 12 & 14	Hypo 15	Hypo 17	Hypo 16	Hypo 20

CATHETER AND ENDOTRACHEAL TUBE SIZES

The outside diameters of these tubes are expressed either in 'Magill' sizes or in French Catheter Gauge (Charrière) numbers; the latter are the same as the circumference of the tube expressed in millimetres.

The sizes of Oxford non-kinkable tubes* have been based on a rational system of internal diameters; for example, tube No. 5 has an internal diameter of 5 mm.

Since that time there has been a general movement to base endotracheal tube sizes on internal diameters; details can be found in '*British Standard 3487:1962*'.

Magill No.	F.C.G. Nearest No.	Outer diam. mm	Internal diam. for oral tubes mm
00	13	4·4	3·2
0A	15	4·8	3·6
0	16	5·5	4·4
1	19	6·3	4·8
2	21	7·1	5·2
3	24	7·9	5·6
4	25	8·3	6·0
5	27	9·1	6·7
6	29	9·5	7·1
7	31	10·3	7·5
8	33	10·7	7·9
9	36	11·9	8·7
10	38	12·7	9·5
11	42	13·5	10·3
12	45	14·4	11·1

* See ALSOP, F. A. (1955). *Anaesthesia* 10, 401.

CALCULATIONS WITH POWERS OF TEN

The use of powers of 10 facilitates arithmetical operations as well as printing of numbers which are not close to 1.

The definition of positive powers of 10 should be familiar:

$$10^0 = 1, \quad 10^1 = 10, \quad 10^2 = 100, \quad 10^3 = 1000, \ldots$$

The definition of *negative* powers of 10 proceeds on similar lines:

$$10^{-1} = 0 \cdot 1, \quad 10^{-2} = 0 \cdot 01, \quad 10^{-3} = 0 \cdot 001$$

Every number can be written as the product of a small number lying between 1 and 10 multiplied by a power of 10.

Examples

(a) $31\,000 = 3 \cdot 1 \times 10\,000 = 3 \cdot 1 \times 10^4$

(b) $0 \cdot 0000062 = \dfrac{6 \cdot 2}{1\,000\,000} = 6 \cdot 2 \times 10^{-6}$

In multiplication the powers of 10 are added, for division they are subtracted:

(c) $100 \times 1000 = 100\,000 \quad$ or $\quad 10^2 \times 10^3 = 10^{2+3} = 10^5$

(d) $\dfrac{1}{1000} = \dfrac{10^0}{10^3} = 10^{0-3} = 10^{-3}$

(e) $\dfrac{1000}{0 \cdot 0001} = 10\,000\,000 \quad$ or $\quad \dfrac{10^3}{10^{-4}} = 10^{3-(-4)} = 10^{3+4} = 10^7$

(f) $1000 \times \dfrac{1}{10} = 100 \quad$ or $\quad 10^3 \times 10^{-1} = 10^{3-1} = 10^2$

The advantage of this representation becomes even more apparent in the following example:

(g) $\dfrac{98\,000 \times 0 \cdot 000458}{0 \cdot 02 \times 0 \cdot 0098} = \dfrac{9 \cdot 8 \times 10^4 \times 4 \cdot 58 \times 10^{-4}}{2 \times 10^{-2} \times 9 \cdot 8 \times 10^{-3}} =$

$\dfrac{9 \cdot 8 \times 4 \cdot 58}{2 \times 9 \cdot 8} \times \dfrac{10^{(4-4)}}{10^{(-2-3)}} = \dfrac{4 \cdot 58}{2} \times \dfrac{10^0}{10^{-5}} = 2 \cdot 29 \times 10^{0-(-5)}$

$= 2 \cdot 29 \times 10^5 = 229\,000$

MULTIPLES OF METRIC UNITS

During the past few decades many powers of 1000 ($= 10^3$) have been designated by special names.* The terms 'milli' (10^{-3}) and 'kilo' (10^3) have been familiar for a long time; others have found increasing use in the fields of micro chemistry, electronics and nuclear science.

milli (m)	:	10^{-3}	kilo (k)	:	10^3
micro (μ)	:	10^{-6}	mega (M)	:	10^6
nano (n)	:	10^{-9}	giga (G)	:	10^9
pico (p)	:	10^{-12}	tera (T)	:	10^{12}
femto (f)	:	10^{-12}			
atto (a)	:	10^{-18}			

* See BRITISH STANDARD (1954) No. 1991 Part 1, London.

COMMON MATHEMATICAL SYMBOLS

Symbols		*Examples*
$<$	less than	$4 < 5$
$>$	greater than	$\frac{1}{5} > \frac{1}{7}$
$\simeq$	approximately equal to	$7.001 \simeq 7$
$\sim$	of the order of	size of atom $\sim 10^{-8}$ cm
$\propto$	proportional to	circumference of circle $\propto$ radius

BIOGRAPHICAL NOTES

ARRHENIUS, Svante August. 1859–1927. Swedish chemist and physicist. The son of a land surveyor, he was educated at Upp'sala and studied later at Stockholm, where he investigated electrolytic solutions. A memoir submitted to the Swedish Academy of Sciences in 1883 foreshadows his famous theory of electrolytic dissociation. His 'rule' for the effect of temperature on the rate of chemical reactions was formulated in 1889.

Nobel Prize for Chemistry awarded to him in 1903 while Professor of Physics at Stockholm. Noted for his fundamental contributions to a variety of fields, including cosmology and meteorology. Worked with Rutherford at Manchester. Devoted much time to popularize science.

'Arrhenius was a true polyhistor and being endowed with a memory both tenacious and accurate he had a marvellous command of scientific facts. Nevertheless, there was little "academic" about him.'*

AVOGADRO, Amedeo. 1776–1856. Italian physicist. Professor of Higher Physics in the University of Turin. Enunciated his 'Law' in a paper entitled, *Essai d'une manière de déterminer les masses relatives des molécules élémentaires des corps, et les proportions selon lesquelles elles entrent dans ces combinaisons* in 1811, *J. de Physique*, **73**, 58–76.

BERNOULLI, Daniel. 1700–82. Swiss mathematician and physicist. Professor of Mathematics at St. Petersburg for seven years. On returning to Basel he became Professor of Anatomy and Botany, and later Professor of Experimental and Speculative Philosophy. His most important work was *Hydrodynamica* (1738).

BOYLE, Henry Edmund Gaskin. 1875–1941. Anaesthetist, St. Bartholomew's Hospital, London. Awarded O.B.E. while serving as anaesthetist in First World War. An original member of the Association of Anaesthetists of Gt. Britain and Ireland, and one of the first pair of examiners appointed for the Diploma of Anaesthetics. Author of *Practical anaesthetics* (1907), London.

BOYLE, The Hon. Robert. 1627–91. Chemist and natural philosopher. Son of the first Earl of Cork. Worked in Oxford and London.

Boyle's 'Law' was published in 1662: *A defence of the doctrine touching the spring and weight of air . . . against . . . Franciscus Linus*, Lond. as an appendix to the 2nd ed. of *New experiments physical-mechanical* (1662), Oxford. Was also an experimental physiologist of distinction; together with Christopher Wren he demonstrated the effects of injecting opium into the veins of dogs. He also found time to study Hebrew, Chaldee and Syriac, and he produced a large body of writings upon theological subjects.

Boyle was a prime mover in founding the Royal Society, but he declined the Presidency because of scruples about taking the oath. A most interesting biography was written by More, L. T. (1944), *The life and works of the Hon. Robert Boyle*, New York.

CATTLIN, William Alfred Newman. 1814–86. Surgeon and dentist. One of the founders of the Odontological Society. While in London he obtained the

* Quoted from: Sir James Walker (1928), *J. Chem. Soc.*, i, 1380.

F.R.C.S. in 1856 and the L.D.S. in 1860. From 1863 onwards in dental practice at Brighton. President of the Odontological Society in 1866.

Clover wrote in 1868: 'Mr. Cattlin of Brighton connects the bottle of gas with a bag holding about 400 cu. in., and allows this small bag to receive a supply during the inhalation. He placed this bag about a foot from the mouthpiece with which it was joined by a large tube.' (MS. notes now in the Nuffield Department of Anaesthetics, Oxford.) The reservoir bag, sometimes mistakenly referred to as rebreathing bag, was, until the end of the nineteenth century, commonly known as Cattlin's bag.

CAVENDISH, The Hon. Henry. 1731–1810. Eminent experimental scientist and bibliophile. Eldest son of Lord Charles Cavendish, and grandson of the third Duke of Devonshire. Studied at Cambridge without taking a degree. Owned a number of houses in London, one of which, in Dean Street, Soho, was filled with his extensive library. He inherited a large fortune in middle life, but continued to live quite simply. His social activities were restricted to the attendance at weekly meetings of the Royal Society, of which he was elected a Fellow in 1760.

He carried out numerous fundamental investigations in the fields of chemistry, electricity, gravitation and astronomy. He was an exceptionally careful experimenter, and was slow in publishing the results of his researches, many of which appeared in the *Philosophical Transactions* between 1766 and 1809. Scientists tended to disregard his findings although these anticipated many later 'discoveries' by Priestley, Davy, Faraday and others. The Physics Laboratory at Cambridge is named after him, and it was here that Lord Rutherford undertook his famous experiments on atomic nuclei.

CELSIUS, Anders. 1701–44. Swedish astronomer. While holding the Chair of Astronomy at Uppsala from 1730 onwards, he travelled extensively for his Government to astronomical observatories in Western Europe. In his investigations on thermometry, he surpassed the inventors of other thermometric scales (Réaumur, Fahrenheit) both in clarity and precision. His scale is the same as the centigrade scale, except that he called the boiling point of water '0', and the freezing point '100'. °C should be pronounced 'degree Celsius'; the use of the name 'centigrade' has been officially abandoned since 1948. The relevant publication by Celsius is: *Observationer om tvenne beständiga grader på en thermometer* (1742), *Vetensk. Acad. Handl.*

CHARLES, Jaques Alexandre César. 1746–1823. French physicist and mathematician. Professor of Physics at Paris for over thirty years.

Charles was interested in aeronautics, and after the Montgolfier brothers had made their ascent in a balloon filled with warmed air, he filled a balloon with hydrogen which successfully ascended from the Champs de Mars on August 2, 1783.

He propounded, but did not publish, his law of the expansion of gases in 1787. Gay-Lussac himself freely acknowledged that Charles had both recognized and demonstrated the constant dilatation of gases for equal increments in temperature.

CLOVER, Joseph Thomas. 1825–82. British Anaesthetist, F.R.C.S. in 1853. Intended to become a surgeon but as he was not robust he decided to adopt what seemed to him the less arduous specialty of anaesthetics, combining this with some general practice.

After John Snow's death in 1858, Clover played the leading part in English anaesthetic practice. He was invariably consulted in connection with the many anaesthetic committees of investigation appointed during the eighteen-sixties and seventies. Although he wrote little he designed many anaesthetic appliances. The quantitative chloroform apparatus was described in 1862. His gas/ether sequence (*Brit. med. J.* (1876), ii, 74) obviated the unpleasantness of ether induction. In the following year he described the famous 'Clover's Inhaler' (*Brit. med. J.* (1877), i, 69–70). This small portable apparatus, later slightly modified by Hewitt (*Anaesthetics and their administration*, pp. 277–8, (1901), London), is still used in some hospitals, and skilfully employed gives adequate results. Ombrédanne's inhaler (*Gaz. Hôp.*, Paris, (1908), **81**, 1095–1100), described over twenty years *after* Clover's death, closely resembles Clover's both in design and appearance.

FAHRENHEIT, Gabriel Daniel. 1686–1736. Born at Danzig the son of a merchant, he received a business education at Amsterdam, but became interested in physics and natural philosophy. As a result he turned to the manufacture of meteorological instruments and became a skilled glass-blower. Most of his thermometric investigations were carried out in 1721 and were published in the *Phil. Trans.*, London (1724). Nominated Fellow of the Royal Society, London, in 1724.

FICK, Adolph Eugen. 1829–1901. Eminent German physiologist and medical physicist. Born at Kassel of a learned family. Although he showed an early interest in mathematics, he studied medicine at Marburg and Berlin, qualifying in 1851. Professor of Physiology at Zürich, and later for thirty-one years at Würzburg. His famous 'principle' was enunciated in the paper *Über Diffusion* in 1855, *Ann. d. Phys. u. Chem.*, **94**, 59–86. A man of wide learning and member of many learned Societies, he was particularly interested in the dynamics of the circulation of blood.

GAY-LUSSAC, Joseph Louis. 1778–1850. Professor of Chemistry and Physics in Paris. His researches on the physical properties of gases belong to his earlier working years, and his memoir on the expansion of gases, *Sur la dilatation des gaz et des vapeurs*, was published in 1802, *Ann. de Chim.* **43**, 137–75. His most important physical paper, *Mémoirs sur la combinaison des substances gazeuses, les unes avec les autres*, appeared in 1809, *Arcueil, Mém. de Phys.*, **2**, 207–34.

During 1804 Gay-Lussac made, for the Académie des Sciences, two balloon ascents in order to study terrestial magnetism above the earth's surface. In the first ascent, with J. B. Piot, a height of 4000 metres was reached, and in the second, alone, he reached 7 016 metres. He also investigated temperature and humidity, and at different heights took samples of air for subsequent analysis. He found that altitude made no difference to the composition of air.

GRAHAM, Thomas. 1805–69. Scottish chemist. Son of wealthy merchant at Glasgow, who wished him to enter the Church. As young Thomas would not agree to do this, parental financial support was withdrawn and he had to live by writing and teaching. Obtained his M.A. degree at the age of 19, became Professor of Chemistry at the Anderson Institute, Edinburgh, in 1830 and at University College, London, in 1837. From 1855 to 1869 he was Master of the Mint. Elected F.R.S. in 1836, and first President of the London Chemical Society in 1841.

His lectures were characterized by accuracy, but he was not a fluent speaker. His manner was nervous and he was not robust in health. Graham's 'Law' was propounded in a paper given to the Royal Society of Edinburgh in 1831 and published two years later: *On the law of the diffusion of gases* (1833), *Phil. Mag.* **2**, 175–90; 269–76; 351–8.

According to this law, the rate of diffusion of fluids through a porous partition is inversely proportional to the square root of their densities—under certain conditions. Graham further studied the laws governing Effusion (passage of gas through minute orifices into a vacuum) and Transpiration (passage of gas under pressure through long, fine capillaries). He also invented Dialysis in which colloids are separated from crystalloids by means of semi-permeable membranes.

HAGEN, Gotthilf Heinrich. 1797–1884. Eminent civil engineer, born at Königsberg. Descended from a family numbering amongst its members numerous scientists and civil servants. From 1831 in Berlin, held various Government posts of high rank during next forty years. Travelled extensively and became foremost hydraulic engineer of the middle nineteenth century.

His meticulous work on the law governing the flow of liquids through narrow tubes entitles him to have his name bracketed with Poiseuille; it was published as *Über die Bewegung des Wassers in engen zylindrischen Röhren* in 1839, *Poggendorff's Annalen der Physik u. Chem.*, **46**, 423–42. The Hagen–Poiseuille Law is valid only for long, narrow tubes and small velocities. For larger velocities the flow becomes turbulent. Hagen appreciated already the transition from laminar to turbulent flow, and his work clearly opens the way for Reynolds' classic investigations on turbulent flow some thirty years later.

HENRY, William. 1774–1836. English chemist and physician. M.D. Edinburgh in 1807.

Son of Thomas Henry, F.R.S., a surgeon-apothecary in Manchester who had discovered a new and lucrative way of manufacturing magnesium oxide ('calcined magnesia').

In 1803 Henry communicated to the Royal Society a paper entitled: *On the quantity of gases*, in which he described experiments showing the quantity of gases absorbed by water at different temperatures and pressures. Henry was for a time physician to the Manchester Royal Infirmary, and wrote a number of papers on medical subjects.

In childhood, Henry's growth was stunted and his health impaired by a severe accident. This, and the fact that his father's chemical business brought in plenty of money, led him in later life to give up medicine and devote himself to pure science. He was the author of a textbook *The elements of experimental chemistry*, (1799), London, which by 1829 had passed through eleven editions.

KELVIN: THOMSON, Sir William, First Baron Kelvin of Largs. 1824–1907. Born at Belfast, the son of the Professor of Mathematics at the Royal Academy Institution. After studying mathematics at Cambridge, he became Professor of Natural Philosophy at Glasgow at the early age of 22, setting up the first physical laboratory in Great Britain. He received numerous honours both in the scientific and social world. He was made a Knight after organizing the successful laying of the first Transatlantic telegraph cable in 1866. He was twice President of the Royal Society, made a Baron in 1892, a Privy Counsellor in 1902 and Chancellor of Glasgow University in 1904.

Lord Kelvin introduced his 'absolute thermometric scale' in 1848. He wrote hundreds of articles dealing with subjects in the field of mathematics, physics and engineering.

LOSCHMIDT, Josef. 1821–95. Austrian physicist. Professor of Physics in Vienna. Enunciated his theory of gases in: *Zur Theorie der Gase*, 1866, *S.B. Akad. Wiss. Wien*, **54**, 646–62.

MARSTON, Robert. 1853–1925. Dentist of Leicester. A man of considerable inventiveness who, in the field of inhalation anaesthesia, designed apparatus which embodied ideas far in advance of his time (see p. 230).

He described his various anaesthetic machines in a handbook, *The anaesthetist's pocket companion*, (1899), Leicester. His other interests included such widely different subjects as dental ceramics, safety signalling devices for railways, and a process for attaching boot soles to uppers. Uncle of A. D. Marston, Senior Anaesthetist to Guy's Hospital, and Past President of the Association of Anaesthetists of Great Britain and Ireland.

POISEUILLE, Jean Léonard Marie. 1799–1869. French physiologist. M.D. Paris, 1828. Published papers on the movement of blood in the veins (1832) and in the capillaries (1839). His famous work, *Recherches expérimentales sur le mouvement des liquides dans les tubes de très petits diamètres* appeared as a series of papers during 1840–1, *C.R. Acad. Sci., Paris*, 11–12.

RÉAUMUR: René Antoine Ferchault Seigneur de Réaumur, des Angles et de Bermondière. 1683–1757. Studied Law and turned then to Technology. Member of the French Academy of Sciences in 1708. Published numerous technical papers before undertaking the construction of his thermometers.

He insisted on the use of one fixed point only (freezing point of water); the other divisions of his alcohol-filled thermometer were calculated from the supposedly constant expansion of alcohol with temperature. The scale which finally became known by his name has little to do with his own, dubious measurements. A similar complaint can be made about the accuracy of Fahrenheit's work, and it was only CELSIUS who introduced precision methods into thermometry.

REGNAULT, Henri Victor. 1810–78. French chemist and physicist. Professor of Physics, Paris, 1841. His many interests included organic chemistry and thermometry.

His researches, *Études sur l'hygrometrie* were published in 1845, *C. R. Acad. Sci., Paris*, 20, 1127–66 and 1220–37. This work on the expansion of gases was carried out in the laboratory of the world-famous porcelain factory at Sèvres, of which he had been appointed director in 1854. During the Franco-Prussian War the results of Regnault's latest researches on gases were destroyed. This, and the death of his son in the fighting, brought Regnault's scientific activity to a close in 1872, although he himself lived until 1878.

REYNOLDS, Osborne. 1842–1912. English engineer and physicist. Born at Belfast, the son of the headmaster of a grammar school. After receiving practical training in mechanical engineering, he studied at Cambridge. In 1868 he was offered the newly-founded Chair of Engineering at Owens College, Manchester, and held this post until his retirement through ill health in 1905. He was elected F.R.S. in 1877.

Reynolds was the first to study the turbulent flow of liquids in great detail, and the particular 'number' determining the transition from laminar to turbulent flow is known by his name (see also under HAGEN). This work, *An experimental investigation of the circumstances which determine whether a motion of water shall be direct or sinuous, and of the law of resistance in parallel channels*, appeared in 1883, *Phil. Trans., London*, 174, 935–82.

SNOW, John. 1813–58. First specialist anaesthetist and pioneer in physiology of anaesthetics. M.D., London, 1844.

When, in December 1846, the news came from America that Morton had successfully used ether for surgical anaesthesia, Snow hastened to investigate the subject, and by January 1847 he had designed an inhaler in which the proportion of vapour taken up by the air drawn over the liquid ether could be regulated. The temperature of the vaporizing chamber was kept high by means of a water-bath, and a valved face-piece was substituted for Morton's clumsy mouth-tube.

As early as 1847 he published a strikingly accurate description of five stages of anaesthesia in his book *On the inhalation of the vapour of ether in surgical operations*, pp. 1–2, London. He carried out many careful experiments on the physiological effects of different percentages of anaesthetic drugs.

Snow is popularly remembered for having given chloroform to Queen Victoria during the birth of two of her children. To anaesthetists he is known by his two classical books, *On the inhalation of the vapour of ether in surgical operations* (op. cit.) and *On chloroform and other anaesthetics*, (1858), London. To physicians he is known for his monograph on cholera, which showed for the first time that this disease was transmitted by drinking-water.

VENTURI, Giovanni Battista. 1746–1822. Italian physicist, statesman and man of letters. Professor of Physics at Modena and later at Pavia. His paper *Recherches expérimentales sur le principe de communication latéral dans les fluides appliqué à l'explication de différents phénomènes hydrauliques*, (1797), Paris, was published in English in 1799, Lond., and as a series during 1798–9, *Nicholson's J. Nat. Philos*, 2–3.

WALLER, Augustus Désiré. 1856–1922. M.D. (Aberdeen) and F.R.S. British physiologist and son of distinguished physiologist. Lecturer to London School of Medicine for Women and afterwards to St. Mary's Hospital, London. First to obtain a human 'electro-cardiogram' (*J. Physiol.*, 1887, **8**, 229–34).

He endorsed the opinion first expressed by John Snow (*On Chloroform . . .* p. 69) and later by Paul Bert (*C. R. Acad. Sci.*, Paris, 1881, **93**, 768–71) that the most important factor in safe chloroform anaesthesia was the limiting of the strength of vapour in the inhaled air. Waller was a Member of the Chloroform Committee (1901) whose final report was made in 1911, *B.M.A. Report on the Special Chloroform Commission*, London.

INDEX